RWN 00007 £23.70

D0242905

Fundamentals of Anaesthesia and Acute Medicine

Paediatric
Intensive Care

Fundamentals of Anaesthesia and Acute Medicine

Paediatric Intensive Care

Edited by
Alan Duncan

Director, Paediatric Intensive Care Unit, Princess Margaret Hospital, Perth, Western Australia

Series editors
Ronald M Jones

Professor of Anaesthetics, St Mary's Hospital Medical School, London

Alan R Aitkenhead

Professor of Anaesthesia, University of Nottingham

Pierre Foëx

Nuffield Professor of Anaesthetics, University of Oxford

WS 410

First published in 1998
by BMJ Books, BMA House, Tavistock Square,
London WC1H 9JR

British Library Cataloguing in Publication Data

A catalogue record for this book is available
from the British Library

ISBN 0-7279-1073-6

Typeset, printed and bound in Great Britain by
Latimer Trend & Company Ltd, Plymouth

Contents

CONTENTS

Contributors

Desmond Bohn MB, MRCP, FFARCS, FRCPC
Associate Director, Paediatric Intensive Care Unit, Hospital for Sick Children, Toronto, Ontario, Canada

Warwick Butt MB, BS, FRACP
Staff Specialist, Intensive Care Unit, Royal Children's Hospital, Melbourne, Victoria, Australia

Alan Duncan MB, BS, FRCA, FANZCA, FFICANZCA
Director, Paediatric Intensive Care Unit, Princess Margaret Hospital, Perth, Western Australia, Australia

Jonathan Gillis MB, BS, FRACP
Head, Intensive Care Unit, Royal Alexandra Hospital for Children, Sydney, Australia

Paul Hutchins MA, BM, BCh, FRACP, MRCP, DCH, FRCPCH
Medical Head of Home Ventilation Program and Head of Children's Assessment Centre, Royal Alexandra Hospital for Children, Sydney, Australia

Niranjan Kissoon MB, BS, FRCP(C), FAAP, FCCM
Professor, College of Medicine, University of Florida; Director, PICU Wolfson Children's Hospital; Director of Research, Department of Paediatrics, University of Florida Health Science Center, Jacksonville, Florida, USA

Geoff Knight MB, BS, FRACP
Staff Specialist, Paediatric Intensive Care Unit, Princess Margaret Hospital for Children, Perth, Western Australia, Australia

Duncan Macrae
Director, Cardiothoracic Intensive Care Unit, Hospital for Sick Children, Great Ormond Street, London, UK

Neil T Matthews
Director, Paediatric Intensive Care, Adelaide Women's and Children's Hospital, Adelaide, South Australia, Australia

Stephen Scuplak MB, BS, FRCA
Registrar, Cardiothoracic Intensive Care Unit, Hospital for Sick Children, Great Ormond Street, London, UK

Frank Shann MD, FRACP
Professor of Critical Care Medicine and Director of Intensive Care, Royal Children's Hospital, Melbourne, Victoria, Australia

Paul Swan MB, BS, FANZCA, FFIANZCA
Staff Specialist, Paediatric Intensive Care Unit, King Faisal Hospital, Riyadh, Saudi Arabia

James Tibballs MB, BS, BMedSci, MEd, FANZCA, FFICANZCA
Deputy Director, Intensive Care Unit, Royal Children's Hospital, Melbourne, Victoria, Australia

Foreword to the Fundamentals of Anaesthesia and Acute Medicine series

The pace of change within the biological sciences continues to increase and nowhere is this more apparent than in the specialties of anaesthesia, acute medicine, and intensive care. Although many practitioners continue to rely on comprehensive but bulky texts for reference, the accelerating rate of biomedical advances makes this source of information increasingly likely to be dated, even if the latest edition is used. The series *Fundamentals of Anaesthesia and Acute Medicine* aims to bring the reader up to date with authoritative reviews of the principal clinical topics which make up the specialties. Each volume will cover the fundamentals of the topic in a comprehensive manner but will also emphasise recent developments or controversial issues.

International differences in the practice of anaesthesia and intensive care are now much less than in the past, and the editors of each volume have commissioned chapters from acknowledged authorities throughout the world to assemble contributions of the highest possible calibre. Three volumes will appear annually and, as the pace and extent of clinically significant advances varies among the individual topics, new editions will be commissioned to ensure that practitioners will be in a position to keep abreast of the important developments within the specialties.

Not only does the pace of advance in biomedical science serve to justify the appearance of an international series of this nature but the current awareness of the need for more formal continuing education also underlines the timeliness of its appearance. The editors would welcome feedback from readers about the series, which is aimed at both established practitioners and trainees preparing for degrees and diplomas in anaesthesia and intensive care.

RONALD M JONES
ALAN R AITKENHEAD
PIERRE FOËX

Preface

If adult intensive care was born of the polio epidemic in the 1950s with the development of artificial ventilation techniques, the major impetus for paediatric intensive care followed the development of polyvinyl chloride endotracheal tubes and their use for prolonged nasal intubation. When Dr Bernard Brandstater presented his early experience with this technique at the Anaesthesiology Society meeting in Austria in 1962, he opened the doors to the widespread application of mechanical ventilation to infants and children. So commenced a remarkable era of progress which has seen both the adaptation of adult techniques to small infants as well as innovations in paediatric intensive care that have impacted on the care of critically ill adults. Techniques such as continuous positive airway pressure, inverse ratio ventilation, the emphasis on the pulmonary circulation and the use of pulmonary vasodilators, as well as a holistic approach to patient and family care, have all emanated from neonatal and paediatric intensive care units.

Topics for this book have been chosen because of their importance to paediatric morbidity and mortality, their prevalence as problems in paediatric intensive care, or because of recent advances or trends in the field. Most chapters cover the basic foundations of the subject although some are of a more scientific and advanced nature. All of the chapters attempt to provide state of the art information on these important topics.

It is increasingly recognised in medicine and other disciplines that it is not only what service or therapy is provided that determines outcome but often, more importantly, the way it is provided. The focus on quality in health care delivery must also be extended to the specialty of paediatric intensive care. Outcome in terms of cost benefit is clearly determined by factors such as the organisation of services, as well as the experience and training of staff working in the area. In times of financial constraints it is essential that paediatric intensive care services are provided in such a way as to guarantee value for money. If this is achieved the community can be assured that the resources committed to this specialty will be rewarded many times over by the quantity and quality of productive lives saved.

ALAN DUNCAN

1: Organisation and outcome of paediatric intensive care

FRANK SHANN

In developed countries, paediatric intensive care has an important impact on the health of children. For example, in Victoria, a state of Australia with a population of 4.5 million people, one child in every 70 (1.5% or 15 per 1000 live births) is admitted to the intensive care unit at the Royal Children's Hospital. If we assume, conservatively, that half these children would die without intensive care, the number of lives saved is 15×0.5 or 7.5 per 1000 live births. Without paediatric intensive care, Victoria's under 15-year-old mortality rate would double from 7.1 to 14.6 deaths per 1000 live births.

Specialised paediatric intensive care units have evolved to cater for the particular needs of critically ill infants and children. This chapter presents the arguments for regionalisation of paediatric intensive care services on the basis of outcome and economic considerations.

Regionalisation of paediatric intensive care

Numerous studies in many specialties of medicine have found that units that look after many cases of a particular disease have better results than units with few cases.[1,2] These studies provide strong indirect evidence that the quality of care is likely to be improved if children are looked after in a few large paediatric intensive care units, rather than in many small units.

Direct evidence that mortality is lower in large specialist paediatric intensive care units comes from three separate studies. A study in Oregon and Washington[3] found that the mortality rate (adjusted for severity of illness) was 102% of expected in three specialist paediatric intensive care units and 139% of expected in 71 general units – the difference was so

1

large that it was statistically significant despite the small number of deaths in the study.

Another study[4] found that high risk patients in six tertiary paediatric units in Holland had a mortality rate that was only 85% of expected, but that mortality was 143% of expected in four non-tertiary units (p<0.05). Low risk patients in the tertiary units had a higher than expected mortality rate, but 60% of the 25 low risk children who died in the tertiary units had incurable disease with no prospect of long term survival – and treatment may have been limited in some of these children.

We have compared the mortality rate of all children who received intensive care in Victoria,[5] a state of Australia, with that of children in the Trent region of the United Kingdom – both areas have a population of about 4 million. Adjusting for severity of illness, the mortality rate was 75% higher in Trent, where children receive intensive care in small paediatric intensive care units or general intensive care units, than in Victoria, where most children receive intensive care in one large tertiary paediatric intensive care unit. The excess deaths in Trent children were equivalent to 43% of the deaths in ICU, and 11% of all deaths in children between the ages of 1 month and 16 years in Trent.

A recent study in the United States of America[5] found no reduction in mortality in larger or busier paediatric intensive care units, but it had sufficient power (β 0.1, α 0.05) to detect only a 40% change in mortality caused by a given risk factor. Further, to determine the effect of the size of an intensive care unit, the important factor is not the number of patients in the study, which was 5415, but the number of intensive care units, which was only 16.

These studies compared large specialist tertiary paediatric intensive care units with smaller non-specialist units, so we cannot tell whether the lower mortality in the large units was due to the greater number of patients in these units, the presence of specialists in paediatric intensive care or the fact that the large units were in tertiary hospitals with more supporting services. However, whatever the explanation for the higher mortality in small units, these studies provide strong evidence for looking after very ill children in large regionalised intensive care units.

Similar considerations apply to the debate about whether children should be looked after in specialist paediatric units or in general intensive care units with a preponderance of adult patients. Many of the diseases of children in intensive care are very different from the diseases of adults, so we must presume that children should be looked after in specialist paediatric units if they are to benefit from the lower mortality found in units looking after many cases of a particular disease.[1,2] Indeed, the American College of Critical Care Medicine and the American Society of Critical Care Medicine,[7] the British Paediatric Association,[8] and the Australian National

Health and Medical Research Council[9] have all said that children should receive intensive care in specialist paediatric units.

There are, of course, some children who need only a brief period of intensive care (for example, after surgery) who can be safely looked after in a general intensive care unit. A useful guideline is that children who need endotracheal intubation for more than 12–24 hours should be looked after in a specialist paediatric intensive care unit.

Large regionalised paediatric intensive care units are likely to provide a higher standard of care and a regionalised system is also very much less expensive. One large intensive care unit costs much less to run than three small ones, because many of the fixed costs of running an intensive care unit are almost independent of size. For example, I have calculated that nursing and medical salaries would total about £37 million if the United Kingdom had 32 paediatric intensive care units each with 500 admissions a year, compared with only £27 million if there were 12 units each with 1300 admissions a year.[10]

If specialist paediatric emergency teams are available, very ill children can be safely transported over long distances to specialist paediatric intensive care units. Transporting children inevitably results in some family dislocation, but this disruption is substantially less than that caused by the excess morbidity and mortality associated with care in non-specialised units.

Staffing

There is evidence that having full time intensive care consultants improves the outcome of both adult[11] and paediatric[6,12] intensive care. It is acknowledged that the medical director and the majority of senior medical staff should be recognised specialists in paediatric intensive care. Specific training programmes in paediatric intensive care are now available in a number of countries including Australia, Canada, and the United States of America. There is merit in every paediatric unit having some full time consultant staff who originally trained in anaesthesia and some who originally trained in paediatrics.

Pollock[6] has shown that mortality is substantially increased (OR 1.84, 95% CI 0.96–3.52) in the first three months after new residents have started in paediatric intensive care units that employ first (p = 0.03) or second (p = 0.0001) year residents. In Melbourne, our house staff work full time in intensive care and they are all registrars with at least four years of experience in paediatrics or anaesthesia; our minimum appointment is for six months and most appointments are for 12–18 months.

3

The quality of the nursing staff available is at least as important as the quality of medical staff in paediatric intensive care. One of the many advantages of regionalisation is that large units are able to run their own training courses in paediatric intensive care nursing; this helps recruit new staff and encourages existing staff to keep up to date.

Number of beds and units

The number of paediatric intensive care beds needed for a given population will depend on the degree of regionalisation (larger units will reduce the number of beds needed because local peaks in demand tend to average out), the proportion of medium dependency (unintubated) patients admitted, and the average length of stay.

TABLE 1.1—*Children from Victoria, Australia, and Trent Region, England, who received intensive care in 1994*[5]

	Victoria	Trent Region
Children 0–15 years	1 011 000	1 833 000
Children in intensive care*	1194	1014
Admissions/100 000 children	118	122
Ventilated 1st hr/100 000	65	50
Days per admission	2.14	3.94
ICU days/year/100 000	253	480
Paediatric ICUs	2	8
Paediatric ICU beds**	11	17

* Excluding neonates <28 days old, but including neonates having cardiac surgery.
** (Fully staffed beds in named paediatric ICUs) + (fully staffed general ICU beds × child admissions/total admissions).

Table 1.1 compares population data from Victoria, Australia, with data from the Trent region of the United Kingdom.[5] In Victoria, paediatric intensive care is highly regionalised with one paediatric and one general intensive care unit (with two paediatric beds) admitting children for a population of 1 000 000 children. In contrast, a similar number of children living in Trent received intensive care in eight paediatric and 11 general intensive care units. Both Victoria and Trent had about 120 admissions to intensive care per 100 000 children per year, but children stayed almost twice as long in intensive care in Trent, so Trent had 90% more intensive care bed days per 100 000 children (table 1.1). The substantially longer length of stay in Trent is almost certainly due to the lack of regionalisation, with many children being looked after in small intensive care units that have consultant, resident and nursing staff with less experience in paediatric intensive care than the staff in Victoria.

If there are 120 paediatric intensive care admissions per 100 000 children per year in a population and each admission lasts 2.5 days, one paediatric intensive care bed will be needed per 100 000 children to achieve 80% bed occupancy (of course, if there are longer stays or lower bed occupancy rates, more beds will be needed). If the minimum size for a regionalised paediatric intensive care unit is 10 beds, one paediatric unit will be needed for every 1 000 000 children. Smaller paediatric intensive care units will be needed in sparsely populated regions of some countries, such as Australia and Canada, and it is sensible to combine medium dependency care with intensive care facilities in these circumstances. Because there are substantial differences in cost and outcome between medium dependency and intensive care patients, paediatric units should report data about their cost, admissions, length of stay, and mortality separately for unintubated and intubated patients.

Predicting mortality in intensive care

It is very important to be able to describe objectively how sick a group of patients is. Severity of illness scores are needed to discover the best way to organise paediatric intensive care (by comparing different units), to monitor the effects of changes in practice (by observing trends within units over time), to assess the relationship between severity of illness and cost, and to monitor the effects of rationing intensive care. In January 1994, an entire issue of *Critical Care Clinics* was devoted to a discussion of outcome prediction in intensive care patients.[13]

Mortality prediction scores, such as PRISM,[14,15] are usually derived by collecting a large number of predictor variables (such as blood pressure and blood gases) from a large group of patients in intensive care and then using logistic regression analysis to derive an equation that predicts which children will die and which will survive. It is then assumed that patients who are more likely to die are sicker than those who are less likely to die. This is a reasonable assumption for many patients, but it is not true for groups of patients that need intensive care but have a very low risk of dying (for example, children with severe croup).

Mortality prediction models are often used to test the standard of care in a particular intensive care unit by calculating the standardised mortality rate (SMR), which compares the actual mortality rate of the unit's patients with the expected rate. For example, if 110 of 1000 patients in the unit died and the risk of death (ranging from 0 to 1) calculated using PRISM for each of the 1000 patients summed to 100, the standardised mortality rate would be 110/100 or 110% of the PRISM standard.

5

Mortality prediction scores are fairly accurate when they are used to describe groups of patients, but they are not yet accurate enough to be used to determine the management of an individual patient. However, it may be possible to improve the accuracy of these scores by observing how an individual patient's score changes with time.[16]

PRISM II is calculated from the most abnormal values of 14 variables over a 24 hour period, and PRISM III requires even more data.[15] Because it is so difficult to collect the large amount of information needed to calculate PRISM, many paediatric intensive care units do not calculate it routinely. Furthermore, worst in 24 hours scores have two methodological problems. First, they appear to be more accurate than they really are: about 40% of deaths in paediatric intensive care occur in the first 24 hours, so the score is really diagnosing death rather than predicting it. Second, such scores blur the differences between units: a child admitted to a good unit who rapidly recovers will have a score that suggests a mild illness, while the same child mismanaged in a bad unit will have a score that suggests severe illness – the bad unit's high mortality rate will be incorrectly attributed to it having sicker patients than the good unit. A new outcome prediction model, the Paediatric Index of Mortality (PIM) score, that uses only admission data, has been developed at the Royal Children's Hospital, Melbourne and it has been tested in six paediatric intensive care units in Australia and one in England.[17]

Outcome in neonates, children and adults

Mortality prediction scores, such as PRISM and PIM, only attempt to predict survival in intensive care or in hospital. However, it is just as important to examine long term mortality and morbidity rates in the survivors of intensive care.

Table 1.2 shows the outcome of neonates, children and adults two years after they had been in intensive care in teaching hospitals of the University of Melbourne. Neonates weighing less than 1000 g at birth and adults had high mortality rates and only 15–20% of them were functionally normal survivors. Children had a much lower mortality rate and 65% were functionally normal survivors.

Paediatric intensive care is highly cost effective because children have short stays in intensive care, a low mortality rate and a low handicap rate.

TABLE 1.2—*Outcome two years after intensive care, Victoria, Australia, 1983*

	Neonates birthweight <1000g[a]	Children >28 days of age[b]	Adults[c]
Dead	60%	15%	55%
Severe handicap	10%	10%	10%
Mild handicap[d]	10%	10%	20%
Functionally normal	20%	65%	15%

[a] Data from references [18] and [19], and Kitchen WH, personal communication.
[b] Data from reference [20] and unpublished data.
[c] Proc 9th Aust and NZ Int Care Soc Meeting, Perth 1984, and Cade JF, personal communication.
[d] Handicapped, but likely to lead an independent life.

Summary

There is strong indirect and direct evidence that children who need intensive care should be looked after in large regionalised specialist paediatric intensive care units, rather than in small paediatric units or with adults in general units. Large regionalised paediatric intensive care units are cheaper and, on average, they achieve lower mortality rates.

The improved quality of care from regionalisation probably results from several factors: the effects of size (practice makes perfect), the presence of full time specialists in paediatric intensive care, the ability to attract full time senior resident staff and trained paediatric intensive care nurses, and the fact that regionalised units are usually located in specialist paediatric teaching hospitals. In general, any child who needs endotracheal intubation for more than 12–24 hours should be looked after in a specialist paediatric intensive care unit.

Most developed countries will have about 120 paediatric intensive care admissions per 100 000 children per year; if each admission lasts 2.5 days, then one paediatric intensive care bed will be needed per 100 000 children for 80% bed occupancy. One 10-bed paediatric intensive care unit will be needed for every million children.

Mortality prediction scores, such as PRISM and PIM, are useful for making comparisons between different intensive care units and for monitoring trends over time within one unit. However, these scores are not yet accurate enough to be used to determine treatment for individual patients.

Paediatric intensive care is highly cost effective because children stay a short time in intensive care, they have a low mortality rate and the survivors have a low handicap rate. In developed countries, paediatric intensive care makes a substantial impact on infant and child mortality.

1 Luft HS, Garnick DW, Mark DH, McPhee SJ. *Hospital volume, physician volume, and patient outcomes*. Ann Arbor: Health Administration Press Perspectives, 1990.
2 Farley DE, Ozminkowski RJ. Volume-outcome relationships and in-hospital mortality: the effect of changes in volume over time. *Med Care* 1992;**30**:77–94.
3 Pollack MM, Alexander SR, Clarke N, Ruttimann UE, Tesselaar HM, Bachulis AC. Improved outcomes from tertiary center pediatric intensive care: a statewide comparison of tertiary and nontertiary care facilities. *Crit Care Med* 1991;**19**:150–9.
4 Gemke RJBJ, Bonsel GJ. Comparative assessment of pediatric intensive care: a national multicenter study. *Crit Care Med* 1995;**23**:238–45.
5 Pearson G, Shann F, Barry P, *et al*. Should paediatric intensive care be centralised? Trent versus Victoria. *Lancet* 1997;**349**:1213–7.
6 Pollack MM, Cuerdon TT, Patel KM, Ruttimann UE, Getson PR, Levetown M. Impact of quality-of-care factors on pediatric intensive care unit mortality. *JAMA* 1994;**272**: 941–6.
7 Thompson DR, Clemmer TP, Applefeld JJ, *et al*. Regionalisation of critical care medicine: task force report of the American College of Critical Care Medicine. *Crit Care Med* 1994; **22**:1306–13.
8 British Paediatric Association. *The care of critically ill children*. London: British Paediatric Association, 1993.
9 National Health and Medical Research Council. *Management of seriously ill children in adult intensive care units*. Canberra: National Health and Medical Research Council, 1983.
10 Sheldon T, ed. *Which way forward for the care of critically ill children?* York: University of York NHS Centre for Reviews and Dissemination, 1995.
11 Fisher M. Intensive care: do intensivists matter? *Intens Care World* 1995;**12**:71–2.
12 Pollack MM, Katz RW, Ruttimann UE, Getson PR. Improving the outcome and efficiency of intensive care: the impact of an intensivist. *Crit Care Med* 1988;**16**:11–17.
13 Schuster DP, Kollef MH, eds. Predicting intensive care unit outcome. *Crit Care Clinics* 1994;**10**:1–246.
14 Pollack MM, Ruttimann UE, Getson PR. Pediatric risk of mortality (PRISM) score. *Crit Care Med* 1988;**16**:1110–16.
15 Pollack MM, Patel KM, Ruttimann VE. PRISM III: an updated pediatric risk of mortality score. *Crit Care Med* 1996;**24**:743–52.
16 Ruttimann UE, Pollack MM. A time-series approach to predict outcome from paediatric intensive care. *Comput Biomed Res* 1993;**26**:353–72.
17 Shann, F, Pearson G, Slater A, Wilkinson K. Paediatric index of mortality (PIM): a mortality prediction model for children in intensive care. *Intensive Care Med* 1997;**23**: 201–7.
18 Doyle LW, Murton LJ, Kitchen WH. Increasing the survival of extremely immature (24- to 28-weeks' gestation) infants – at what cost? *Med J Aust* 1989;**150**:558–68.
19 Kitchen WH, Doyle LW, Ford GW, *et al*. Changing two-year outcome of infants weighing 500 to 999 grams at birth: a hospital study. *J Pediatr* 1991;**118**:938–43.
20 Butt W, Shann F, Tibballs J, *et al*. Long-term outcome of children after intensive care. *Crit Care Med* 1990;**18**:961–5.

2: Acute respiratory emergencies

NIRANJAN KISSOON

Introduction

Respiratory system compromise leading to hypoxia is the most common life threatening emergency in children. It may be due to either primary respiratory diseases (acute respiratory emergencies) or respiratory embarrassment secondary to insults to other organ systems. For example, respiratory compromise may occur in trauma, shock, and acute brain injury and may contribute to the morbidity (secondary injuries) associated with these diseases. The major importance and pivotal role of respiratory system dysfunction as a contributor to morbidity and mortality in children is highlighted in the Advanced Pediatric Life Support Course of the American Academy of Pediatrics and the American College of Emergency Physicians, as well as the Pediatric Advanced Life Support Course of the American Heart Association.[1,2] In these courses, lectures and workshops which address respiratory insufficiency and failure and advanced airway management are the major focus.

The universal approach to resuscitation with attention to airway and breathing as first steps is predicated on the recognition of the deleterious effects of respiratory insufficiency. The natural progression of inadequately treated respiratory insufficiency is respiratory failure leading to cardiopulmonary failure and cardiopulmonary arrest (fig 2.1). Cardiopulmonary arrest has a dismal outcome in children with death or hypoxic cerebral damage occurring commonly. Recognition and management of acute respiratory emergencies prior to respiratory collapse offers the best chance of a favourable outcome. This chapter addresses the common acute respiratory emergencies and their management (table 2.1).

9

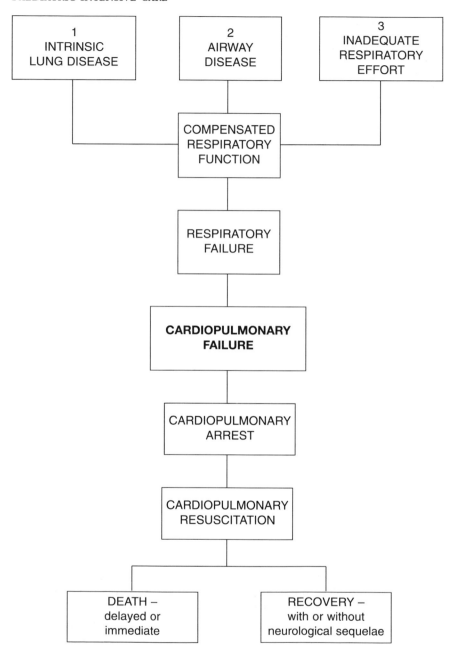

Common diseases in groups 1–3 are outlined in table 2.1

FIGURE 2.1—*Natural progression of acute respiratory emergencies*

TABLE 2.1—*Acute respiratory emergencies**

1. Intrinsic lung disease
   - Pneumonia
2. Airway diseases
   - Lower
     Bronchiolitis
     Severe bronchial asthma
   - Upper
     - Infections
       Acute laryngotracheobronchitis (croup)
       Supraglottitis
       Diphtheria
       Bacterial tracheitis (pseudomembranous croup)
       Pharyngeal and retropharyngeal abscess
       Tonsillitis and peritonsillar abscess
   - Accidents and trauma
     Glottic, subglottic or oesphageal foreign body
     External trauma to neck
     Burns to upper airway
     Iatrogenic
       Postintubation
       Postinstrumentation
     Angioedema
3. Inadequate respiratory effort
   - CNS depression from head injury, coma, status epilepticus, drug overdose
   - Peripheral nervous system dysfunction from spinal cord trauma, Guillain-Barre syndrome, botulism, myasthenia gravis
   - Increased chest wall compliance from flail chest
   - Respiratory muscle fatigue from excessive work of breathing, shock states
   - Respiratory muscle failure from muscular dystrophies

* Groups 1 and 2 relate primarily to the respiratory system and will be discussed in detail. Group 3 presents as respiratory emergencies secondary to non-respiratory system disease.

Pathophysiology and developmental anatomy

Children are predisposed to respiratory compromise as compared to adults because of anatomical and physiological differences of the respiratory system. A decreased alveolar number and diffusion area is one of several factors that places the child at a disadvantage. For instance, while there is a wide variation in the number of alveoli at birth, the average is 50 million as compared to 400 million in the average adult.[3] Of greater importance is the alveolar surface area which is $2.8 \, m^2$ at birth, $32 \, m^2$ at 8 years, and $75 \, m^2$ in the adult.[4] Children are also likely to sustain pathological decreases in alveolar number since alveolar and airway development are susceptible to *in utero* as well as early postnatal injuries. For example, regional lung dysplasia may be due to ventilator treatment of lung diseases in children, bronchopulmonary dysplasia, meconium aspiration, and viral infections. Dysplasia will result in decreased pulmonary reserve and, therefore, an increased susceptibility to acute respiratory decompensation.

11

The circular configuration of the thorax with the perpendicular attachment of the ribs to the vertebral column is a further disadvantage to children as it limits elevation of the ribs during inspiration. As the child develops the erect posture, the cross-sectional configuration of the chest becomes elliptical so that elevation of the rib cage occurs in the advantageous "bucket handle" movement. Elastic recoil of the chest also increases with age. It is assumed that the increase in recoil pressure results from progressive ossification of the rib cage, improvement in intercostal muscle tone, and the development of a negative pressure on the abdominal side of the diaphragm. In many childhood diseases (asthma, bronchiolitis, bronchopulmonary dysplasia) diaphragmatic contractility is also impaired as hyperinflation reduces diaphragmatic fibre length and force output.[5] The smaller diaphragmatic muscle mass of infants, fewer oxidative fatigue resistance fibres, soft cartilaginous rib cage, and inhibition of intercostal muscle activity during rapid eye movement sleep leads to inefficient ventilation and predisposes the child to diaphragmatic fatigue and apnoea.[6]

As resistance to airflow is related to the fourth power of the airway radius, small changes in the airway diameter have a profound effect on airway resistance in the child. The age at which an infant is no longer an obligate nose breather is uncertain. However, children with choanal atresia may have life threatening difficulties despite a patent oropharynx and an upper respiratory tract infection with copious nasal secretion may lead to mild to moderate respiratory distress in anatomically normal children. Upper airway compromise in children may also be due to anatomical factors such as micrognathia, neck flexion, tracheomalacia or subglottic stenosis. In addition, the relatively weak cartilaginous support in infants and young children may lead to dynamic compression of the trachea due to forced expiratory flows in asthma and bronchiolitis. The airway enlarges in diameter and length with age. However, the growth of the distal airway lags behind that of the proximal airway during the first five years of life, a phenomenon which may explain why viral infections of the lower airway pose more of a threat to infants and young children.[7]

Children are also at an increased risk of atelectasis due to small airway disease or mucous plugs. This occurs because the adult lung contains anatomical channels that allow ventilation distal to an obstructed airway, or "collateral ventilation". The interalveolar pores of Kohn appear between the first and second years of life, while Lambert's channels provide communication between bronchi and adjacent alveoli beginning at 8 years of age.[8] Without these channels, atelectasis or emphysematous changes may occur more commonly and lead to ventilation-perfusion mismatching.

Acute or chronic hypoxia in utero or in the early postnatal period may also delay the normal structural adaptive changes which lead to a fall in pulmonary vascular resistance. Patients with congenital heart disease with large left to right shunts (elevated pulmonary blood flow and pressure) have increased pulmonary vascular reactivity and abnormal smooth muscle growth and differentiation. These shunts may be important in the pathogenesis of progressive pulmonary vascular disease and pulmonary hypertension and may lead to a vicious cycle of right heart failure, further aggravation of hypoxia, and increased ventilation-perfusion mismatching. In addition, congenital heart disease with cardiomegaly or dilated pulmonary arteries may cause bronchial obstruction and lung overexpansion.

In summary, anatomic and physiologic factors as well as developmental abnormalities of the respiratory system place the infant and young child at a disadvantage as compared to older children and adults. The resultant decrease in respiratory reserve, coupled with an increased metabolic rate in childhood, leaves little room for deliberation when faced with a respiratory emergency.

An approach to acute respiratory emergencies

The child in acute respiratory distress should be approached in a calm, confident manner with minimal intrusion. In order to decrease anxiety, the child should initially be left to assume a position of comfort, usually in a parent's arms or lap. If, at any time during observation, the clinician suspects the need for airway support (including positioning, bag valve mask ventilation, and intubation), the child may need to be taken from the parents to the appropriate treatment area. Management strategies in children with respiratory emergencies depend on an estimation of the severity of respiratory insufficiency (evidence of hypoxia and hypercapnia) as well as a knowledge of the natural history of the presumptive diagnosis (table 2.2).

Assessment of severity of respiratory insufficiency

The assessment of severity of respiratory distress requires examination of overall clinical status as well as evaluation of target organ systems. It is important to appreciate that most diagnoses and therapeutic decisions in the child with acute respiratory distress can be made from a thorough history and physical examination. Laboratory monitoring in most cases is used to confirm the clinical impression. In respiratory emergencies, prompt and aggressive treatment should not be delayed by laboratory investigations. Laboratory evaluation, however, may aid in diagnosis and prognosis, guide and assess therapy, alert the caregiver to changes in status, and detect complications.

13

TABLE 2.2—*Clinical evidence of compromised gas exchange*

Evidence for hypercapnia*

Headache	Wheezing
Drowsiness, coma	Decreased air entry by auscultation
Sweating	Asymmetric air entry by auscultation
Tachycardia	Excessive work of breathing
Hypertension	Paradoxical chest wall motion
Peripheral vasodilation	Paradoxical abdominal wall motion
Stridor	Apnoeic episodes

Evidence for hypoxaemia*

Dyspnoea	Tachycardia
Confusion	Hypertension
Agitation	Peripheral vasoconstriction
Restlessness	Rales by auscultation
Tachypnoea	Murmur by auscultation
Retractions	Dysrhythmias
Nasal flaring	Bradycardia
Grunting	Hypotension
Sweating	Cyanosis

* In many instances, hypercapnia and hypoxaemia coexist and a clearcut separation based on signs and symptoms is not possible.

Respiratory monitoring may indicate the need for emergency therapy to prevent respiratory failure, the progression of illness despite therapy, an improvement related to therapeutic intervention, the ability to maintain spontaneous ventilation or, in some situations, irreversible loss of respiratory function.

The physical examination of the child in respiratory distress is discussed first as the history may not be immediately available and early intervention is frequently based on physical findings only.

Physical examination

General assessment

An appreciation of the variability of respiratory rate and heart rate in relation to age and clinical state is important in the overall assessment of respiratory distress. The normal respiratory rate of the child is inversely related to age with rates greater than 50 being abnormal in the infant and greater than 30 abnormal in the child.[1,2] The respiratory rate has its greatest variability in newborn and young infants and may be increased due to a variety of reasons including anxiety, fear, fever, pain, and sepsis. The heart rate is initially rapid at birth (120/min) and gradually decreases as the child approaches adolescence. Respiratory distress, with or without hypoxia, is one of the most common causes of tachycardia in children. Sinus tachycardia can also result from anxiety, fever, pain, blood loss, and any other insults which result in increased sympathomimetic activity.

Since the major pathophysiological derangement in respiratory insufficiency is hypoxaemia, it is important for the physician to recognise its global effects. An initial assessment of the child should detect evidence of diaphoresis, pupillary dilation, and fear, which are all features of the "fight or flight" adrenergic response to hypoxia (table 2.2). Posture provides a clue as to the degree of respiratory difficulty. The child who is alert, lying comfortably or playing is in minimal difficulty. However, the child who prefers to sit in a tripod position is in moderate to severe difficulty and is attempting to derive maximal diaphragmatic excursion since the diaphragm is approximately 4 cm higher in the supine position.

Central nervous system assessment

Of all vital organ systems, the central nervous system is the least tolerant of hypoxia. Central nervous system assessment does not entail a full neurological examination initially, but is limited to assessment of global neurological function such as alertness, cooperation, and motor activity. The child who is alert, cooperative, and active is not compromised to any great degree. However, the child with respiratory insufficiency who is restless or irritable or manifests any signs of confusion (such as inability to recognise parents) or has a decreased level of consciousness should be considered to be in respiratory failure. While seizure is an uncommon presenting sign, generalised seizures in a child with acute respiratory distress signify central nervous system oxygen deficiency and require aggressive treatment.[9]

Respiratory system assessment

The pattern of breathing, including respiratory rate, rhythm, and effort, is important in assessing the respiratory system. An abnormally high breathing frequency, or tachypnoea, is commonly seen with asthma, bronchiolitis, and pneumonia, but can also be seen with metabolic acidosis, fever, agitation or psychological disturbances. Tachypnoea is the expected compensatory response in lower airway disease and the finding of a normal or decreased respiratory rate, bradypnoea, may be an ominous sign signalling decompensation. The older child may be able to communicate the subjective experience of breathing difficulty, or dyspnoea. The child with moderate distress may be able to speak in phrases or partial sentences, whereas the severely affected child may be unable to speak or often can only speak in single words or short phrases. Grunting due to decreased lung compliance

15

is also common in lower airway disease, but may be absent in the child who is becoming fatigued.

Increased respiratory effort and work of breathing may be evaluated by assessment of accessory muscle use (sternomastoid, intercostal, and scalene muscles), subcostal, sternal, and intercostal retractions, nasal flaring, and the rate and depth of the respiratory effort. Children in moderate to severe respiratory distress will present in the initial stages with marked accessory muscle activity, as well as subcostal and intercostal retraction. Nasal flaring only may indicate mild respiratory distress, but use of sternomastoid and other accessory muscles signifies a markedly increased respiratory effort. The presence of poorly coordinated breathing (lack of coordination between thoracic and diaphragmatic muscles of respiration) is an ominous sign. In its extreme form, there is failure of synchronisation and the chest moves inward during inspiration. Decreased work of breathing in the child with moderate to severe respiratory distress may indicate extreme fatigue and imminent collapse.

Assessment of cyanosis

The colour of the skin and mucous membranes of the child in acute respiratory distress may be normal, pale or cyanotic, depending on severity and other factors. Central cyanosis suggests severe desaturation of haemoglobin but may not be recognised in the presence of anaemia, poor perfusion, hypercapnia or poor lighting in the examination room.[10] In addition, the evaluation of cyanosis is subjective.[11] If present, therefore, cyanosis is an important sign of compromised oxygenation but if it is absent, this should not be construed as indicating adequate oxygenation. An objective measure of oxygenation, pulse oximetry, is now widely available.

Cardiovascular system assessment

Tachycardia is the usual physiological response to respiratory insufficiency. However, a normal heart rate or bradycardia in the presence of hypoxaemia signifies severe myocardial oxygen deprivation. Pulsus paradoxus is a valuable sign in assessing the severity of airway obstruction in status asthmaticus.[12] Pulsus paradoxus of greater than 20 mmHg is associated with moderate to severe airway obstruction. However, its usefulness is limited to older children and adults, as it is difficult to elicit in the young child. This may be due to the use of inappropriately sized (too large) blood pressure cuffs or difficulty in auscultation of heart sounds due to noisy breathing.

The physician should be able to make an overall assessment of the severity of respiratory compromise based on the above features. Other signs and symptoms and historical features will be necessary to obtain a definitive diagnosis. A complete chest examination may provide clues to the diagnosis. For example, percussion will detect hyperresonance in asthma but not if pneumonia or severe atelectasis is present. Palpation of the chest wall will detect the presence of crepitations from surgical emphysema or tracheal deviation due to a pneumothorax. Finally, auscultation may reveal minimal or absent breath sounds (silent chest) indicative of severe air flow obstruction, widespread crackles in bronchiolitis, or unequal sounds in pneumonia or pneumothorax.

Laboratory investigations

In an acute respiratory emergency, the history and physical examination are sufficient to make a provisional diagnosis and guide initial therapy (including the need for airway support). The role for further laboratory investigations is more limited. Ideally, arterial blood gases should be used to provide an objective measure of pulmonary gas exchange (oxygen saturation and carbon dioxide content). Its usefulness in the young child may be limited if sampling proves difficult. The pain and anxiety associated with attempts at obtaining arterial gases may lead to sampling errors or cause further deterioration. This is most likely to occur in children with a severely compromised upper airway but also in any child with limited respiratory reserve. The arterial blood gas has limited usefulness in the initial assessment of younger children with upper airway obstruction.

Pulse oximetry, a non-invasive method of estimating circulating oxygen, can be used on either an intermittent or a continuous basis.[13] This monitor has the advantage of not requiring calibration before use. It also provides continuous readings and frequent changes of application site are not required. However, the disadvantage of pulse oximetry is that it does not reflect a decreasing PaO_2 until the PaO_2 is less than 80 mmHg. For patients with an S_aO_2 below 75–80%, values may not provide an accurate reflection of arterial oxygen saturation. In addition, the accuracy of oximetry can be affected by patient movement, compression of the sensor on the oximeter, low perfusion states, dysfunctional haemoglobin (methaemoglobinaemia), nail polish, and infrared heat lamps.

Chest radiography may be useful in confirming or refuting a diagnosis but should not delay treatment if the child is in respiratory failure. It is relatively contraindicated in severe upper airway obstruction, especially suspected epiglottitis. However, it is commonly used in patients in acute respiratory distress who are not in extremis. Radiographic examination should ideally be done at the bedside or the child should be accompanied to the radiology suite by personnel skilled in provision of assisted ventilation and carrying appropriate equipment. Investigations such as estimation of

17

peak expiratory flow rates are limited to the cooperative asthmatic in mild to moderate respiratory distress to establish baseline severity and as a guide to therapy. Peak expiratory flow rate measurements should not, however, delay therapy in severe asthma.

Search for definitive diagnosis

Upper airway emergencies (table 2.1)

Concurrent with assessment of the severity of respiratory distress, specific signs and symptoms and historical factors pinpointing specific diseases should be sought. For example, the features differentiating between croup,

TABLE 2.3—*Differentiating features between croup, bacterial tracheitis, and epiglottitis*

	Croup	Bacterial tracheitis	Epiglottitis
Aetiology	Viral	Staphylococcus α Haemolytic streptococci	*H. influenzae* Type B
Site of obstruction	Subglottic	Subglottic	Supraglottic
Age	6 months to 3 years	All ages	2–6 years
Clinical features			
Symptoms/signs			
Onset	Gradual (days)	Gradual	Sudden (hours)
Fever	37–38°C	38°C+	38°C+
Sound	Barky/stridor	Barky/stridor	Muffled/gutteral
Dysphagia	0	±	2+
Drooling	None	None	Present
Posture	Recumbent	Sitting	Sitting (tripod)
RR	Rapid	Normal	Initially normal
Retractions	Present	Present	Absent early
Facies	Normal	Anxious	Anxious, distressed, toxic
*X ray**			
	Subglottic narrowing Distention of hypopharynx Tapering of trachea (Steeple sign)	Subglottic narrowing Ragged tracheal mucosal surface	Enlarged epiglottis Distention of hypopharynx

* *X* rays should not be attempted if the diagnosis of epiglottitis is strongly suspected on clinical grounds.

epiglottitis, and bacterial tracheitis (table 2.3) are often distinctive. However, at times these conditions may be difficult to differentiate and may also be confused with a foreign body aspiration. In the assessment of the child with croup, estimation of the severity and the anticipated progression needs

TABLE 2.4—*Clinical croup score*

Parameter	0	1	2
Inspiratory breath sounds	Normal	Harsh, with rhonchi	Delayed
Stridor	None	Inspiratory	Inspiratory and expiratory
Cough	None	Hoarse cry	Bark
Retractions, flaring	None	Flaring and suprasternal retractions	Flaring, suprasternal intercostal retractions
Cyanosis	None	In air	In 40% oxygen

From Downes JJ, Raphaely RC. *Anesthesiology* 1975;**43**:238–50.
Mild croup usually has a score of less than 2, moderate croup a score of 2–4, and severe croup a score of 5 or greater.[57]

to be made in order to determine further management. The clinical croup score (table 2.4) has been recommended as a tool to aid in the decision making process, but it should not be used to replace good clinical judgment. In making decisions regarding triage of patients with croup, emphasis should be placed on the age of the child and on the ability of the parents to assess and respond appropriately if the child's condition deteriorates. In the child less than one year of age, the threshold for hospitalisation should be lower.

Foreign bodies in children lodge most commonly in the major bronchi.[14] Initially, the child may have coughing, gagging, choking, stridor, wheezing, hoarseness, dysphonia, drooling or cyanosis. The initial symptoms may resolve and a symptomless interval which lasts from hours to days or months may occur. The symptoms are determined by the location of the foreign body in the respiratory tract and the degree of obstruction. Total obstruction at the level of the trachea or larynx will rapidly produce respiratory failure and an inability to assist ventilation artificially. Partial obstruction in the larynx can cause inspiratory stridor, aphonia, drooling, gagging, and poor gas exchange, whereas partial obstruction of the trachea may present with inspiratory stridor, choking, and coughing. Partial obstruction of the bronchus results in wheezing and coughing.

Retropharyngeal abscess, although uncommon, is mainly seen in children less than 3 years of age. It presents with a preceding history of an upper respiratory tract infection or sore throat, fever, stridor, toxic appearance, meningism, and difficulty in swallowing secretions. The child may lie with the neck extended. The diagnosis is suggested by widening of the soft tissue space between the cervical vertebrae and air column on lateral *x* ray of the neck and is confirmed by examination under anaesthesia. Tonsillitis or peritonsillar abscess may also cause airway obstruction. The usual symptoms include trismus, pain on talking, muffled voice, drooling, and dysphagia. Diphtheria usually presents with a sore throat, low grade fever, and signs of airway obstruction due to a thick pharyngeal membrane. The associated palatopharyngeal incoordination may also lead to swallowing difficulties.

Orofacial trauma may result in mechanical obstruction of the airway due to teeth, blood, and fragments of bone or haematoma at the base of the tongue. External trauma to the neck may result in stridor, voice change, subcutaneous emphysema, and severe respiratory distress. Internal trauma of the airway is usually less obvious and may result from intubation, endoscopy or chemical burns. Airway obstruction more commonly occurs in children with preexisting subglottic stenosis. Predisposing conditions for acquired subglottic stenosis include prior intubation (particularly with an endotracheal tube of excessive diameter), neck trauma, burns, high tracheostomy site, traumatic intubation, and infection.[15] Angioneurotic oedema may cause upper airway obstruction and usually involves localised skin swelling, as well as oedema of the face, hand, and feet.

Lower airway emergencies

Asthma, the most common lower airway emergency, manifests as expiratory wheezing. Most children will have a history of reactive airway disease and will already be receiving treatment. The diagnosis, however, can be difficult on the first presentation or in a child with atypical symptoms. A family history of reactive airway disease, a history of recurring symptoms, and a good response to bronchodilators all support the diagnosis. One should remember the aphorism that "all that wheezes is not asthma", although asthma is the most common cause. The severity of symptomatology in asthmatics can be categorised into mild, moderate, and severe by features outlined in table 2.5.

Bronchiolitis usually presents with an upper respiratory prodrome which includes copious nasal discharge, restlessness, cough, and fever. The onset of lower airway involvement is characterised by tachypnoea, tachycardia, and chest retractions. Auscultation of the lungs reveals wheezing with occasional fine crackles. Other causes of wheezing that should be borne in mind, especially in the young child, are bacterial pneumonia, chlamydia pneumonitis, anatomical abnormalities such as a vascular ring, foreign body, and congestive heart failure.

Treatment of airway emergencies

When respiratory insufficiency is diagnosed, the initial response should be provision of supplemental inspired oxygen and, if indicated, assisted

TABLE 2.5—*Assessment of the severity of acute asthma*

	Mild	Moderate	Severe
History	Intermittent wheezing On no chronic medications Few hospitalisations	On chronic medications ≤2 treatments at home Regular hospitalisation No ICU admissions	On chronic medications ≥2 treatments at home ICU admission(s) Intravenous β-agonist Previous ventilations
Physical examination			
CNS	Absence of CNS signs Speaks in full sentences Minimal use of accessory muscles	Anxious, speaks in phrases or partial sentences Use of accessory muscles	Coma, seizures Speaks only in single words or short phrases Signs of chronic respiratory insufficiency
Respiratory system	No cyanosis in room air Good air entry with wheezes	Cyanosis in 40% oxygen Decreased air entry with wheezes	Cyanosis in 100% oxygen Silent chest
Cardiovascular system	↑ HR PP<10 mmHg	↑↑ HR PP 10–20 mmHg	↑↑↑ or ↓ HR PP>20 mmHg
PEFR	70–90% of predicted or of baseline function	50–70% of predicted or of baseline function	<50% of predicted or of baseline function
FEV$_1$/-FVC	85%	75%	45%
Pulse oximetry[x]	S$_a$O$_2$ >95%	S$_a$O$_2$ 90–95%	S$_a$O$_2$ <90%
Blood gases[x]	PaO$_2$>80 PaCO$_2$<35	↓ PaO$_2$ (60–80) N or ↑ (PaCO$_2$<50)	↓ PaO$_2$<60 ↑ PaCO$_2$>50

FVC	Forced vital capacity	↑ Increased
FEV$_1$	Forced expiratory volume 1 s	↓ Decreased
PEFR	Peak expiratory flow rate	HR Heart rate
x	At sea level in room air	PP Pulsus paradoxus
N	Normal	

Categorisation into mild, moderate or severe respiratory compromise should ideally be based on an overall assessment of the patient and not on a single parameter.

21

ventilation using a bag valve mask device. Endotracheal intubation may be necessary for a variety of reasons, the most common being the provision

TABLE 2.6—*Indications for endotracheal intubation*

1. Cardiopulmonary resuscitation
2. Need to maintain a patent airway
   - Airway obstruction (croup, epiglottitis)
   - Ineffective cough and gag reflex (altered sensorium)
3. Need to improve respiratory effort
   - Poor effort
   - Central (drugs, infection, trauma)
   - Spinal cord (trauma)
   - Chest wall deformity (kyphosis)
   - Normal effort but overwhelming demand
     - Upper airway disease (croup, epiglottitis)
     - Lower airway disease (bronchiolitis, asthma, pneumonia)
4. Need to control other systems
   - Elevated intracranial pressure – hyperventilation
   - Shock – remove respiratory effort
   - Drug overdose – airway protection during gastric lavage

of ventilation to alleviate respiratory failure (table 2.6). In fact, respiratory failure accounts for 50% of admissions to critical care units and is the third most common cause of death in infants.

Endotracheal intubation

A thorough knowledge of the anatomy and physiology of the paediatric respiratory system is crucial for effective management of the airway (table 2.7). Successful intubation can only be guaranteed when the medical personnel and patient are properly prepared and the appropriate equipment is available (table 2.8).[16] The need for intubation should be anticipated and it should be performed as a semielective procedure, rather than waiting until there is cardiorespiratory collapse and the need to perform a crash intubation.

Intubation should be conducted by the most experienced person available in a calm and orderly fashion. All patients should have cardiorespiratory and pulse oximetry monitoring. Under some conditions, such as the non-fasting state, patients with head trauma and possibly increased intracranial pressure, and in severe respiratory distress such as asthma, intubation may be achieved using the rapid sequence induction technique. The suggested sequence for rapid sequence induction is outlined in fig 2.2. While the scope of this chapter precludes an indepth discussion of intubation techniques, interested readers may obtain further information from recent literature and advanced life support courses.[1,2,16,17] One should be aware that rapid sequence induction should not be used or should be used very cautiously

TABLE 2.7—*Differences in the paediatric airway when compared with that in the adult*

Anatomic differences	Clinical significance
Proportionally larger head	Increases neck flexion and obstruction
Smaller nostrils	Increases airway resistance
Larger tongue	Increases airway resistance
Decreased muscle tone	Airway obstruction by tongue
Epiglottitis – longer, stiffer, more horizontal	Increases airway obstruction
Larynx more anterior	Difficult to perform blind intubation
Cricoid ring is narrowest portion	Cuffed tubes not recommended
Shorter trachea	Increases right mainstem intubation
Airway more narrow	Increases airway resistance

Physiologic differences	Adult	Infant
RR (breath/min)	15	40
Tidal volume (ml/kg)	6	6
Vital capacity (ml/kg)	70	35
Total lung capacity (ml/kg)	86	63
O_2 consumption (ml/kg/min)	3.5	6.4

TABLE 2.8—*Sequence of intubation*

- Have drugs and equipment available
- Use sniffing position to align the airway
- Preoxygenation:
    Awake: 100% by mask
    Apnoeic: 100% bag and mask
- Sedation
- Preoxygenation – establish ability to ventilate
- Administer muscle relaxant
- Open mouth
- Insert laryngoscope and sweep tongue to left
- Suctioning may be required
- Visualise cords
- Insert endotracheal tube from right side
- Check correct tube position

under conditions in which intubation may be difficult, such as significant facial oedema (angioedema), upper airway trauma, distorted laryngotracheal anatomy or airway anomalies.

Once the endotracheal tube is inserted, it is important to ascertain its position, as right mainstem intubation is a common complication. Proper position of the tube is judged by the following: direct visualisation between cords, auscultation of chest and epigastrium, symmetric chest movement, stable vital signs, endotracheal carbon dioxide monitoring and, more recently, magnetic detectors.[18] Confirmation of tube length requires immediate chest radiography. If the endotracheal tube position in the

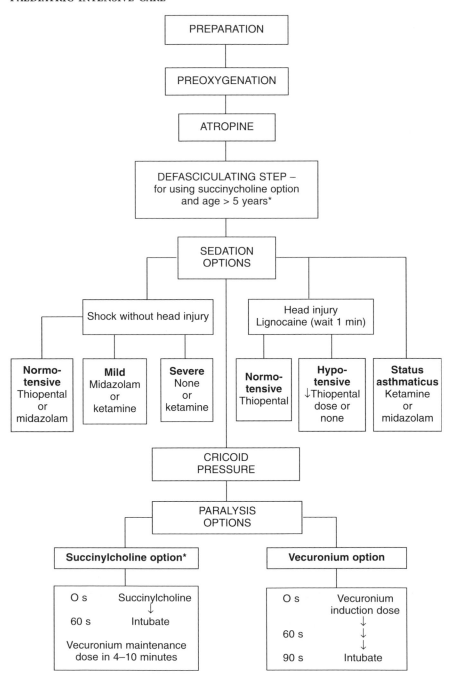

FIGURE 2.2—*Suggested sequence and options for rapid sequence induction*

trachea cannot be confirmed by these methods and the patient's condition is deteriorating, the tube should be removed and bag valve mask ventilation commenced. Intubation can then be reattempted after adequate reoxygenation.

Upper airway emergencies

Intubation for upper airway obstruction (table 2.1) should follow the general principles outlined for endotracheal intubation and requires the coordinated efforts of a skilled team. If the child becomes obtunded or is unable to ventilate adequately prior to intubation, bag valve mask ventilation should be initiated. In spite of the degree of obstruction, many of these patients can be effectively ventilated using a bag valve mask apparatus. If this is effective, then awaiting more experienced personnel is advisable as inexperienced manipulation of the airway may cause trauma and further increase the degree of obstruction. If bag valve mask ventilation is ineffective, intubation should be attempted by the physician present who is most skilled in the procedure. If this fails, needle cricothyroidotomy should be attempted.

A needle cricothyroidotomy consists of placing a catheter into the tracheal lumen through the cricothyroid membrane. The procedure involves placing the patient in the supine position with the head slightly extended and in the midline. Using aseptic techniques, the cricothyroid membrane is identified between the thyroid and cricoid cartilages. The trachea is stabilised using the thumb and forefinger of one hand to prevent lateral displacement during the procedure. The skin is punctured in the midline through the lower half of the cricothyroid membrane using a 12–14 gauge over the needle catheter attached to a 5–15 ml syringe. The needle should be advanced caudally at a 45° angle while applying negative pressure to the syringe. Entry into the tracheal lumen is accompanied by aspiration of air. The stylet should be withdrawn and the catheter advanced further and secured to the patient's neck. The hub of the catheter might then be attached to oxygen tubing with a side hole connected to an oxygen source capable of delivering at least 50 psi at the nipple. Intermittent ventilation can be achieved by occluding a side hole cut in the oxygen tubing with the thumb for one second and releasing for four seconds. Tidal volume is determined by oxygen flow rate. Adequate oxygenation can be maintained using this technique for 30–45 min.

The treatment of severe croup, bacterial tracheitis and epiglottitis are outlined in the algorithm in fig 2.3. The patient should initially be provided with oxygen in a non-threatening manner and nursed in the parent's arms. In patients with severe croup, racemic adrenaline (0.25–0.50 ml of a 2.25% solution diluted 1:8 and aerosolised) should

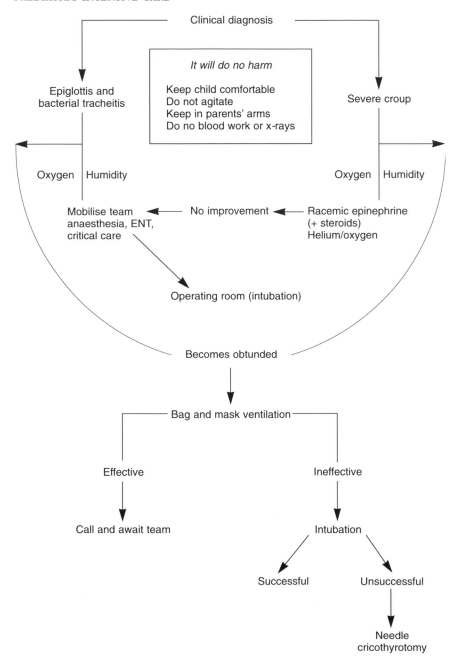

Clinical diagnosis

It will do no harm

Keep child comfortable
Do not agitate
Keep in parents' arms
Do no blood work or x-rays

Epiglottis and
bacterial tracheitis

Severe croup

Oxygen | Humidity

Oxygen | Humidity

Mobilise team ◄— No improvement ◄— Racemic epinephrine
anaesthesia, ENT,   (+ steroids)
critical care   Helium/oxygen

Operating room (intubation)

Becomes obtunded

Bag and mask ventilation

Effective

Ineffective

Call and await team

Intubation

Successful

Unsuccessful

Needle
cricothyrotomy

FIGURE 2.3—*Algorithm for the management of epiglottitis, bacterial tracheitis and severe croup*

26

be administered to provide relief of the obstruction. Several treatments with racemic epinephrine may suffice. However, in those refractory to adrenaline, helium, a low density inert gas, may be tried. Helium is substituted for nitrogen to decrease the force necessary to move the gas through the airways. When provided with a mixture of 20–30% oxygen and 70–80% helium in an intensive care unit setting, patients with croup refractory to adrenaline have shown improvement, with immediate recurrence of symptoms if the mixture was removed.[19] Helium-oxygen mixtures are also useful in patients in whom racemic adrenaline is contraindicated (for example, those with tetralogy of Fallot).[19] The limitations of helium-oxygen mixtures include the high expense of helium, the high concentrations required (minimum 60%), and the temporising rather than curative property of the treatment.[19]

Several recent studies have reported substantial improvement in children with croup treated with steroids.[21,22] Benefit has been demonstrated with oral, intramuscular, and inhaled administration. A single dose of nebulised steroids (2 mg of nebulised budesonide) may therefore be tried in patients with mild or severe croup while injected forms may be appropriate for severe cases (0.6 mg/kg dexamethasone).[20,21,22] If there is a favourable response, the child may be transferred to the critical care unit for further monitoring and management (nothing by mouth, humidity, and oxygen). The use of oral or intramuscular dexamethasone has eliminated the need for intubation in most cases. However, children who do not respond to therapy and who are becoming exhausted and obtunded should be considered for emergency intubation. Intubation is best conducted following inhalation anaesthesia with personnel skilled in airway support in attendance.

The suspicion of a diagnosis of epiglottitis necessitates transportation of the child to the operating or resuscitation room accompanied by the parent and appropriate personnel as well as equipment to secure an emergency airway. Following an inhalation anaesthetic, nasotracheal intubation should be performed and antibiotics administered (cefotaxime 150 mg/kg/day intravenously every eight hours for 2–3 days followed by chloramphenicol 100 mg/kg/day orally every six hours for a further 3–4 days). Blood and supraglottic swab specimens should be sent for culture.

In patients with bacterial tracheitis, marked respiratory distress and toxicity may demand urgent endotracheal intubation. Laryngoscopy reveals a normal epiglottis with subglottic oedema and copious mucopurulent secretions from the trachea. *Staphylococcus aureus* is the most common organism. As in patients with epiglottitis, broad spectrum antibiotic therapy (cefuroxime 75–200 mg/kg/day or nafcillin 50–100 mg/kg/day every six hours and chloramphenicol 100 mg/kg/day every six hours) should be prescribed.

Traumatic injuries caused by foreign bodies, iatrogenic instrumentation injuries, and chemical or thermal burns are also common causes of upper respiratory airway obstruction. Acute airway injury due to chemical or thermal burns necessitates intensive care admission for close monitoring for signs and symptoms of airway compromise. Endoscopic examination of the airway and oesophagus may be indicated in some patients. Intravenous fluids, oxygen, and racemic epinephrine may relieve obstructive symptoms and alleviate the need for mechanical airway support. Early relief of airway obstruction is strongly indicated, particularly in airway burns. Corticosteroids, although used by some physicians, are probably of no benefit.

Foreign body removal requires close teamwork between the intensive care practitioner, pulmonologist or surgeon, and anaesthesiologist. The use of inhaled bronchodilators, postural drainage, and percussion is not recommended for foreign body removal because dislodgment of a distal foreign body into the subglottic space may cause severe or total airway obstruction.[23] Patients with complete upper airway obstruction due to an impacted laryngeal or tracheal foreign body will present with an inability to speak or generate airflow, cyanosis, and possibly cardiorespiratory arrest. The airway should be opened by grasping both the tongue and the lower jaw between the thumbs and fingers and lifting (tongue-jaw lift). If a foreign body is visualised, it should be removed. Blind finger sweeps are not recommended since they may push a foreign body further into the airway. If this manoeuvre fails in a child, the Heimlich manoeuvre should be attempted.[1,2,24]

In the conscious (standing or sitting) victim, the Heimlich manoeuvre is performed in the following manner.

1. Stand behind the victim with arms directly under the victim's axillae, encircling the victim's torso.
2. The thumb side of one fist should be placed against the victim's abdomen in the midline slightly above the umbilicus and well below the tip of the xiphoid process.
3. The fist should be grasped with the other hand and a series of quick upward thrusts administered.
4. Each thrust should be a separate, distinct movement, intended to relieve the obstruction. Abdominal thrusts should be continued until the foreign body is expelled or the patient loses consciousness.
5. If the victim loses consciousness, the airway should be opened using a tongue-jaw lift and the obstructing object removed with a finger sweep, if visualised.
6. Rescue breathing should be attempted after proper head positioning. If the airway remains obstructed in the unconscious victim the Heimlich manoeuvre should be repeated as outlined below.

In the unconscious victim, the Heimlich manoeuvre is performed in the supine position as follows.

1. Jaw lift should be attempted and any foreign object removed by finger sweep.
2. If rescue breathing is unsuccessful, one should kneel beside the victim or straddle the victim's hips.
3. The heel of one hand should be placed on the child's abdomen in the midline slightly above the umbilicus and well below the rib cage and xiphoid process while the other hand is placed on top of the first.
4. Both hands should be pressed into the abdomen with a quick upward thrust directed upward in the midline for five distinct thrusts.
5. The airway should then be opened by grasping both tongue and lower jaw and lifting the mandible (tongue-jaw lift) and the foreign body, if visualised, removed by a finger sweep.
6. The manoeuvre should be repeated until ventilation is successful.

For the infant less than 1 year old, the Heimlich manoeuvre (subdiaphragmatic thrusts) is not recommended because of the potential for liver injury. Back blows, chest thrusts, and the use of gravity should be instituted.[1,2]

The emergency medical services should be activated after approximately one minute of attempting foreign body expulsion and rescue efforts resumed. In situations in which the emergency airway equipment is unavailable and the Heimlich manoeuvre has failed to dislodge a foreign body in the upper airway, endotracheal intubation may be tried in the unconscious patient. The foreign body may then be advanced into a mainstem bronchus (usually right) and ventilation administered through the endotracheal tube withdrawn into the trachea. Alternatively, the foreign body may be extracted if it becomes impacted into the lumen of the endotracheal tube which is then removed from the airway.

The child suspected of having an allergic reaction and who complains of hoarseness, dysphagia or a lump in the throat should be promptly treated with adrenaline, even if the oropharyngeal examination is normal. Adrenaline (1:1000 dilution) is administered in a dose of 0.01 ml/kg to a maximum of 0.3 ml/kg intramuscularly if hypotension or airway compromise exists. This dose should be repeated at 10–20 min intervals, depending on the patient's response. Standard supportive measures including intravenous fluids, supplemental oxygen, and cardiac monitoring should be provided for these patients. If complete airway obstruction occurs or if respiratory distress worsens despite parenteral adrenaline, the patient should be intubated orally. Nebulised racemic adrenaline may be attempted while preparing for intubation although its benefits, if any, are transient. If supraglottic oedema obscures the airway, cricothyrotomy (in older children) or needle cricothyroidotomy (in children younger than 6 years) with percutaneous transtracheal ventilation may be performed prior to airway access by surgical means or further attempts at intubation by skilled personnel.

Lower airway emergencies

Acute severe asthma is the most common lower airway emergency encountered in the paediatric population. The history and physical examination (table 2.5) will enable the clinician to identify those who are severely ill or at high risk of further deterioration. The initial arterial oxygen saturation using pulse oximetry is useful in determining the severity of disease and outcome of therapy. In one study, although no cut-off could be established (because trends were gradual), a saturation of less than or equal to 91% had a substantially higher likelihood of poor outcome (admission or return to the emergency department).[25] Historical factors placing a patient at high risk for life threatening asthma are as follows.

- Previous severe asthma (respiratory failure requiring intubation, hypoxic seizures)
- Frequent need for hospitalisation to control asthma
- Dependence on corticosteroids (inhaled or oral)
- Non-compliance or abuse of medications
- Labile asthma with pronounced diurnal airway obstruction
- Brittle asthma with unexpected rapid deterioration of pulmonary function
- Chronic asthma with depressive symptoms and manipulative use of asthma[26]

Patients admitted to general hospital wards have a higher mortality from asthma than those admitted to intensive care units, despite the presumption that ward patients were less severely ill on admission.[27] Indications for paediatric critical care admission for children with status asthmaticus are outlined in table 2.9.[28,29]

While there are minor differences in drug preference in the treatment of severe asthma, the most commonly used drugs are outlined in table 2.10. Humidified oxygen should be administered to maintain PaO_2 above 80 mmHg or oxygen saturation above 92%. Reversal of bronchospasm may be achieved by β-adrenergic receptor simulation which leads to bronchial smooth muscle relaxation. Several β-agonists, both selective (β_2) and non-selective (β_1), have been utilised in the treatment of the severely asthmatic child. Non-selective β_1-agonists include adrenaline, ephedrine, and isoprenaline while selective β_2-agonists include isoetharine, metaproterenol, terbutaline, salbutamol, phenylterol, bitolterol, pirbuterol, and salmeterol.[30]

30

TABLE 2.9—*Indications for paediatric critical care admission for status asthmaticus*

- Disturbed consciousness
- Exhaustion
- Recumbent position accompanied by diaphoresis
- Markedly decreased air entry
- Interrupted speech
- Elevated or rising carbon dioxide tension
- Air leak syndrome
- Severe hyperexpansion
- Previous history of respiratory failure
- Drug toxicity, particularly theophylline or sedatives
- Worsening or failure to improve on standard therapy
- Cardiac or respiratory arrest
- Metabolic acidosis
- Peak flow rates 100 l/min or less or falling rates despite therapy
- Inability to provide adequate staffing on general wards

The importance of β-agonists is such that selective β_2-agonist administration is often the first line therapy for children with status asthmaticus.[31]

Salbutamol is a selective β_2-adrenergic agonist with pharmacological properties similar to terbutaline.[32,33] When salbutamol is administered by nebulisation, it produces significant bronchodilation within 15 min and lasts for 3–4 hours. The cardiovascular effects of salbutamol are considerably less than those of isoprenaline in doses producing comparable bronchodilation. The frequency of administration of nebulised β_2-agonists continues to be controversial. Most investigators recommend that these drugs be given every 20–30 min and not more frequently than every 20 min, a recommendation that is also supported by the drug manufacturers.[34] A recent study suggests that continuous nebulisation of β_2-adrenergic agonists is more effective than intermittent nebulisation in the treatment of severe status asthmaticus.[35]

Some children treated with nebulised β_2-agonists such as salbutamol may not improve and progress to respiratory failure. Intravenous sympathomimetics (isoprenaline, terbutaline, and salbutamol) may be used in these patients in an attempt to avoid mechanical ventilation. Tachycardia, myocardial ischaemia, cardiac muscle enzyme elevation, and death have been associated with intravenous isoprenaline and hence this agent is less favoured compared to the selective β_2-agonists. At equipotent doses, selective β_2-agonists are probably as effective as isoprenaline in reversing hypercarbia with less cardiac risk.[36] Intravenous administration of β_2-agonists may result in more adverse effects than continuous nebulisation. All patients with respiratory failure therefore should have continuous monitoring of heart rate, respiratory rate, pulse oximetry, and arterial pressure via an indwelling arterial line. In addition, frequent blood

TABLE 2.10—*Drug therapy in severe asthma*

Drug	Dosage	Comment
Nebulised β-agonists		
Salbutamol	0.1–0.3 mg/kg/h	Given continuously
Anticholinergic agents		
Nebulised ipratropium bromide	125–250 µg q 3–6 h	Available only as metered red dose inhaler in the United States
Intravenous β-agonists		
Terbutaline	Loading dose of 10 µg/kg over 30 min followed by continuous infusion of 1–10 µg/kg/min	
Salbutamol	As above	As above
Subcutaneous β-agonist		
Adrenaline	0.01 mg/kg of 1:1000 sol q 20 min × 3 doses	
Steroids		
Methylprednisolone	1 mg/kg q 4–6 h	
Hydrocortisone	5 mg/kg q 4–6 h	
Methylxanthines		
Aminophylline	Loading dose of 10 mg/kg (maximum 500 mg)	Monitor serum levels
Magnesium sulphate	30–70 mg/kg IV over 30 min once only	Not FDA approved for this use; monitor serum level (see text)
Sedatives		
Lorazepam	0.05–0.1 mg/kg q 4–6 h prn	For emergence reaction after ketamine
Ketamine	4 µg/kg/min by continuous infusion	

gases, glucose, and serum electrolyte monitoring should be performed. Haemodynamic effects seen with intravenous β_2-agonist therapy include tachycardia, dysrhythmias, hypertension, and possible myocardial ischaemia. Metabolic side effects include hypoglycaemia, hypokalaemia, rhabdomyolysis, lactic acidosis and hypophosphataemia.

Stimulation of cholinergic receptors in the airway by a variety of stimuli may result in reflex bronchoconstriction which can be blocked by anticholinergic agents. Currently, at least five drugs (atropine, ipratropium bromide, oxytropium bromide, atropine methonitrate, and glycopyrrolate bromide) are in use or are being actively investigated as anticholinergic bronchodilators. Ipratropium bromide is the only anticholinergic agent currently approved by the United States Food and Drug Administration as a bronchodilator. In a number of relatively small studies in children, the concomitant use of inhaled ipratropium bromide and a selective β_2-agonist has been shown to produce a significant improvement in lung function, compared to treatment with aerosolised β_2-agonists alone. Ipratropium bromide or other anticholinergic agents should only be used to augment the bronchodilator effect of a selective β_2-agonist and not as the sole bronchodilator.[37]

Theophylline, a methylxanthine derivative that functions at least in part as a bronchodilator, has been used widely for many years in the treatment of acute asthma. Although a few reports cast doubt on its efficacy when administered with β-agonists during the acute asthmatic episode, theophylline is still a useful drug in acute asthma.[38] It is still widely accepted in many institutions as one of the first line drugs for acute asthma as well as chronic maintenance therapy. However, recently it has been used less frequently in North America and mostly in children who respond poorly or fail to improve on maximum β-agonist therapy.

Corticosteroid administration is important in the treatment of status asthmaticus because inflammation is central to the pathophysiology of asthma. Acute administration of intravenous or intramuscular methylprednisolone or oral prednisone in the emergency department can reduce hospitalisation rates and prevent relapse of symptoms if continued.[39] Although the standard recommended dose of corticosteroid (methylprednisolone 2–4 mg/kg/day every six hours IV) will maintain a minimal plasma steroid concentration of 100–150 mg/ml, the ideal preparation, dose, and dosing interval of corticosteroid have not been determined. There has been a recent tendency to use higher doses with shorter dosing intervals in children with severe disease.[40] Corticosteroids should be administered immediately to any asthmatic in moderate or severe distress and should be strongly considered in any acutely ill patient with a history of severe attacks, frequent hospitalisations or multiple courses of steroid use. Patients with a history of prolonged, debilitating symptoms, especially those who have been resistant to aggressive inhalation therapy, are also candidates for corticosteroids.

Other therapies such as sodium bicarbonate, sedatives, anaesthetic agents, and magnesium sulphate have also been used in acute severe asthma with varying success. The role of bicarbonate therapy is still controversial and is usually restricted to partial correction of metabolic acidosis (when base excess exceeds -5), in patients who have responded to inhaled bronchodilators but continue to hyperventilate and experience dyspnoea.[41] Bicarbonate is also used to buffer respiratory acidosis especially when utilising controlled hypoventilation in the intubated child.

Sedatives may be used to decrease anxiety and provide bronchodilation in the paediatric intensive care environment where monitoring is ideal and expertise is immediately available. Ketamine is a dissociative anesthetic with excellent sedative and analgesic properties. It also relaxes smooth muscles directly, as well as possessing sympathomimetic actions. Ketamine (0.5–1.0 mg/kg over 5 min then infused at 1.0–2.5 mg/kg/hour) has been shown to be beneficial in intubated asthmatic children who were not responding to maximal bronchodilator therapy by decreasing peak inspiratory pressures, increasing chest wall excursions, and decreasing arterial carbon dioxide tension.[42] Ketamine has also been administered to non-intubated asthmatic children who have failed conventional management and to facilitate intubation.[43] Side effects of ketamine include arrhythmias due to catecholamine sensitisation, increased airway secretions and, rarely, laryngospasm. Benzodiazepines (diazepam 0.1–0.2 mg/kg/hour or lorazepam 0.1 mg/kg loading then 0.025 mg/kg/hour) should be administered concomitantly in the intubated child to ameliorate emergence reactions. Inhaled anaesthetic agents (halothane, isoflurane, and ethrane) have also been tried as bronchodilators with varying success.[44]

Magnesium sulphate is now being used with increasing frequency in the child with acute asthma not responding to conventional therapy. Documentation of objective improvement from uncontrolled studies has been difficult because of the concurrent administration of other bronchodilators. Our recent experience of using a one-time dose of 40–50 mg/kg intravenously over 20 min in four patients was associated with a 20–90% improvement in peak expiratory flow rate and a 14–25% decrease in $PaCO_2$.[45] While individual variations are commonly observed, a serum magnesium level of 4 mg/dl or higher is usually necessary to achieve a significant bronchodilation. The onset of action of intravenous magnesium is within minutes of starting the infusion and lasts approximately two hours. Our ongoing studies have suggested that a loading dose of 60–70 mg/kg intravenously and a continuous infusion of 20–40 mg/kg/hour is needed to maintain optimal serum levels. Side effects of magnesium infusions are mild and include transient sensations of facial warmth, flushing or malaise. Significant adverse effects have not been reported.[44,46]

Management of a severe attack

Patients in moderate to severe distress should receive nebulised therapy at least every 20–30 min or continuously until improvement is noted or side effects limit administration. If nebulised therapy is not immediately available, subcutaneous adrenaline should be administered. The asthmatic in severe respiratory distress who does not respond to treatment with frequent nebulised β-agonists presents a management challenge. In such patients, intravenous β-agonists have been used successfully to reverse bronchospasm and avert the need for mechanical ventilation. Intravenous steroids should also be administered in such patients. The use of other therapeutic modalities, as outlined in table 2.10, depends on the patient's condition, other medications, and personal preference of the treating physician.

Mechanical ventilation

The indications for mechanical ventilation in status asthmaticus should be considered carefully and are as follows.

- Failure of maximal pharmacologic therapy
- Cyanosis and hypoxaemia (PaO_2 of less than 60 mmHg) unrelieved by oxgen therapy
- $PaCO_2$ greater than 65 mmHg and rising more than 5 mmHg per hour or accompanied by severe acidaemia
- Minimal chest movement or minimal air entry
- Severe retractions
- Deteriorating mental status, lethargy or agitation
- Recumbent position and severe diaphoresis
- Respiratory or cardiac arrest

The goal of mechanical ventilation is to rest the inspiratory muscles and provide adequate gas exchange until the severe airway obstruction can be reversed pharmacologically.

There have been no studies demonstrating the superiority of one mode of ventilation over another. As these patients are usually paralysed or anaesthetised, the control mode of ventilation is preferred. In the conventional ventilation technique, the tidal volume is set at 10–12 ml/kg and minute ventilation is gradually increased by adjusting either the frequency or inspiratory flow rates to normalise $PaCO_2$ gradually. Concern about the adverse effects of high peak airway pressure has popularised the use of controlled hypoventilation as an alternative ventilation strategy.[47] Mechanical ventilation should be limited to as short a time as possible until the bronchodilators and steroids are producing their effect.[48]

Bronchiolitis

In many healthy infants, bronchiolitis is a self-limiting illness and can be managed safely at home. However, patients who are unable to tolerate feeding require hospital admission and intravenous fluids to maintain hydration. Patients should be monitored closely and those with hypoxia given supplemental oxygen therapy. Patients with underlying cardiopulmonary disease, especially infants with bronchopulmonary dysplasia, usually require hospitalisation. Because of the similarities between bronchiolitis and asthma, and because bronchoconstriction may play a role in the illness, common clinical practice also includes the use of β-agonist therapy. However, there is no convincing evidence that bronchodilators produce clinically significant improvement in infants with viral bronchiolitis.[49] The mainstay of therapy, therefore, is oxygen, minimal handling, and fluid management. If β-agonist therapy is to be used (doses similar to asthma), it should be combined with careful monitoring of heart rate and oxygen saturation and should not be continued if deterioration or no clinical benefit is noted. A recent report on the use of racemic adrenaline suggests that it is superior to salbutamol in infants with bronchiolitis and deserves consideration as a treatment option in infants whose symptoms are poorly responsive to β-agonists.[50]

Patients in severe respiratory distress, especially those who are hypercarbic, should be considered candidates for admission to a paediatric intensive care unit. The need for intubation and ventilation is usually based on clinical criteria (respiratory muscle fatigue). Optimal ventilation is achieved utilising high tidal volumes (10–15 ml/kg), slow intermittent mandatory ventilation (16–22 breaths per minute), allowing a prolonged expiratory time.[51]

Ribavirin, a broad spectrum antiviral agent, was approved in 1986 by the United States Food and Drug Administration for treatment of serious respiratory syncytial virus infection in hospitalised children. The American Academy of Pediatrics recommends its administration in infants who are at high risk for severe or complicated infection and those who are severely ill or mechanically ventilated for respiratory syncytial viral infection.[52,53] The recommendations, however, are not widely endorsed by paediatric intensivists and hence indications for its use are still being widely debated.

Pneumonia

A significant percentage of infantile pneumoniae result in hospitalisation and as many as 25% of hospitalised children require intensive care.[54] Viral pneumonia, including respiratory syncytial virus, is a frequent cause of admission to the paediatric ICU for respiratory failure. Other common causes are parainfluenza virus and adenovirus. Pneumonia caused by adenovirus can be especially severe and may result in chronic disability due to bronchiolitis obliterans. The clinical features of non-bacterial pneumonia are quite variable and include lethargy, irritability, and vomiting. Respiratory tract findings include tachypnoea, intercostal retraction, crackles and wheezes. The aetiological agent may be confirmed by rapid diagnostic tests using immunofluorescent staining techniques and direct fluorescent antibody or enzyme-linked immunosorbent assays for viral antigens.

The treatment for most non-bacterial pneumonitis is supportive care. Non-bacterial pneumoniae with specific therapy include *Chlamydia trachomatis* and *Mycoplasma pneumoniae*. Erythromycin (40–50 mg/kg/day in four doses, orally, rarely intravenously) effectively eradicates these organisms from the respiratory tract and prevents disease transmission although its effect on the clinical course of the disease is less certain. Intravenous trimethoprim sulphamethoxazole (20 mg/kg/day trimethoprime, 100 mg/kg/day sulphamethoxole in four doses) provides effective treatment in *Pneumocystis carinii* pneumonia.

Primary bacterial pneumoniae are an infrequent cause of admission to paediatric intensive care units, except when patients have significant underlying disease. Extrapulmonary manifestations of bacterial pneumonia such as fever, vomiting, and obtundation may result in admission to the paediatric intensive care unit. Primary bacterial pneumoniae are commonly caused by *Streptococcus pneumoniae*, *Haemophilus influenzae*, and *Staphylococcus aureus*. Chills and fever associated with tachypnoea, intercostal retraction, and decreased breath sounds over the affected area are the classic presenting features. In younger infants and children, non-specific complaints may predominate. Pleural effusions are fairly common and are occasionally the major feature of the disease.

Empirical management of severe bacterial pneumonia should include therapy for penicillinase producing organisms such as *Staphylococcus aureus* and β-lactamase producing *Haemophilus influenzae*. Usually a semisynthetic penicillin (amoxicillin clavulinate 40 mg/kg/day in three doses) in combination with a second generation cephalosporin (cefuroxime 75–150 mg/kg/day in three doses) is effective. Cefuroxime alone is also recommended as the initial antibiotic as it is effective against the common pathogens and is safe in children. In some areas, methicillin resistance to *Staphylococcus aureus* is prevalent and in such instances vancomycin (60 mg/kg/day in three doses) is recommended instead of a semisynthetic penicillin. In the newborn period (<6 weeks) a combination of ampicillin (75–100 mg/kg/day in four doses) and gentamicin (5 mg/kg/day in a single dose) is appropriate. Antibiotic therapy should be guided by the sensitivity profile of the region. The general principles of treatment (hydration, antipyretics, and provision of ventilatory support) are similar to other severely ill children. If wheezing is present, aerosolised or oral β-agonists may be administered.

Critical care transport

Respiratory deterioration due to primary respiratory disease (croup, epiglottitis, bronchiolitis or asthma) or secondary to other organ dysfunction (seizures, shock, head trauma) is a frequent reason for critical care transport.[55] Respiratory compromise can be subtle and is the commonest cause of preventable morbidity during interhospital transport even in low risk patients with no primary lung disease. If there is any doubt of the patient's ability to protect their airway or to breathe adequately, intubation and assisted ventilation should be instituted prior to transport. Failure to anticipate the need for airway control and ventilation may be disastrous because intubation in a cramped transport vehicle is fraught with complications and is likely to fail. Airway obstruction is also common in children with decreased level of consciousness or coma who have no oral airway or endotracheal tube in place. All patients should therefore be afforded non-invasive monitoring of oxygenation and ventilation for early detection of compromised function. Established protocols of treatment of primary respiratory disease such as epiglottitis, croup, and asthma should be available and strictly adhered to during transportation.

Agitation resulting in accidental extubation is a feared complication during transport. Occlusion of endotracheal tubes by secretions is also a particular problem in infants less than 4 months old and in those with respiratory tract infections.[56] Protocols for the appropriate use of sedatives, proper securing of tubes, and tracheal toilet should be available and strictly followed. Acute gastric dilation is a common finding in the critically ill child and may predispose the patient to aspiration and further respiratory compromise, especially during the changes in ambient pressure experienced during air transport. A nasogastric tube should therefore be inserted prior to transport.

1 Chameides L, Hazinski MF, eds. *Pediatric advanced life support*. Chicago: American Heart Association, 1994.
2 Silverman BK, ed. Advanced pediatric life support course. Dallas: American Academy of Pediatrics, American College of Emergency Physicians, 1993.
3 Langston C, Kida K, Reed M, Thurlbeck WM. Human lung growth in late gestation and in the neonate. *Am Rev Respir Dis* 1984;**129**:607–13.
4 Dunnil MS. Postnatal growth of the lung. *Thorax* 1962;**17**:329–33.
5 Sharp JT. The chest wall and respiratory muscles in airflow limitation. In: Roussos C, Macklem PT, eds, *The thorax, part B*. New York: Dekker, 1985:1155–201.
6 Lopes JM, Muller NL, Bryan MH, Bryan AC. Synergistic behavior of inspiratory muscles after diaphragmatic fatigue in the newborn. *J Appl Physiol* 1981;**51**:547–51.
7 Thurlbeck WM. Postnatal growth and development of the lung. *Am Rev Respir Dis* 1975;**111**:803–44.
8 Macklem PT. Airway obstruction and collateral ventilation. *Physiol Rev* 1971;**51**:368–436.
9 Newcombe RW, Akhter J. Respiratory failure from asthma: a marker for children with high morbidity and mortality. *Am J Dis Child* 1988;**142**:1041–4.

10 Nowak RM, Tomlanovich MC, Sarkar DD, Kvale PA, Anderson JA. Arterial blood gases and pulmonary function testing in acute bronchial asthma. Predicting patient outcomes. *J Am Med Assoc* 1983;**249**:2043–6.
11 Tremper KK, Barker SJ. Pulse oximetry. *Anesthesiology* 1989;**70**:98–108.
12 Galant SP, Groncy CE, Shaw KC. The value of pulsus paradoxus in assessing the child with status asthmaticus. *Paediatrics* 1978;**61**:46–51.
13 Maunder RJ, Hudson LD. Respiratory monitoring in the intensive care unit. In: Schumaker WC, Abraham E, eds, *Diagnostic methods in critical care: automated data collection and interpretation.* New York: Dekker, 1987:33–45.
14 Freidman EM. Foreign bodies in the paediatric aerodigestive tract. *Pediatr Ann* 1988;**17**: 640–7.
15 Holinger PH, Kutnick SL, Schild JA, Holinger LD. Subglottic stenosis in infants and children. *Ann Otol Rhinol Laryngol* 1976;**85**:591–9.
16 Kissoon N, Singh N. Airway management and ventilatory support. In: Reisdorff EJ, Roberts MR, Wiegenstein JG, eds, *Pediatric emergency medicine.* Philadelphia: WB Saunders, 1993:51–67.
17 Walls R. Rapid-sequence intubation in head trauma. *Ann Emerg Med* 1993;**22**:1008–13.
18 Bhende MS, Karr VA, Wiltsie DC, Orr RA. Evaluation of a portable infrared end-tidal carbon dioxide monitor during paediatric inter-hospital transport. *Paediatrics* 1995;**95**: 875–8.
19 Duncan PG. Efficacy of helium-oxygen mixtures in the management of severe viral and post-intubation croup. *Can Anaesth Soc J* 1979;**26**:206.
20 Klassen TP, Feldman ME, Watters LK, Sutcliffe T, Rowe PC. Nebulized budesonide for children with mild-to-moderate croup. *N Engl J Med* 1994;**331**:285–9.
21 Landau LI, Geelhoed GC. Aerosolized steroids for croup. *N Engl J Med* 1994;**331**:322–3.
22 Husby S, Agertoft L, Mortensen S, Pedersen S. Treatment of croup with nebulized steroid (budesonide): A double blind, placebo controlled study. *Arch Dis Child* 1993;**68**:352–5.
23 Humphries CT, Wagner JS, Morgan WJ. Fatal prolonged foreign body aspiration following an asymptomatic interval. *Am J Emerg Med* 1988;7:611–13.
24 Heimlich HJ. A life-saving maneuver to prevent food choking. *JAMA* 1975;**234**:398–401.
25 Geelhoed GC, Landau LI, Le Souef PN. Evaluation of SaO₂ as a predictor of outcome in 280 children presenting with acute asthma. *Ann Emerg Med* 1994;**23**:1236–41.
26 Birkhead G, Attaway NJ, Struck RC, Townsend MC, Teutsch S. Investigation of a cluster of deaths of adolescents from asthma: evidence implicating inadequate treatment and poor patient adherence with medications. *J Allergy Clin Immunol* 1989;**84**:484–91.
27 Karetzky MS, Asthma mortality: an analysis of one year's experience, review of the literature, and assessment of current modes of therapy. *Medicine* (Baltimore) 1975;**54**: 471–84.
28 Jaimovich D, Kecskes SA. Management of reactive airway disease. *Crit Care Clin* 1992; **8**:147–62.
29 Meeker DP, Goldstein RH. Severe asthma: which patients need intensive care? *J Crit Illness* 1987;**2**:18.
30 Weinberger M. Antiasthmatic therapy in children. *Pediatr Clin North Am* 1989;**36**:1251–84.
31 Becker AB, Nelson NA, Simons FE. Inhaled salbutamol (albuterol) versus injected epinephrine in the treatment of acute asthma in children. *J Pediatr* 1983;**102**:465–9.
32 Katz RW, Kelly HW, Crowley MR, Grad R, McWilliams BC, Murphy SJ. Safety of continuous nebulized albuterol for bronchospasm in infants and children. *Paediatrics* 1993; **92**:666–9.
33 Schuh S, Parkin P, Rajan A, et al. High versus low dose frequently administered nebulized albuterol in children with severe acute asthma. *Paediatrics* 1989;**83**:513–18.
34 Polter G. Nebulized β-adrenergic agents in the treatment of acute paediatric asthma. *Pediatr Emerg Care* 1986;**2**:250.
35 Papo MC, Frank J, Thompson AE. A prospective, randomized study of continuous versus intermittent nebulized albuterol for severe status asthmaticus in children. *Crit Care Med* 1993;**21**:1479–86.
36 Bohn D, Kalloghlian A, Jenkins J, Edmonds J, Barker G. Intravenous albuterol in the treatment of status asthmaticus in children. *Crit Care Med* 1985;**12**:892–6.

37 Greenough A, Yuksel B, Everett L, Price JF. Inhaled ipratropium bromide and terbutaline in asthmatic children. *Respir Med* 1993;**87**:111–14.

38 DiGiulio GA, Kercsmar CM, Krug SE, Alpert SE, Marx CM. Hospital treatment of asthma: lack of benefit from theophylline given in addition to nebulized albuterol and intravenously administered corticosteroids. *J Pediatr* 1993;**122**:464–9.

39 Chapman KR, Verbeek PR, White JG, Rebuck AS. Effect of a short course of prednisone in the prevention of early relapse after emergency room treatment of acute asthma. *N Engl J Med* 1991;**324**:788–94.

40 Hill JH. Acute severe asthma. In: Blummer JL, ed, *A practical guide to pediatric intensive care*. St. Louis: Mosby, 1990:317.

41 Bouachour G, Tirot P, Varache N, Harry P, Alguier P. Metabolic acidosis in severe acute asthma: effect of alkaline therapy. *Rev Pneumonol Clin* 1992;**48**:115–19.

42 Rock MG, Reyes de la Rocha S, L'Hommedieu C, Truemper E. Use of ketamine in asthmatic children to treat respiratory failure refractory to conventional therapy. *Crit Care Med* 1986;**14**:514–16.

43 Straub PG, Hallam PL. Ketamine by continuous infusion in status asthmaticus. *Anaesthesia* 1986;**44**:1017–19.

44 DeNicola LK, Monem GF, Gayle MO, Kissoon N. Treatment of critical status asthmaticus in children. *Pediatr Clin North Am* 1994;**41**:1293–324.

45 Pabon H, Monem G, Kissoon N. Safety and efficacy of magnesium sulfate infusions in children with status asthmaticus. *Pediatr Emerg Care* 1994;**10**:200–3.

46 Monem GF, Kissoon N. Magnesium sulfate therapy in asthma. *Pediatr Ann* 1996; **25**: 136–44.

47 Darioli R, Perret C. Mechanical controlled hypoventilation in status asthmaticus. *Am Rev Respir Dis* 1984;**129**:385–7.

48 Mountain R, Sahn SA. Clinical features and outcome in patients with acute asthma presenting with hypercapnia. *Am Rev Respir Dis* 1988;**138**:535–9.

49 Kissoon N. Bronchodilator therapy in wheezy infants: a commentary. *Pediatr Emerg Care* 1993;**9**:121–2.

50 Sanchez I, De Koster J, Powell RE, Wolstein R, Chernick V. Effect of racemic epinephrine and salbutamol on clinical score and pulmonary mechanics in infants with bronchiolitis. *J Pediatr* 1993;**122**:145–51.

51 Frankel LR, Leviston NJ, Smith DW, Stevenson DK. Clinical observations on mechanical ventilation for respiratory failure in bronchiolitis. *Pediatr Pulmonol* 1986;**2**:307–11.

52 American Academy of Pediatrics Committee on Infectious Diseases. Use of ribavirin in the treatment of respiratory syncytial virus infection. *Paediatrics* 1993;**92**:501–4.

53 Report of the Committee on Infectious Diseases. American Academy of Pediatrics, PO Box 927, 141 Northwest Point Boulevard, Elk Grove Village, Illinois 60009–0927. 23rd edition, 1994:570–5.

54 Stagno S, Brasfield DM, Brown MB, *et al.* Infant pneumonitis associated with cytomegalovirus, chlamydia, pneumocystis, and ureaplasma: a prospective study. *Paediatrics* 1981;**68**:322–9.

55 Kissoon N. Triage and transport of the critically ill child. *Crit Care Clin* 1992;**8**:37–57.

56 Kanter RK, Thompkins JM. Adverse events during interhospital transport: physiologic deterioration associated with pretransport severity of illness. *Paediatrics* 1989;**84**:43–8.

57 Singh N, Kissoon N. Croup and epiglottitis. In: Surpure JS, ed, *Synopsis of pediatric emergency care*. Boston: Andover Medical Publishers, 1993:23–32.

3: New ventilation strategies

DESMOND BOHN

Introduction

The concept that mechanical ventilation could temporarily replace spontaneous breathing only began to gain widespread acceptance in the 1930s with the introduction of negative pressure breathing apparatus. Although these devices were remarkably effective in the treatment of diseases associated with weakness or paralysis of the respiratory muscles (pump failure), they were not effective in diseases involving the pulmonary parenchyma (lung failure). The demonstration that positive pressure ventilation (PPV) was effective for the treatment of acute respiratory failure was first demonstrated 40 years ago during the poliomyelitis epidemic in Europe and Scandinavia when patients were tracheostomised and manually ventilated with gases delivered by a simple anaesthetic circuit.[1] This in turn led to the development of the first mechanical positive pressure ventilators by Engstrom in Scandinavia and Emerson in North America and ushered in the era of intensive care medicine.

In the succeeding interval we have seen major technological advances in ventilator design without a similar improvement in the survival of the pulmonary disease processes they were designed to treat. We are now in an era where we have a virtual cornucopia of choices of ventilator management strategies for the treatment of acute respiratory failure (ARF) in both adults and children. It is difficult to evaluate the efficacy of these therapies because few, if any, have been subjected to any sort of clinical trial and most published experience has been based on rescue therapy in a high mortality group of patients with hypoxia and pulmonary barotrauma. With all these innovations it is hard to say what now distinguishes conventional from non-conventional ventilation. For the purpose of this review, conventional ventilation will be defined as either pressure or volume controlled ventilation delivered at physiological rates and tidal volumes. Other modes of oxygenation and CO_2 exchange, be they delivered by conventional machines or alternative devices, will be defined as non-conventional.

While it is disappointing that the advances in ventilator technology have not resulted in improved survival in ARF, we have come to recognise the reality that when it comes to dealing with patients with the type of parenchymal lung disease typified by diffuse atelectasis and hypoxaemia, positive pressure ventilation is as likely to be part of the problem as part of the solution. One of the basic principles adopted in PPV in the past 40 years is that we should attempt to mimic normal physiology and this has governed our choice of ventilator settings until comparatively recently. This has decreed that the objective is to achieve normocarbia and normoxia with tidal volumes and respiratory rates which were appropriate for the normal lung. While this strategy is fundamentally sound and without hazard in the normal lung, the same does not necessarily apply in the diseased lung. With the increasing realisation of the importance of ventilator induced lung injury, alternative ventilation strategies are being explored in the management of ARF which are based more on the recognition that the ventilation strategy needs to be adapted to the underlying pathophysiology of the lung rather than slavishly following the principle of mimicking normal physiology. This new approach demands that we rethink some of the traditional teaching about normal respiratory physiology and concentrate on understanding the underlying pathophysiology of this type of lung disease as well as being aware of the increasing evidence for secondary lung injury produced by mechanical ventilation.

The pathophysiology of acute respiratory failure

For the purposes of this review we will ignore ARF caused by neuromuscular or central nervous system diseases which come under the broad heading of failure of respiratory pump. Such diseases have elevated $PaCO_2$, minimal if any intrapulmonary shunting and are easily managed with conventional ventilation settings. We will concentrate on diseases that produce acute "lung failure" which are typically associated with diffuse atelectasis, permeability oedema, low lung compliance, and intrapulmonary shunting. We shall use as our paradigm the infant respiratory distress syndrome (IRDS) in premature infants and the adult (now commonly termed acute) respiratory distress syndrome (ARDS) in all other age groups. Although these are separate and distinct diseases in terms of causality, the lung has only a limited repertoire of response to injury in any age group and in this instance the pathophysiological changes in the lung are similar.

In the case of ARDS we will follow the agreed European/North American Consensus Conference definition of bilateral infiltrates on chest x ray, absence of cardiac failure and a PaO_2/FiO_2 ratio <200.[2]

In the non-diseased state the total cardiac output passes through the pulmonary capillaries which are either juxtaposed to the alveoli (intraalveolar) or contained within the interstitial space (extraalveolar) with minimal leakage of fluid. This is because in the normal state the junctions between the capillary endothelial cells are permeable to fluid flux and they are impermeable to protein and solutes. The small amount of fluid that leaks into the interstitial space is reabsorbed by the lymphatics. The epithelial lining is impermeable to both fluid and solutes. This normal state of affairs can be perturbed by inhalational injury to the epithelial lining (aspiration, smoke inhalation, etc.), by systemic diseases that damage the integrity of the endothelial (sepsis, trauma, embolism, etc.) or by primary surfactant deficiency which results in a number of pathological changes within the lung. Any of these insults can activate neutrophils and cause them to migrate to the lung where they attach to the endothelium and open the tight junctions, resulting in leakage of fluid and protein initially into the interstitial space and subsequently into the alveolus. The leakage of this proteineous material containing fibrin results in inhibition of surfactant activity and the formation of hyaline membranes around the alveolar lining. Epithelial injury results in damage to the surfactant producing type 2 cells. There is frequently plugging of the pulmonary microcirculation with platelet thrombi and this, together with the release of thromboxane, produces a rise in pulmonary vascular resistance and pulmonary hypertension. This phase of ARDS is frequently referred to as the exudative phase. The gradual leakage of fluid into the interstitial space causes the lung to lose some of its elasticity, the earliest symptom being tachypnoea as FRC falls and the lung becomes stiffer. The initial blood gas abnormality is characteristically hypoxaemia and hypocarbia, the $PaCO_2$ only rising above normal later in the illness as respiratory muscle fatigue sets in. A second proliferative phase of ARDS follows which is characterised by fibroblast infiltration into the interstitial space and the laying down of fibrous tissue, the harbinger of the development of chronic lung disease. At this stage there is gross destruction of air spaces and dilation of terminal bronchi, leading eventually to a honeycomb appearance to the lung.

In the 1970s pathologists frequently referred to this constellation of findings as "respirator lung". Clinicians argued that the ventilator allowed time for the full expression of the underlying disease and that these lesions had nothing to do with the ventilator. The only damage that was unequivocally due to the ventilator was the constellation of air leak syndromes known collectively as barotrauma. Anything else was attributed to oxygen toxicity. In reality it is difficult for a pathologist looking down a microscope at a section of lung tissue to define where the primary lung disease stops and ventilator induced injury begins. The rebuttal to the argument about the ventilator itself being responsible for the pathological changes was provided in a paper by Nash *et al.*[3] entitled "Respirator lung: a misnomer". They ventilated normal goats for two weeks with either air or 100% oxygen; those on oxygen all died, those on air all survived without damage. They concluded that "Mechanical positive pressure ventilation, at physiological inspiratory pressures, does not in and of itself cause morphologic pulmonary alterations". The caveat to this comforting conclusion is that the term "physiological inspiratory pressures" was taken to mean a peak inspiratory pressure of 12 cmH$_2$O and sick lungs obviously need substantially higher pressures. The obvious benefits that developing ventilator technology offered in terms of the treatment of acute respiratory failure have tended to mask the potential dangers of PPV; it is difficult to believe, when using PPV to treat pulmonary oedema, that it also causes pulmonary oedema. However, the evidence is now overwhelming that PPV can produce severe pathology in the normal lung and contribute substantially to pathology in the abnormal lung. More importantly, having at least partially understood the cause of the injury, we are developing tactics to minimise the damage. In order to understand the rationale for the use of non-conventional ventilation strategies we should first review the evolution of positive pressure ventilation as well as the now abundant evidence for positive pressure induced lung damage in both normal and injured lungs.

The evolution of positive pressure ventilation in acute respiratory failure

Since the early days of the use of mechanical ventilation it has been recognised that positive pressure respiration does not mimic normal breathing. If this were so, patients with normal lungs could be ventilated on an FiO$_2$ of 0.21 at the same tidal volumes and respiratory rates seen in spontaneous breathing. It was Bendixen[4] in 1963 who showed that during general aneasthesia, mechanical ventilation in patients with normal lungs was associated with a fall in PaO$_2$ and a rise in PaCO$_2$. He ascribed this change to the development of atelectasis due to the loss of the normal intermittent "sighing" present in the unanaesthetised, spontaneously breathing human. He proposed the use of an intermittent large tidal volume breath or "sigh" to overcome this problem which then became a design feature of ventilators of that period. It was not until a decade later that

Froese and Bryan[5] showed that the major cause of atelectasis with the induction of anaesthesia and muscle relaxation was a loss in lung volume due to the cephalad movement of the diaphragm. To compensate for this physiological aberration we have resorted to increasing the inspired oxygen concentration and delivered tidal volumes to well in excess of those used in spontaneous respiration.

However, in diseased lungs, what seemed like a medical imperative, i.e. to normalise blood gases in patients with diffusely atelectatic, low compliant lung disease by using ever larger tidal volumes, rarely resulted in survival. It wasn't until the 1970s that it was first shown that by maintaining a positive expiratory pressure, oxygenation could be improved. Ashbaugh[6] showed that positive end expiratory pressure (PEEP) was effective in ventilated adult patients with ARDS and Gregory[7] went on to show that a similar strategy, continuous positive airway pressure (CPAP), could be used successfully in spontaneously breathing newborn infants with hyaline membrane disease. During the succeeding 20 years the use of positive pressure ventilation with PEEP has proved successful in improving oxygenation in both ARDS and IRDS. The question is how much PEEP is required. The answer is the level that improves oxygenation with the least adverse effect on haemodynamics. Suter and Fairley[8] increased PEEP until they got the highest compliance; the "best PEEP" varied from 0 to 15 cmH$_2$O, the magnitude of the PEEP depending on the severity of the loss of lung compliance. Further increase in PEEP decreased both the compliance and oxygen transport. One of the major difficulties in setting a PEEP level or indeed any ventilatory parameter in ARDS is the non-homogeneity of the disease process. This became strikingly clear with the advent of thoracic CT scans. In ARDS the disease looks diffuse on the plain film, but on the CT scan there is a collection of densities in the dependent parts of the lung, with the non-dependent lung looking more or less normal (fig 3.1).

Furthermore, these densities, which presumably represent atelectatic or flooded units, are mobile as their location can change with posture. It is clear that the pressures required to open the dependent regions of the lung may overdistend the non-dependent regions. Although the application of PEEP is consistently associated with improved oxygenation in ARF, the recognition that mortality from oxygenation failure has not been reduced significantly in the past 20 years despite major improvements in ventilator technology has led to a search for alternative rescue therapy in an attempt to improve oxygenation in the situation where the lung is already damaged from a combination of underlying disease and ventilator therapy. In order to evaluate critically whether these innovations represent a useful option in ARF, we must discuss the role that positive pressure ventilation plays in the development of acute lung injury.

45

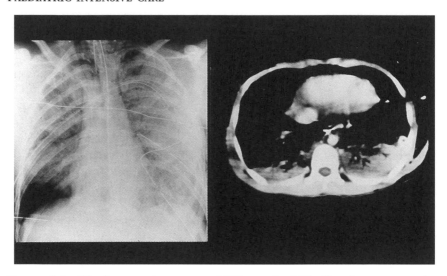

FIGURE 3.1—*Simultaneous chest x ray and CT scan of a child with pulmonary contusion. Although the chest might be interpreted as showing little or no aerated lung the CT shows that all the oedema and haemorrhage is located in the dependent regions with the rest of the lung appearing normal*

Ventilator induced lung injury

Barotrauma is the term most commonly used to describe damage to the lung from the ventilator and is usually understood to refer to a constellation of air leak syndromes, the incidence of which rises almost linearly with the peak pressure. We need another word for barotrauma as this merely reflects the end stage of the more subtle but equally serious epithelial and endothelial injury leading to pulmonary oedema and protein leak induced by mechanical ventilation and high inspired oxygen levels.

The first clear study of the problem was a classic paper by Webb and Tierney.[9] Rats with normal lungs were mechanically ventilated with room air for a target period of one hour. Those ventilated at pressures of 45 cmH$_2$O developed severe hypoxaemia and decreased compliance and died with post mortem evidence of extensive alveolar and perivascular oedema (fig 3.2). Those ventilated at 30 cmH$_2$O had reasonable gas exchange, no change in compliance, and all survived. Animals ventilated at 14 cmH$_2$O showed no abnormality. Thus a clear dose response was established for the induction of lung injury. Dreyfuss[10] added a time dimension: in normal animals after five minutes of PPV at 45 cmH$_2$O there was perivascular oedema with no visible epithelial lesions; after 20 min at the same pressure there was widespread alveolar flooding with swelling and

46

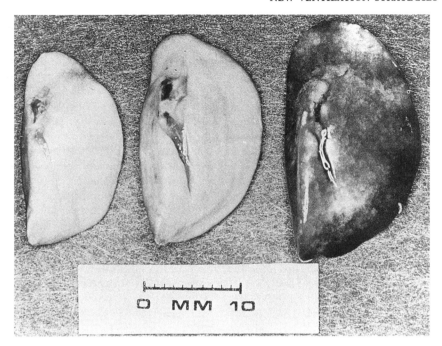

FIGURE 3.2—*Excised lungs of animals ventilated at differing airway pressures showing increasing damage with increasing PIP. Reproduced with permission from ref* [9]

disruption of the epithelium. These studies can be criticised because they were done in rodents with highly compliant chest walls or in open chest animals. However, Kolobow[11] met this criticism by ventilating normal sheep at 50 cmH$_2$O and produced severe and often lethal lung damage within 24 hours. One might also take issue with these studies in that they appear to use unreasonably high pressures, but they were done in normal lungs, attempting to simulate what would happen in the sick lung where the injury is by no means uniform and the regions of relatively normal lung tissue are frequently subjected to high peak airway pressures. If half the alveoli are closed, the volume distention of the open units had to more or less double to maintain normocarbia. When Tsuno[12] showed that ventilating sheep at 30 cmH$_2$O for 48 hours resulted in severe (but not lethal) lung damage, there was real cause for concern.

The relationship between pressure and volume during PPV is illustrated in fig 3.3. During inspiration no change in lung volume occurs until a pressure of 10 cmH$_2$O is reached, at which time there is rapid increase in volume. This first point or "knee" on the P/V curve is frequently referred to as the inflection point. The steep part of the curve levels out when the lung approaches total lung capacity (TLC) and any further application of

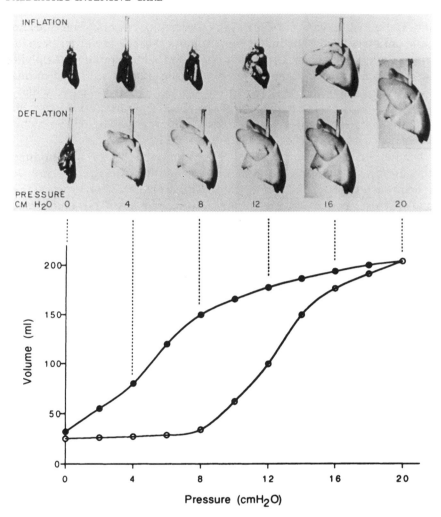

FIGURE 3.3—*Pressure volume curve of the excised lung. There is no increase in lung volume until a pressure of 10 cmH₂O is reached. Note that for any given pressure the lung volume on the expiratory limb of the P/V curve is higher than the inspiratory. Adapted with permission from Radford EP. Static mechanical properties of the mammalian lung. In: Fenn WO, ed, The handbook of physiology. Washington: American Society of Physiology, 1964:429–49.*

pressure merely results in overdistention. Assuming a normal P/V curve, the generally accepted upper limit to define TLC is 30 cmH₂O as further increments of pressure produce no significant increase in volume. If 30 cmH₂O is the "upper limit" in the normal lung, it must represent substantial overpressure in an atelectatic or flooded lung. The deflation

48

limb of the P/V curve is different in that derecruitment of alveoli does not occur until well below the inflection point and that for any given pressure lung volume is higher in inspiration compared with expiration. Applying these principles in the setting of ARF would suggest that limitation of tidal volume would prevent overdistention at the top of the P/V curve while a PEEP level to maintain lung volume above the lower inflection point would avoid the cyclical collapse and reexpansion of terminal lung units which is responsible for much of the ventilator induced injury.

The important variable is not airway pressure but transpulmonary pressure, that is, the difference in pressure between the alveolus and the pleural space (it should be noted that mouth pressure does not necessarily equal alveolar pressure because of flow resistive pressure drops in the small airways).

Dreyfuss[13] showed that the protein leak into the lung was as large when the same tidal volume was generated by negative pressure ventilation as with positive pressure. Furthermore, he showed that if high positive pressures were used but the volume expansion of the lung was restricted by a body cast, there was no protein leak. The conclusion from this study was that the volume distention of the lung was important in producing the lung injury. Similarly, Hernandez[14] produced a protein leak in an isolated rabbit lung using trivial pressures ($15\,cmH_2O$) while it required $45\,cmH_2O$ to produce a similar leak in the intact rabbit and again this could be prevented by limiting expansion with a body cast.[15]

While most of the evidence in the literature stresses the dangers of peak airway pressure, the level of end expiratory pressure is also crucial in ameliorating that injury. This was clearly demonstrated by Webb and Tierney[9] who showed that normal rats ventilated at $45/0\,cmH_2O$ developed severe hypoxaemia and died with both alveolar and perivascular oedema while those ventilated with $45/10\,cmH_2O$ only had perivascular oedema and survived. Similar observations were made by Dreyfuss[13] who showed a marked reduction in both oedema and protein leak when $10\,cmH_2O$ of PEEP was applied.

We now have a significant body of experimental data which suggests that in normal animals cyclical lung distention delivered by PPV with peak inspiratory pressures of $30\,cmH_2O$ or above can produce permeability oedema and pathological changes which are similar to ARDS and that these changes can be at least partially prevented by PEEP.

Given the fact that patients with this type of lung disease require positive intrathoracic pressure to reverse their hypoxaemia, these studies would suggest that the ideal strategy to avoid ongoing injury would be to prevent lung overdistention by limiting the peak inspiratory pressure while maintaining a lung volume at an end expiration with PEEP sufficient to prevent alveolar derecruitment. There are several experimental studies comparing the degree of injury using low tidal volume/high PEEP with low PEEP/high tidal volume ventilation, high PEEP, and low PEEP strategies. Corbridge,[16] in an acid aspiration model, showed a significantly lower shunt fraction and less pulmonary oedema with a high PEEP (10 cmH$_2$O) low tidal volume strategy compared to a normal tidal volume low PEEP (3 cmH$_2$O), with the same peak pressure.

Sandhar et al.[17] had very good results in a surfactant depletion model created by repetitive lung lavage. They first measured the inflection point on the P/V curve which is the pressure at which lung volume starts to increase (around 11 cmH$_2$O in this study). They then set the PEEP above the measured inflection point on the inflation limb of the P/V curve and compared this with a group with a PEEP of 3 cmH$_2$O. Mean airway pressures were matched by altering the I:E ratio. They found much better gas exchange and few, if any, hyaline membranes in the high PEEP group. The problem with this high PEEP strategy is that in the abnormal lung the "opening pressure" is about 10–15 cmH$_2$O. If peak pressure is also limited, the tidal volume may be insufficient to contol PaCO$_2$. Therefore both Corbridge and Sandhar had to increase respiratory rate to maintain normocarbia. This leads to a residual anxiety that the differences in damage may be due to other factors such as alteration in pulmonary haemodynamics or cardiac output.

This issue was addressed by Muscedere[18] who injured the lung by surfactant depletion and brief mechanical ventilation. The animals were sacrificed and a static P/V curve measured to define the inflection point on the inflation limb of the curve (which was around 15 cmH$_2$O). The lungs were then ventilated in air with a fixed tidal volume of 2 ml for two hours. One group was ventilated with no PEEP, the next with a PEEP of 4 cmH$_2$O, i.e. below the inflection point, the next had a PEEP set above the inflection point. A control group had no post mortem ventilation and were statically inflated for two hours. Those with no PEEP or PEEP below the inflection point had a marked decrease in compliance, whereas those ventilated above the inflection point had a significant increase in compliance. The pathology was of particular interest as both the no PEEP and the PEEP below the inflection point had severe hyaline membrane formation, with an important difference in distribution: those with no PEEP had lesions mainly in respiratory and membranous bronchioles, whereas those with PEEP below the inflection point had lesions predominantly in the alveolar ducts. In marked contrast, those ventilated above the inflection point had no more damage than the control group that had no post mortem ventilation. However, in those ventilated above the inflection point a small but significant number of pneumothoraces developed. There are two important messages in this study: first, the injury was clearly related to the degree of end expiratory pressure and second, the group subjected to the highest pressures had the greatest "volutrauma" while those ventilated above the inflection point had the least injury.

Alternative ventilation strategies

The non-conventional ventilation strategies available for the treatment of ARF include those that use standard tidal volumes and rates but vary the inspiratory time (prolonged I:E ratio), those that use reduced PIP and tidal volume while maintaining a normal $PaCO_2$ by either ventilating dead space (high frequency ventilation), reducing the dead space (intratracheal pulmonary ventilation) or allowing the $PaCO_2$ to rise (pressure limited ventilation–permissive hypercapnia). In addition to these there are adjuncts to mechanical ventilation (surfactant and nitric oxide) as well as providing PPV by mask (non-invasive ventilation). Finally, one can eliminate the secondary injury altogether by removing the ventilator and providing extracorporeal oxygenation. The characteristics of these various alternative strategies are summarised in table 3.1.

Increased inspiratory time ventilation

Mechanical ventilation that attempts to follow physiological principles demands that inspiratory time is considerably shorter than expiration, usually in a ratio of 1:2 or 1:3. An alternative method of improving oxygenation in hypoxic pulmonary failure has been prolongation of inspiration to the extent of reversal of the I:E ratio (IRV) in an attempt to overcome the regional inhomogeneity of differing lung units. In order to evaluate critically the efficacy of this therapy we need to understand the differing principles between pressure and volume modes of ventilation.

The first mechanical ventilators introduced into clinical medicine were all pressure limited and time cycled. These were largely replaced with the development of volume ventilators except in neonates and infants where mechanical ventilation is still managed using the pressure control mode because of the problem of triggering and the variable leak around the endotracheal tube in the infant. In adults and older children volume control is the most frequently chosen mode.

The two types of ventilation differ very significantly in terms of the pattern of gas flow into the lung, change in lung volume as well as the pressure waveform generated within the airway. In volume control ventilation, with the opening of the inspiratory valve, the gas flow into the lung rises rapidly to its peak, maintains a plateau during inspiration and

51

TABLE 3.1—*Alternative ventilation strategies*

Ventilation mode	Flow	Airway pressure	Main features	Disadvantages
Volume control (VC)	Variable according to rate of gas flow. Commonly rapid constant with plateau but can be decelerating at slow gas flow	Compliance and resistance dependent. Gradual rise to peak followed by plateau	Guaranteed minute volume	Not leak compensated. High airway pressures in severe lung disease
Pressure control (PC)	Decelerating	Square wave. Preset pressure	More even distribution of gas flow. Leak compensated	Varying TV and MV according to compliance
Pressure control inverse ratio ventilation (PC-IRV)	Decelerating	Square wave	Lower PIP	Auto-PEEP. Cardiovascular compromise
Pressure regulated volume control	Decelerating	Square wave	Lowest airway pressure with guaranteed minute volume	PIP can vary below preset level
Pressure limited ventilation	Decelerating	Square wave	Low tidal volume. Reduced secondary injury	Hypercapnia
Intratracheal pulmonary ventilation (ITPV)	High constant gas flow		Reduced dead space	High gas flow can lead to humidifier "blow out"
Airway release ventilation (ARV)	High constant gas flow	CPAP with intermittent release	Spontaneous respiration	Useful only in mild lung injury
High frequency ventilation	High constant gas flow	Sustained MAP	Very low TV. Reduced secondary injury	Underestimation of MAP and less than ideal humidity on HFJV

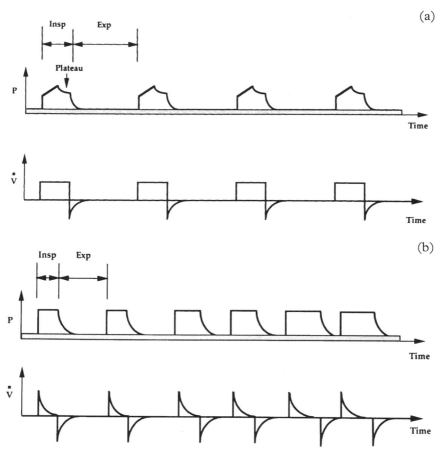

FIGURE 3.4—*Pressure and flow profiles during volume preset (a) and pressure preset (b) with increasing inspiratory time*

then falls abruptly to zero with the opening of the expiratory valve (fig 3.4a). Airway pressure shows a small immediate rise due to the resistance of the endotracheal tube and rises ramplike as the resistive forces in airways are overcome. During the expiratory phase gas flows out of the lung in a decaying exponential curve. In pressure control ventilation (fig 3.4b) gas flow into the lung increases quickly with the opening of the inspiratory valve as airway pressure rapidly rises to its preset value with gas flows of up to 200 l/min. During the remainder of the inspiratory cycle gas flow declines exponentially in order to maintain airway pressure at its preset level (decelerating gas flow). Airway pressure is maintained at a plateau level for the duration of the inspiratory cycle before rapidly falling to the

53

end expiratory level as the inspiratory valve closes. In the conventional approach in both modes expiration is typically longer than inspiration in the ratio of 1:2 or 1:3.

When comparing the two different modes of ventilation in the same model of lung disease, the airway pressures used to inflate the lung will be different. With pressure control ventilation the peak airway pressure is set by the operator and the tidal volume delivered will depend on the compliance and resistive characteristics of the patient's lung. In volume control ventilation the tidal volume delivered by the ventilator is fixed and the airway pressure generated is dependent on those same compliance and resistive properties. There is a school of thought which says that there are significant advantages in switching from the more traditional approach of volume control to pressure control in the setting of severe lung disease as this may cause less severe secondary lung injury. In order to examine the validity of this claim we need to understand the concept of mean airway pressure and the factors that govern it.

During the inspiratory phase of mechanical ventilation, positive pressure is used to overcome resistance in the endotracheal tube and airways and not only inflate the terminal lung units, but maintain them in the open position during this phase of the respiratory cycle to allow for diffusion of oxygen. In the setting of ARF, high airway and alveolar pressures are required to expand alveoli and maintain them inflated during inspiration. In addition, in order to prevent lung collapse with the onset of expiration, airway pressure is prevented from declining to zero by the application of PEEP. Therefore positive pressure within the lung is governed by a combination of PIP, PEEP, inspiratory and expiratory time as well as gas flow rate. This can be expressed as the mean airway pressure (MAP) and represents the pressure measured at the airway averaged over time. The mathematical formula for this is:

$$MAP = \frac{PIP \times t_i + PEEP \times t_e}{T_{tot}} \; cmH_2O)$$

where t_i is the inspiratory time, t_e is the expiratory time and T_{tot} the duration of the respiratory cycle.

There is obviously a direct relationship between MAP and mean alveolar pressure but as we have seen previously in the P/V curve, the relationship between airway pressure and lung volume is not a straight line due to hysteresis properties of the lung. With the conventional settings of volume control positive pressure ventilation, we most frequently alter MAP by changing PIP or by increasing PEEP. An alternative approach is to increase MAP by using the third variable in the formula, namely prolonging the inspiratory time so that the conventional ratio for I:E is increased from

1:2 to 1:1 or actually reversing it to 2:1 or longer. The physiological consequences of this approach are that the alveoli are held open longer during the respiratory cycle which, in the setting of lung oedema and atelectasis, will directly influence oxygenation. It may have serious adverse effects when injudiciously applied in that the high MAP and the short expiratory time may trap gas in the terminal lung units with alveolar pressure remaining positive at end expiration. This phenomenon, known as auto-PEEP, can lead to pulmonary barotrauma and lung rupture. In addition, increases in MAP result in increased intrathoracic pressure which can be transmitted to vascular structures and reduce cardiac output. In reality we should measure mean lung volume rather than mean airway pressure because it is that which determines the balance between best oxygenation and least overdistention.

There is, then, a physiological basis for believing that there may be advantages to increasing MAP by prolonging inspiratory time even to the point of reversing the conventional I:E ratio in order to improve oxygenation in ARF. This, in fact, is the rediscovery of an old technique first advocated by Reynolds[19] over 20 years ago for improving oxygenation in infants with IRDS ventilated using the pressure control mode in the days before the widespread use of PEEP. We shall now examine the experimental and clinical evidence which would suggest that this approach may improve outcome in acute lung injury, first using the volume control mode and then the pressure control mode.

Inverse ratio ventilation can be delivered in either the pressure control or volume control mode. In most mechanical ventilators designed primarily for adult use where volume control is the primary mode, this can be achieved by slowing the inspiratory flow rate, by adding an inspiratory pause or by decelerating the inspiratory flow to a ramp pattern. In ventilators with the pressure control option, switching to this mode produces a square wave pressure profile the length of which can be extended so that expiratory time is reduced. In either situation MAP will rise directly proportional to the duration of inspiration. The expectation is that this sustained increase in MAP may recruit collapsed lung units more effectively than transient increases associated with conventional settings. Sustained alveolar inflation also appears to decrease dead space and therefore improve the efficiency of alveolar ventilation, allowing for lower tidal volume settings. Experience with this mode of ventilation suggests that recruitment of lung volume is both time dependent and most likely to occur in the early exudative phase of acute lung injury. The inherent hazard of the technique, particularly in the pressure control mode, is that inadvertent auto-PEEP is not recognised.

When comparing the two options of pressure or volume control inverse ratio ventilation, the former has the theoretical advantage in that the decelerating gas flow pattern allows for better mixing and the sustained square wave is more likely to recruit collapsed alveoli. On the other hand, others would argue that the high initial gas flow at the beginning of inspiration may result in greater sheer stress damage to already damaged lung tissue.

Most experience with inverse ratio ventilation in the setting of acute lung injury has been limited to the pressure control mode with inverse ratio (PC-IRV). Published series are generally short term studies (less than one hour) or anecdotal reports that compare oxygenation and ventilator settings when switching from volume control to PC-IRV in patients with acute lung injury. The majority show that peak inspiratory pressure can be reduced without a reduction or even an improvement in alveolar ventilation, that there were (mostly) modest increases in PaO_2 related to the increase in MAP when the level of extrinsic PEEP was reduced. In the studies where it was measured, the level of intrinsic PEEP was significant. It is debatable whether raising MAP by applying square wave pressure with prolonged inspiration and significant amounts of intrinsic PEEP is less damaging to an injured lung than raising the level of extrinsic PEEP. Certainly none of these studies showed any change in mortality with the switch to PC-IRV. It should also be emphasised again that in these studies ventilation protocol was *pressure controlled* and not *pressure limited*; in other words, the accepted convention was a tidal volume of 10–15 ml/kg with the target of a normal $PaCO_2$. As we will see in the next section, this conventional wisdom is now being challenged.

A further difficulty in interpreting the significance of these findings is the fact that the patients in these studies had been on volume control ventilation at high PIP and FiO_2 levels for prolonged periods prior to being switched. In order to show that PC-IRV is superior to volume control in the setting of ARDS, one would have to demonstrate a difference not just in gas exchange but in mortality. This would require that patients with similar severity of illness be enrolled into a randomised trial of both types of ventilation induced injury. Two recently published studies are worthy of comment in that they address some of these issues. Rappaport[20] randomised patients with severe ARDS (PaO_2/FiO_2 ratio <150) to receive either VCV or PC-IRV for at least 72 hours and then to death or weaning and extubation. Although the numbers were small the duration of ventilation was shorter and the static lung compliance was higher in the PC-IRV group. The second study by Lessard[21] was again a short term study comparing blood gas, respiratory mechanics and haemodynamics in adult ARF patients when switching from VC to PCV and PCV-IRV with different I:E ratios. In this study, where tidal volume was kept constant in all modes of ventilation, the authors were unable to demonstrate any improvement with either PCV or PC-IRV, at the same time showing that an I:E ratio of 3:1 (expiratory time 0.75 s) was associated with significant auto-PEEP even when extrinsic PEEP was reduced to zero.

A review of the published data on pressure control and inverse ratio ventilation in ARDS would have to conclude that it remains to be proven whether there is improved outcome compared to volume control in the setting of acute lung injury. In situations where a trial of prolonged inspiratory time ventilation is being undertaken, the following guidelines should be considered.

- The inspiratory time should be slowly increased in 0.1–0.2-s increments rather than selecting a fixed I:E ratio.
- The target should be improved oxygenation without an adverse effect on cardiac output (oxygen delivery) rather than PaO_2 alone.
- The likelihood of intrinsic PEEP (auto-PEEP) must be considered and measured.
- The maximum improvement in oxygenation is likely to be achieved by extending the inspiratory time to an I:E ratio of 1.5:1 without further benefit from further extension.

Pressure limited ventilation (permissive hypercapnia)

The traditional approach to mechanical ventilation has always been targeted on the objective of a normal PaO_2 and $PaCO_2$ and the accepted practice has been to use tidal volumes of 10–15 ml/kg to achieve this. With the increasing recognition that these volumes can injure the already damaged lung has come the realisation that ventilation with reduced tidal volume with a pressure limited target rather than $PaCO_2$ may be a safer option. The origin of this revolutionary approach can be traced back to a landmark paper by Darioli and Perret[22] published in 1984 entitled "Mechanical controlled hypoventilation in status asthmaticus". In it they described a series of adult patients ventilated using the volume control mode but with tidal volumes of 8–12 ml/kg, a low inspiratory flow rate and a rate of 6–10 cycles/min. They set the maximum PIP at 50 cmH$_2$O. If this was exceeded with the initial settings the tidal volume was reduced further and the $PaCO_2$ allowed to rise. All patients survived, the duration of ventilation was short (<3 days) and this in an era where 10–20% mortality was the norm for ventilation support in status asthmaticus. Even more importantly, they enunciated the principle that normocarbia should not be the objective in this situation as the measures required to achieve it are potentially harmful if not lethal. They defined the objective to be correction of hypoxaemia while ignoring hypercarbia up to the level of 90 mmHg (12 kpa).

The next important study that served to support this position was the paper published in 1990 by Hickling.[23] He hypothesised that simply reducing the tidal volume and allowing the CO_2 to rise would be equally effective in preventing ventilation induced lung injury. This revolutionary concept was put to the test in 50 patients with ARDS as defined by a lung injury score of >2.5 and a PaO_2/FiO_2 ratio of <150. The ventilation strategy used was SIMV volume controlled ventilation with the target of a PIP of less than $30\,cmH_2O$ when this could be easily achieved and always less than $40\,cmH_2O$ with a tidal volume as low as 5 ml/kg if necessary. In many instances this resulted in significant degrees of hypercarbia but no attempt was made to correct this. Sodium bicarbonate was not used to correct the acidosis. The oxygenation strategy was increasing levels of PEEP with the objective of reducing the FiO_2 to <0.6. Patients were allowed to breathe spontaneously. Severity of illness data as defined using the Apache II Score were collected. The remarkable result was that the hospital mortality in this series was 16% compared with a predicted mortality of 39% using this scoring system. Despite criticism that these were retrospective data and did not conform to the gold standard of proof by a randomised controlled clinical trial, no single study has done more to influence ventilation practices in the past 20 years. Both these studies have used the volume control mode with limitation of tidal volume as a method of reducing the PIP. The alternative option as a method of preventing volume distention of the injured lung is to use the pressure control mode with limitation of the PIP. It has been suggested that this may be preferable for, as well as allowing for a decelerating gas flow pattern, it guarantees that the preset PIP will not be exceeded. This has led to a renewed interest from adult intensivists in a mode of ventilation that was abandoned 20 years ago except in neonatal ARF.

Based on the accumulated experimental data from animals and the admittedly limited human experience, a pressure limited permissive hypercapnia strategy would seem to make eminent sense as long as we accept that hypercarbia per se, while not desirable, is not intrinsically harmful. While few would argue that modest elevations of $PaCO_2$ in the range of 50 mmHg are of little concern, levels of >100 mmHg cause great anxiety to a generation of critical care physicians trained to strict adherence to the physiological norm. What, then, is the basis for these concerns and how do we weigh them up against the potential for doing harm by continuing the practice of ventilating to a normal $PaCO_2$? Acute elevations in CO_2 result in the rapid development of an intracellular acidosis. A rising hydrogen ion concentration produces an increase in pulmonary vascular resistance and in cerebral blood flow, which may be harmful in cerebral injury or pulmonary hypertension. There is also evidence, some of it conflicting, that acidosis impairs myocardial performance. These statements ignore the very effective renal bicarbonate retention that rapidly compensates for a falling pH during a respiratory acidosis as long as the kidney is functioning normally. In both the permissive hypercapnia series reported above there was very effective renal compensation and in neither was bicarbonate used to correct a respiratory acidosis. In Hickling's study CO_2s of over 100 mmHg were permitted with pHs dropping as low as 7.1 without the administration of bicarbonate. The remarkably improved survival would suggest that acidosis had little adverse effect on myocardial performance. There is also evidence in the literature that in children at least, very high (>200 mmHg) levels of $PaCO_2$ are not associated with adverse consequences as long as oxygenation is maintained.[24]

If we accept that pressure limited ventilation with low tidal volumes and permissive hypercapnia is unlikely to be harmful and is at least as effective as pressure control in ARDS, do we have any evidence to prove that it may in fact lower mortality? Although the retrospective studies published to date suggest that this is true, there is at present only one published prospective study comparing this approach with a standard ventilation technique. Amato,[25] in a randomised controlled clinical trial in adult patients with ARDS, compared a standard VC mode with a ventilation strategy that used a low tidal volume combined with a PEEP level set above the inflection point in order to reduce the FiO_2 to <0.5. Although the numbers in the study were relatively small they were able to show significantly better oxygenation, compliance and greater numbers of patients successfully weaned from mechanical ventilation in the low tidal volume group. They were unable to demonstrate a significant difference in mortality due to the fact that there were an unusually high number of deaths from non-respiratory causes after the patients were extubated.

Although these studies are far from conclusive, the results are impressive enough to generate considerable interest in the use of pressure limited ventilation for severe ARF. This does require us to rethink our priorities in terms of oxygenation and CO_2 elimination.

Algorithm for pressure limited ventilation in ARF

The following is an outline of the strategy used in our intensive care unit for the management of patients with severe ARDS and oxygenation failure who constitute a group with a potential for high mortality. The definition of severe ARDS is based on data from paediatric patients which suggests that the requirement for FiO_2 ≥ 0.5 and a PEEP ≥ 5 cmH$_2$O for more than 12 hours predicts a mortality of >40%.[26] It has as its basis the prevention of lung overdistention by the use of PEEP and low tidal volumes together with the objective of reducing the FiO_2 to the lowest level

59

compatible with adequate oxygenation. A balance has to be struck between what would be *desirable* in all situations (low PIP and low FiO_2) and what would be *tolerable* in situations of severe lung disease in order not to aggravate the lung injury. This approach clearly separates ventilation (CO_2 elimination), dictated by PIP and ventilator rate, from oxygenation, which is determined by PEEP and FiO_2. The basis for this protocol is as follows.

Ventilation: *Desirable objective*   PIP <30 cmH_2O, normal pH or compensated respiratory acidosis (pH >7.2)

                Tolerance   PIP <35 cmH_2O, pH 7.10

Oxygenation: *Desirable objective* FiO_2 <0.5, SaO_2 90%

                Tolerance SaO_2 85%

The strategy to achieve this would be as follows:

1. Pressure limited ventilation to a maximum PIP of 35 cmH_2O.
2. Ignore hypercarbia and target the pH rather than the $PaCO_2$ with the objective of a compensated respiratory acidosis (pH >7.2) but a tolerance for a pH down to 7.10.
3. Increase the PEEP to a level that enables you to reduce the FiO_2 to 0.5 or less, compatible with a saturation of 90% (PaO_2 60 mmHg (8 kpa)).

Ventilation strategy (fig. 3.5a)

Ventilation (as in CO_2 elimination) is controlled by PIP and respiratory rate. The objective is to limit PIP to a maximum of 35 mmH_2O, ignoring the $PaCO_2$ as long as there was an appropriate pH compensation (pH >7.20). Patients are managed with a pressure limited mode (pressure control or pressure limited volume control). The initial pressure setting is no higher than 30 cmH_2O with a ventilation rate of 20–40/min, depending on age. If the first blood gas shows an uncompensated respiratory acidosis (pH <7.10) on two consecutive readings two hours apart the PIP is increased to 35 cmH_2O. Once the target PIP of 35 cmH_2O is reached, the pH and PaO_2 are measured. If the pH is <7.20 at or below the target PIP, the pressure is reduced to the target PIP of 30 cmH_2O regardless of $PaCO_2$ level. If the pH falls below 7.10 on PIP 35 cmH_2O, the respiratory rate may be increased by 5/min. If this fails to restore the pH to >7.20, 2 mmol/ kg of intravenous bicarbonate may be given. If the pH is consistently <7.20 at a PIP of 35 cmH_2O, consider increasing the tolerance to pH 7.10 rather than increasing the PIP.

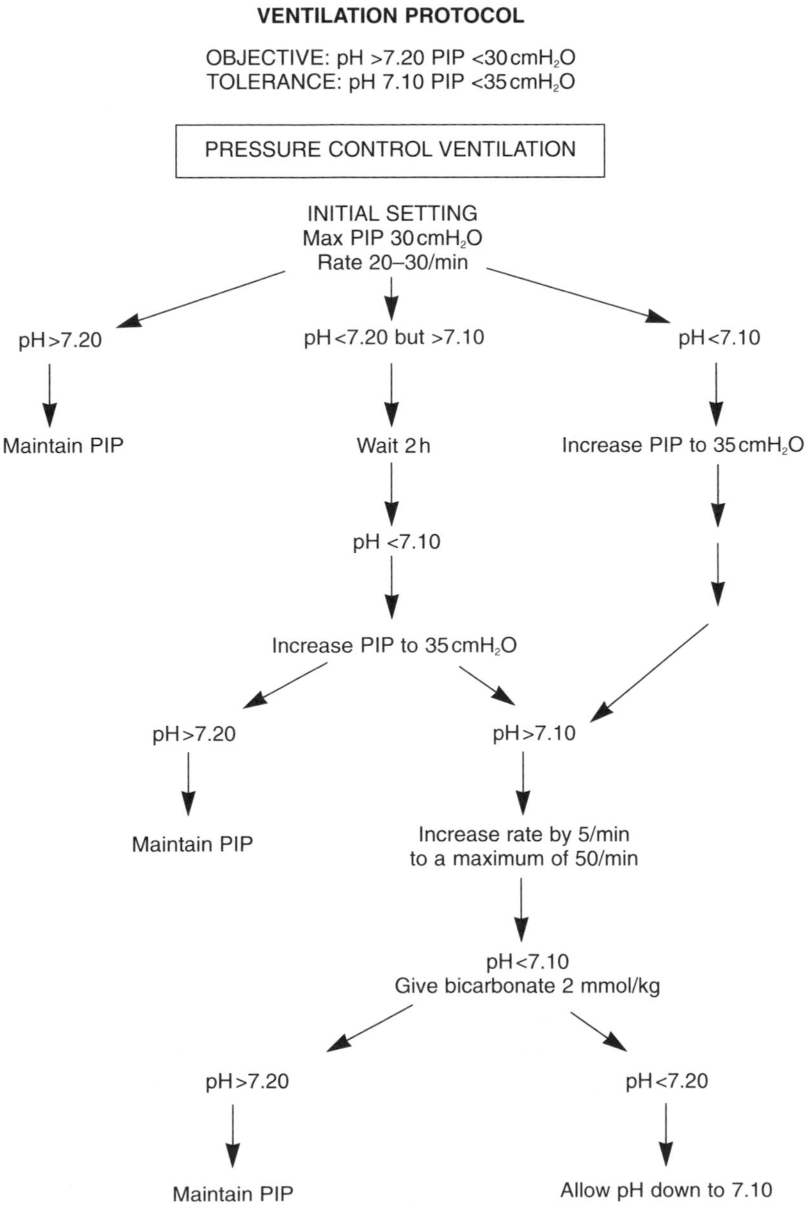

VENTILATION PROTOCOL

OBJECTIVE: pH >7.20 PIP <30cmH₂O
TOLERANCE: pH 7.10 PIP <35cmH₂O

FIGURE 3.5a—*Suggested ventilation strategy for pressure limited ventilation (permissive hypercapnia) for severe ARDS*

Oxygenation strategy (fig 3.5b)

The principal determinants of PaO_2 in mechanically ventilated patients with acute respiratory failure are combinations of inspired oxygen concentration and PEEP. The combination of PEEP, PIP, and inspiratory time dictate the MAP. As high inspired oxygen concentrations have been identified as producing secondary lung injury, the objective is to use the lowest FiO_2 consistent with a PaO_2 >65 mmHg (6.5 kpa) or an arterial saturation >90%. To guarantee full oxygenation and adequate saturation at the outset the FiO_2 is set at 0.8 initially together with a minimum PEEP of 6 cmH_2O. The FiO_2 is then reduced in increments of 0.05 as long as the PaO_2 remains above 65 mmHg or the saturation remains above 90% with a target FiO_2 of 0.5 or less. If the FiO_2 cannot be reduced to this level without PaO_2 dropping to less than 65 mmHg or the saturation to <90%, the FiO_2 is maintained at the lowest level while PEEP is added in increments of 2 cmH_2O until PaO_2 increases to above 65 mmHg. PEEP will continue to be added in increments of 2 cmH_2O while the FiO_2 is reduced to a maximum of 0.5. PEEP up to a level of 15 cmH_2O is used. If the PaO_2 cannot be maintained above 65 mmHg or the saturation above 90% by the addition of the maximum level of PEEP (15 cmH_2O), FiO_2 may be increased in increments of 0.05 until a target PaO_2 and saturation are reached. If an FiO_2 of >0.75 is required then consideration should be given to tolerating an SaO_2 of 85–90%.

High frequency ventilation

The concept that tidal volume could be reduced while maintaining minute ventilation with rapid rates was first introduced in the 1970s as a ventilatory support technique used during surgical procedures involving the upper airway which were made more feasible by having a relatively motionless surgical field. This was subsequently redesigned as a support mode for the management of patients with acute respiratory failure as a way of mitigating the effects of pulmonary barotrauma and proved particularly useful in the management of patients with bronchopleural fistula. There are various forms of high frequency ventilation now being used in clinical medicine, the characteristics of which are summarised in table 3.2. This review will concentrate on the two most commonly used in clinical medicine, namely high frequency oscillatory ventilation (HFOV) and high frequency jet ventilation (HFJV). Both have been used to treat patients with IRDS and ARDS with the objective of minimising lung injury by using small tidal volume ventilation while maintaining oxygenation using a high open lung volume strategy.

62

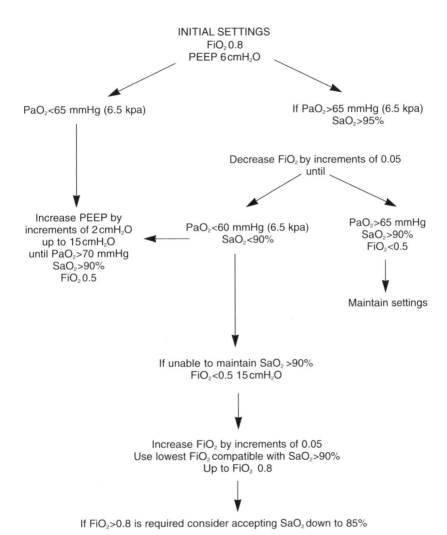

FIGURE 3.5b—*Suggested oxygenation strategy for pressure limited ventilation (permissive hypercapnia) for severe ARDS*

TABLE 3.2—*Types of high frequency ventilation*

Type	Rate	Expiratory phase	Application
High frequency positive pressure ventilation (HFPPV)	60–120/min	Passive	Surgical procedures, IRDS, ARDS
High frequency oscillatory ventilation (HFOV)	60–900/min	Active	IRDS, ARDS in children
High frequency jet ventilation (HFJV)	60–300/min	Passive	IRDS, ARDS

There is little rationale for considering HFV as just "another ventilator" which happens to operate at faster rates and lower airway pressures than conventional ventilators, without a clear understanding of the situations where these features may be a considerable advantage in patient management. There are several situations where a case can be made for considering using HFV in preference to CMV.

- To improve oxygenation by recruiting lung volume while avoiding cyclical lung distention with high PIPs (the "open lung" strategy).
- To achieve more effective CO_2 elimination in situations where this may be particularly important, e.g. persistent pulmonary hypertension of the newborn (PPHN).
- To minimise the effect of secondary or therapy induced lung injury in situations of diffuse parenchymal lung disease with hypoxia.
- To minimise the effect on CVS function by reducing airway pressures.
- To improve operating conditions in certain procedures on the airway and lung.

High frequency oscillatory ventilation (HFOV)

The discovery that a high frequency sine wave was capable of moving CO_2 out of the lung was first made serendipitously during experiments in paralysed animals designed to measure thoracic impedance. Following this original observation, the same technique was shown to produce excellent gas exchange in normal animals using tidal volumes well below dead space. The principle that oxygen would diffuse down a concentration gradient had been well established 20 years before when it was shown that arterial oxygen saturation could be maintained over periods of apnoea as long as 20 min if a high flow of gas was delivered directly into the airway. This technique, known as apnoeic oxygenation, was used to advantage during anaesthesia for laryngeal surgery where oxygen and volatile anaesthetic

64

agents at high flows were delivered via a catheter placed through the vocal cords. The technique was limited in duration by the inevitable rise in $PaCO_2$ that occurred with apnoea. However, it was noted that some CO_2 elimination would occur due to the washout of dead space and that improved the nearer the catheter was placed to the carina. It was also demonstrated that cardiac contraction enhanced the diffusion of CO_2 up the trachea towards the carina, a phenomenon referred to as cardiogenic mixing.

The application of the high frequency sine wave to the airway solved the problem of hypercarbia by further enhancing the diffusion of CO_2 due to extremely efficient mixing of gases within the lung. Although the δ P (difference between peak and end expiratory pressures) is given when measured at the peak of the airway in this system, this does not reflect alveolar pressure, which is very low. Although there is some bulk flow, this is insufficient for alveolar ventilation and the enhanced gas exchange is accounted for by accelerated diffusion.

The first oscillators used to demonstrate this were either adapted from a loudspeaker design or engineering prototypes using a piston within a cylinder driven by a high speed electric motor at speeds of up to 25 Hz. The original animal experiments were performed at 15 Hz (900/min) with fresh gas flows in the circuit of up to 10–15 l/min with attempts to use an expiratory valve in the circuits. At these high flow rates the system was inherently hazardous because of the potential to overpressure the lung. In order to overcome this problem, an open-ended long piece of small calibre tubing known as a low pass filter was incorporated which allowed for flushing of the circuit and elimination of CO_2. As the expiratory phase of HFOV is active, the reservoir of fresh gas flow in the low pass filter prevented entrainment of ambient air during expiration. Although 15 Hz was the preferred frequency in these original experiments, this is not necessarily the optimal setting. At slower speeds the tidal volume of each oscillation increases and more convective flow occurs.

Following the development of those pioneering prototypes, HFOV has progressed from being a physiological curiosity to an alternative mode of ventilation with potential advantages in the management of ARF. In this type of lung disease the conventional ventilator cycle not only produces a convective flow of gas to sweep CO_2 out of the lung, but it has to produce a pressure within the lung in excess of alveolar "opening pressure" in order to achieve oxygen exchange. In the low compliant, atelectatic lung, such as is seen in acute lung injury, airway pressure during the expiratory phase of the respiratory cycle falls below closing pressure, unless high levels of positive end expiratory pressure (PEEP) are used. It is this constant opening and closing of terminal airway units under high pressure that results in further injury to the already damaged lung. HFOV offers an entirely different ventilation strategy for dealing with this form of lung disease. In the first instance, high volume cycling is not necessary to eliminate CO_2 as numerous studies attest to the excellent $PaCO_2$ control with HFOV. Increasing airway pressure by adjusting fresh gas flow can then be used as a device to raise MAP above alveolar opening pressure and maintain lung volume at that level, where the small airway pressure swing around the mean will be less injurious to the lung by avoiding the continual cycle of inflation and collapse of terminal lung units.

In order to establish whether or not HFOV is less injurious to the lung in situations such as these, several groups of investigators have attempted to produce a valid animal model of acute lung injury and then to assess the effects of ventilation on the damaged lung. The Toronto group has chosen to use the surfactant depleted lung produced by repeated saline lavage. They have been able to show quite conclusively that by both blood gas and pathological criteria, HFOV causes less damage to the injured lung than CMV at matched mean airway pressures, using what they have termed their "open lung strategy". They found that when they lavaged the animals and rendered the lung surfactant depleted and poorly compliant, they were initially unable to demonstrate any difference between the modes of ventilation until they used a sustained inflation or "sigh" manoeuvre of $30 \, cmH_2O$ for 15 seconds.[27] Following this they were able to achieve excellent oxygenation in the HFOV group animals while in the CMV group the animals again became hypoxic and went on to die from pressure related complications. Post mortem histology of the lungs in this study also showed some striking differences. Those treated with CMV had changes consistent with severe lung damage as seen in ARDS, namely hyaline membrane formation, PMN infiltration, and oedema formation, while the lung histology in the HFOV group was normal. This study led to an appreciation of the fact that in the presence of the diffusely atelectatic lung, either mode of ventilation was equally injurious unless the lung volume was increased above its opening pressure by a sustained inflation and maintained at that level. In the case of HFOV, this was readily achieved while the lung became rapidly atelectatic again on CMV, despite the use of PEEP.

The group from San Antonio, Texas, has chosen to use another model of lung injury very analogous to IRDS.[28] Their model is the premature baboon which shows all the characteristics of IRDS, with severe hyaline membrane formation in the lung. They compared the outcome in baboons treated with HFOV with those treated with CMV and showed that the mortality was clearly higher in CMV treated animals, who typically showed the effects of severe pulmonary barotrauma at post mortem. The HFOV treated animals, on the other hand, survived for much longer with better gas exchange, required lower FiO_2 and airway pressures and had little evidence of pulmonary barotrauma at post mortem. The importance of this approach has been emphasised in the recent study by McCulloch[29] in the animal lung lavage model, which showed that HFOV at a high lung volume (HFO-A/Hi) produced superior gas exchange and less barotrauma when compared to both HFOV at low lung volume or CMV (fig 3.6). In

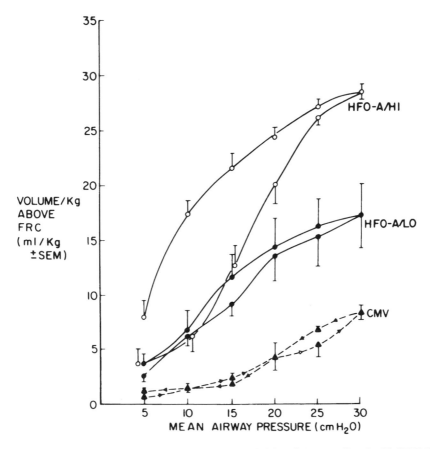

FIGURE 3.6—*Pressure volume curves of surfactant deficient lungs ventilated with HFOV at low and high volumes compared with controls where conventional ventilation was used. Reproduced with permission from ref* [29]

addition, hysteresis and compliance were better in the HFO-A/Hi based on analysis of the P/V curve of the lung.

At the same time as these animal studies were being performed, reports of the use of HFOV in infants with IRDS were appearing in the literature which suggested that effective gas exchange could be maintained at lower mean airway pressures than used on CMV. However, in all these studies, the switch to HFOV had only been made after CMV had been used for a substantial period and failed, so all these infants had substantial degrees of underlying ventilation induced lung injury. The question was raised whether the early introduction of HFOV in neonates with IRDS who required ventilation would decrease the incidence of ventilation and oxygen induced chronic lung injury. In order to answer these questions, the National Institutes of Health sponsored a multicentre randomised trial in North America comparing HFOV with CMV in infants of 750–2000 g birthweight who required positive pressure ventilation in the treatment of respiratory failure in the first 24 hours of life and had been treated with CMV for less than 12 hours (HiFi study).[30] All premature infants in the 750–1250 g group were eligible for enrolment, while in the 1250–2000 g infants the ratio of PaO_2/FiO_2 had to be <100 on at least MAP 9 cmH_2O. Eleven major neonatal centres in North America participated and 673 preterm infants were enrolled. The major endpoint of the study was the incidence of BPD. There was a crossover category where infants could be changed from one mode of ventilation to another after randomisation, which was then defined as a treatment failure. The crossover criteria were:

- $PaCO_2$ >65 mmHg (8.7 kpa) and PaO_2 <45 mmHg (6 kpa) on FiO_2 1.0 and MAP of at least 15 cmH_2O (4.7 kpa)
- $PaCO_2$ <35 mmHg on FiO_2 and MAP at least 15 cmH_2O
- $PaCO_2$ >75 mmHg (10 kpa).

The results showed that there was no difference in outcome between HFOV and BPD in the two groups according to the established criteria of the requirement for supplemental oxygen and abnormal chest x ray findings persisting to the 28th day. More disturbing was the reported finding that there was a statistically increased incidence of intraventricular haemorrhage (IVH) in the HFOV treated group.

It is very difficult to reconcile these disappointing results in terms of BPD with the very clear superiority of HFOV demonstrated in the two previously mentioned animal models of lung injury. It is even more difficult to understand the higher incidence of IVH associated with the use of HFOV in the multicentre trial. A breakdown of the data by study centre showed that the incidence of IVH varied considerably from centre to centre with a much higher incidence in outborn units with sicker patients. There has been some criticism of the design of the trial, particularly centred around the inexperience of many of the centres manifested by the high number of crossovers in the study.

The validity of the conclusions drawn from the HIFI study were further called into question following the publication of a study from Japan where a similar group of premature infants were enrolled in a randomised clinical trial comparing HFOV with CMV in IRDS.[31] Ninety premature infants were enrolled and although both groups received surfactant replacement therapy, the result was remarkable in respect of the very high survival and the outstandingly low incidence of BPD in both groups. The rates of IVH were also very low and the same with CMV as with HFOV. The study was then terminated.

What conclusions should we draw from these very different results? While it may be comforting to conclude that Japanese infants are inherently more resilient than North American infants, this would be ignoring the less comfortable consideration that Japanese neonatologists have a better understanding of the pathophysiology of IRDS than their North American colleagues and they have developed a ventilation strategy that recognises the importance of ventilation induced lung injury or, to put it more simply, it matters not what you do but how you do it.

The ventilation protocol in the Japanese study placed emphasis on the "open lung" approach and included a sigh to re-expand the atelectatic lung. There is no doubt that this is a key part of the strategy for improving oxygenation in the diffusely atelectatic lung. Fig 3.7 shows an example of how the aggressive volume recruitment manoeuvre with a sustained high MAP over a period of 20 min improved both the PaO_2 and the radiological appearance of a newborn infant with meconium aspiration. The mean airway pressure can then be reduced to 15–16 cmH$_2$O to prevent lung overdistention.

HFOV is now making a major comeback as an alternative ventilation strategy in IRDS. There are now several published single institution randomised or rescue studies demonstrating decreased barotrauma in very low birthweight infants, decreased incidence of BPD in IRDS and a reduction in the requirement for ECMO therapy in term infants with ARF and an OI >40.[32-36] In addition, the ease of control of CO_2 makes HFOV an attractive option in PPHN where the induction of a respiratory alkalosis can reverse right to left ductal shunting without the necessity to hyperventilate with high peak inspiratory pressures which lead to pulmonary barotrauma.

The use of HFOV has now extended outside the newborn period with the demonstration of its efficacy as a rescue therapy for older children (up to 35 kg) with ARF complicated by pulmonary barotrauma. This was followed by a randomised controlled clinical trial of CMV and HFOV in children outside the newborn period with hypoxaemia despite high mean airway pressures or air leak.[37] The study was a randomised crossover design and the HFOV strategy used the open lung approach with a MAP setting 5 cmH$_2$O above that used on conventional ventilation. However, the conventional ventilation mode did not use a pressure limited strategy. The survival was higher in the HFOV group when the numbers of patients who were randomised into that arm and did not cross, together with patients who were crossed over from CMV to HFOV, were taken into account.

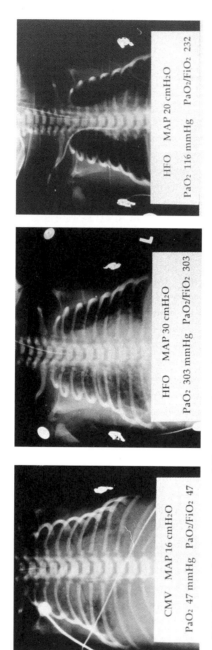

FIGURE 3.7—*Consecutive chest x rays and blood gases of a newborn infant with meconium aspiration syndrome treated with HFOV using an "open lung" strategy. The x rays and blood gases were done before and after switching from conventional ventilation to HFOV with an initial high mean airway pressure. The patient was maintained on HFOV at a reduced mean airway pressure and the x ray repeated 12 hours later*

Despite this promising result, it still remains to be determined whether the use of HFOV in children with ARF will show better outcomes than conventional ventilation using a pressure limited strategy with high PEEP.

High frequency jet ventilation (HFJV)

High frequency jet ventilation was first developed in clinical anaesthesia to provide small tidal volume ventilation for procedures involving the larynx and tracheobronchial tree where the ability to achieve a normal CO_2 with low airway pressures provided ideal operating conditions. Although HFJV and HFOV operate on the same physiological principles of very small tidal volumes delivered at high rates, they should not be considered as merely two variations on the same theme. HFJV uses a high pressure gas source to deliver small tidal volumes at frequencies of 1–5 Hz. Apart from the slower rates used in HFJV, the other major difference is that expiration is passive in the former while it is active in HFOV. The published experience with jet ventilation in ARF is considerably less than oscillation and mostly documents its use as rescue therapy in adult patients with either hypoxaemia despite high PEEP or established air leak. The rationale for the switch is usually the avoidance of further barotrauma by the use of smaller tidal volumes while maintaining a high mean airway pressure, but with lower peak airway pressures. Most of the published experience consists of small numbers with anecdotal reports where this strategy has proved successful, without convincing evidence that the same objective could not have been achieved with conventional ventilation. Improvements in oxygenation can be obtained by driving up the MAP but this usually involves some compromise to cardiovascular function because of the transmitted pressure. The single randomised crossover trial comparing HFJV with CMV in adults with ARF showed no difference in survival.[38] There are, however, trials in children which suggest a benefit. A rescue study published by Smith[39] has shown comparable gas exchange with lower measured airway pressures when patients with ARDS complicated by barotrauma switch from conventional to HFJV. A randomised controlled clinical trial of HFJV in neonates with pulmonary interstitial emphysema (PIE) has shown an improvement in PIE and lower mortality rate in infants treated with HFJV compared to conventional ventilation.[40]

There are some technical safety concerns about the adequacy of humidification in this system as well as reported cases of tracheal damage (necrotising tracheobronchitis) that have been reported in severely ill newborn infants. In addition, the airway pressures measured from the catheter within the trachea during HFJV probably represent a serious underestimate of true MAP because of the Bernoulli effect and consequently there is likely to be a significant amount of auto-PEEP present.

Intratracheal pulmonary ventilation (ITPV)

The trend to using increasingly smaller tidal volume settings in ARF has stimulated research into efforts to reduce dead space during mechanical ventilation. Delivering a high fresh gas flow (1.5–3 l/min) via a catheter placed at the carina has been shown to produce a normal $PaCO_2$ during prolonged apnoea, a technique known as constant flow ventilation. However, the drawbacks are that the gas flows required are prohibitively high as well as the potential for the development of pneumothorax if the airway became obstructed. Kolobow[41] has used the concept of minimal tidal volume to develop the novel technique of intratracheal pulmonary ventilation (ITPV) which incorporates the use of conventional mechanical ventilators and endotracheal tubes. In this system a high fresh gas flow exits from the tip of a catheter placed through an ET tube so that the delivery point is just above the carina, thus eliminating most of the dead space (fig 3.8). The ET tube acts as an expiratory port only. The air and oxygen supply lines for the mechanical ventilator are disconnected and the machine functions only as an electromechanical system for opening and closing the expiratory valve. Using this system, one can achieve very efficient CO_2 clearance with a tidal volume that is a fraction of physiological dead space with very low airway pressures.

The original design incorporated a diffuser head at the tip of the tracheal catheter which, while it allowed for improved gas mixing within the trachea, did result in high airway pressures at end expiration when using high fresh gas flows through small endotracheal tubes. The design of the tracheal catheter has recently been modified to a reverse thrust system whereby the delivered gas exits into the trachea from side holes rather than the tip (fig 3.9). The gas flow in the trachea during inspiration, when the expiratory valve is closed, is towards the carina. No fresh gas enters the ET tube during this phase. During expiration, with the expiratory valve on the ventilator open, gas continues to flow distally through the catheter, creating a Venturi effect within the ET tube and enhancing expiratory gas flow. This system has been extensively tested in experimental animals where normal levels of CO_2 have been maintained for prolonged periods even when all lobes of the lung except for the left upper have been removed. Measurements of carinal pressure have shown that there is no inadvertent PEEP; in fact, a high fresh gas flow may result in a negative carinal pressure due to the Venturi effect. Clinical experience is as yet limited to rescue

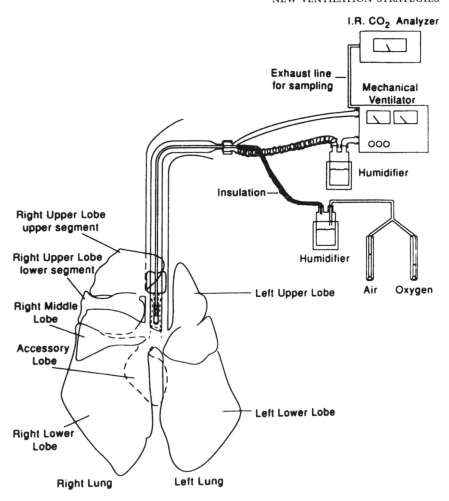

FIGURE 3.8—*Diagram of the ventilator circuit used for intratracheal pulmonary ventilation (ITVP). Reproduced with permission from ref* [41]

therapy in infants with congenital diaphragmatic hernia and an adult with ARF who could not be weaned from ECMO. There are still some safety problems to be resolved before the system can be subjected to human trials as the high gas flows have the potential to cause an inadvertent PEEP if the system is not used correctly. More particularly, the inability of commercially available humidifiers to tolerate the very high gas flow rates commonly used has been a major problem.

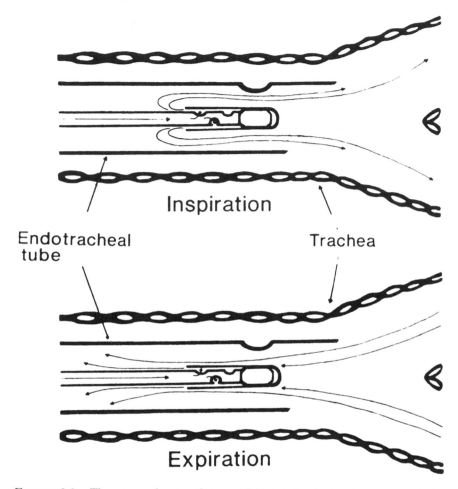

Inspiration

Endotracheal
tube

Trachea

Expiration

FIGURE 3.9—*The reverse thrust catheter used in intratracheal pulmonary ventilation (ITPV). Reproduced with permission from ref* [41]

Another variation on this theme is the technique of tracheal gas insufflation to enhance CO_2 elimination during pressure control ventilation.[42] This differs from ITPV in that the continuous gas flow catheter is placed alongside the ET tube with the tip located just above the carina. The increased fresh gas flow washes out the tracheal anatomic dead space while still using a conventional ventilator. Given the decreased emphasis on the importance of hypercarbia in ARF, the clinical relevance of this technique is questionable.

Airway pressure release ventilation (APRV)

Airway pressure release ventilation was first described by Downs[43] in 1987 for the management of ARDS. He reasoned that spontaneous breathing with CPAP in this situation would be preferable in that it would avoid the secondary lung injury from high airway pressures as well as the adverse effect on venous return produced by conventional ventilation. However, this would not be tolerated by many patients because the low lung compliance produced increased work of breathing and consequently respiratory muscle fatigue. To overcome this problem he devised a system which would provide CPAP at a level which would not depress cardiac function, deliver mechanical breaths without excessive levels of mean airway pressure and allow for spontaneous breathing.

In APRV the CPAP level is adjusted to optimise expiratory lung volume and the airway pressure release is used to augment CO_2 elimination. The patient breathes spontaneously at a raised pressure with periodic reductions which deflate the lungs and eliminate CO_2. The pressure profile of prolonged sustained positive pressure with short periods of pressure release during expiration resembles IRV with the difference being spontaneous rather than controlled breathing. The technique has been tested in experimental models of acute lung injury and seems to produce comparable oxygenation to conventional ventilation over the short term. Experience in humans with ARDS is limited but the data would suggest that there may be a benefit in patients with moderate degrees of lung injury who are capable of spontaneous respiration. In a comparative study of APRV compared to volume controlled inverse ratio ventilation where each was used for a 24 hour period in adult patients with moderate ARDS, the PaO_2/FiO_2 ratio and venous admixture was significantly better during APRV.[44]

Non-invasive ventilation

Non-invasive ventilation refers to techniques for increasing alveolar ventilation without endotracheal intubation. Historically the use of negative pressure ventilation predated endotracheal intubation and positive pressure by many years and still has a place in the management of patients with respiratory failure due to neuromuscular disease. However, the application of the technique is somewhat limited by the tendency for patients to develop obstructive sleep apnoea because of incoordination of upper airway muscles and by the fact that the devices are frequently uncomfortable to wear.

Applying positive pressure to the airway without an endotracheal tube with cither a nasal or face mask is increasingly used in less severe forms of acute or acute on chronic respiratory failure. This is also rediscovering an old technique. The initial application of positive expiratory pressure by Gregory in 1971[7] was done with a sealed head box and the use of nasal CPAP is a well established mode of therapy in ARF in newborn infants. Its use has been successfully extended to older infants with acute exacerbations of viral lung disease as well as neuromuscular diseases. Renewed interest in the technique in adults has been stimulated by the development of nasal CPAP masks to treat nocturnal sleep apnoea and studies which show that nocturnal non-invasive ventilation can reverse the daytime blood gas abnormalities and improve the symptoms in a select group of patients with chronic respiratory failure. The most obvious advantage is the avoidance of endotracheal intubation with less incidence of tracheal injury, ventilator associated pneumonia and the avoidance of sedating and paralysing drugs.

There are now several adult studies on the use of non-invasive modes of ventilation in patients with chronic cardiorespiratory failure which show symptomatic improvement in patients due, at least in part, to resetting the sensitivity of the respiratory centre to $PaCO_2$. The results of these studies vary considerably in the type of patient connection (nasal versus full face mask) and in mode of ventilation (pressure support versus assist control). The success of the technique is very dependent upon the delivery of an adequate tidal volume which is difficult to achieve if there is not an adequate seal. Although the nasal mask had advantages in terms of patient comfort and lower dead space, adequate tidal volume delivery may prove problematic as some of the insufflated gas will leak through the mouth unless it is kept closed. This may prove particulary difficult during sleep. Attempts have been made to overcome this by taping the mouth but a preferable arrangement would seem to be a full face mask fixed to provide an adequate seal. Some of the most interesting studies have been done in patients with congestive heart failure where significant improvements in symptoms are due to the effect of the raised intrathoracic pressure producing decreased afterload on the left ventricle.[45]

There are now at least two published randomised controlled clinical trials of the efficacy of non-invasive ventilation in acute on chronic respiratory failure. Bott[46] found that with nasal mask, volume ventilation in the assist control mode resulted in a lower $PaCO_2$ and reduced mortality when compared with standard (non-ventilation) treatment. Brochard[47] demonstrated similar superior results when pressure support was used with a face mask in a larger randomised controlled trial where the mortality, frequency of complications, intubation rate and hospital stay were all reduced.

The conclusions that can be drawn from the published data on the various types of non-invasive ventilation are that positive pressure delivered by either nasal or face mask has advantages over negative pressure ventilation for patients with neuromuscular disease, chest wall deformities and central hypoventilation syndromes as long as airway secretions are not excessive and upper airway function is intact. Mask positive pressure ventilation can also be successfully used in acute on chronic respiratory failure and as a method of reducing afterload on the left ventricle in patients with congestive heart failure.

Adjuncts to positive pressure ventilation

Prone position ventilation

There is now a recognition that the standard supine position for nursing the critically ill patient may be less than ideal in patients with ARF. Froese and Bryan showed over 20 years ago that during positive pressure ventilation there was a cephalad movement of the dorsal part of the diaphragm and loss of lung volume in people with normal lungs ventilated in the supine position. With positive pressure ventilation in the supine position there is preferential perfusion of dependent lung regions and CT images of patients with ARDS have shown that this is the most prominent area for haemorrhage and oedema formation. Several studies have now described the practice of turning hypoxic patients with ARF to the prone position with improvement in oxygenation and decreases in intrapulmonary shunt, although this finding is not universal.[48]

The proposed mechanisms for this improvement are increased FRC, change in regional diaphragm motion, redistribution of blood flow to less injured lung units and improved secretion clearance. Studies of experimental lung injury have shown that when turning to the prone position, preferential perfusion does not shift to the ventral part of the lung and that oedema is more uniformly distributed along the gravitational axis. There was also no change in FRC or regional diaphragm movement. The explanation for the decreased shunting seen with the prone position seems to be that the gravitational distribution of pleural pressure is much more uniform in the prone position. In the supine position the gravitational forces result in pleural pressure becoming positive in the dependent lung regions and dorsal lung units are below closing volume. This finding suggests that transpulmonary pressure may not exceed airway pressure in this region, resulting in lung collapse. The gravitational pleural pressure differences in the thorax are much less in the prone position, resulting in less of the lung below closing volume and decreased shunt.

The clinical and physiological studies seem to suggest that there may be a benefit from changing from the supine to the prone position when ventilating patients with hypoxaemia due to ARDS. Whether this will benefit all patients has yet to be demonstrated and there are certain caveats to this technique. Ventilating in the prone position makes nursing and the observation of patient disconnection more difficult. There is also the increased risk of neck injury when turning paralysed patients.

Surfactant replacement therapy

Surfactant deficiency as the cause of ARF in premature newborn infants was first described over 30 years ago. The lack of surfactant causes an increase in surface tension forces at alveolar level and the diffusely atelectatic lung that is so typically seen in this disease. If these surface tension forces are reduced with the administration of surfactant, then the tendency for these alveoli to collapse will be reduced and ventilation can be applied at lower peak airway pressures. With the development of naturally occurring and synthetic surfactants this has now become a reality.

Few therapies in the treatment of ARF in any age group have undergone such extensive study as surfactant replacement therapy in IRDS. There are now over 30 published randomised controlled trials of either synthetic or naturally occurring surfactant given at the time of delivery or shortly thereafter. These have been reviewed in a meta-analysis by Jobe[49] which showed that surfactant replacement therapy has reduced the mortality in premature infants with IRDS. As well as this, most controlled trials have been able to demonstrate a reduction in the complications associated with the premature infant lung such as pneumothorax, intraventricular haemorrhage and patent ductus arteriosus. The data on the incidence of bronchopulmonary dysplasia are less convincing. Some studies have shown a reduction in the incidence while others have not. Be that as it may, surfactant replacement therapy remains one of the few unqualified success stories in the treatment of ARF over the past 20 years.

On the other hand, the place of surfactant replacement therapy outside the newborn is less clear. Since the first descriptions of ARDS in the 1960s it has been recognised that there were surfactant abnormalities in the lungs of these patients without clear evidence of deficiency. There is abundant experimental and clinical evidence to show that surfactant is inactivated in ARDS outside the newborn period, probably secondary to the protein leak into the alveolus. Samples of bronchoalveolar lavage fluid taken from adult patients with ARDS and post mortem lung lavage studies in patients dying of ARDS have shown changes in the surfactant protein and phospholipid concentration and altered surface tension behaviour of the fluid. Although the administration of surfactant can be shown to improve oxygenation and compliance in experimental models of ARDS and there are non-randomised clinical trials which have shown benefit, especially in the non-premature newborn with ARF, the recently published randomised controlled trial of nebulised Exosurf in adult patients with sepsis induced ARF demonstrated no benefit.[50] Although this result was disappointing, it may be premature to dismiss surfactant replacement therapy as ineffective in adult ARF. It is now realised that not all surfactants are equally efficacious and that the synthetic varieties which do not have any of the surfactant proteins (A, B or C) may be less than ideal in this situation. It may well be that nebulisation of naturally occurring compounds will prove to be more beneficial as the administration of these in liquid form results in non-uniform distribution and the installation of substantial amounts of fluid into the lung.

Liquid ventilation

One of the most interesting and revolutionary concepts in the treatment of ARF in the past 20 years has been the development of a strategy that replaces a gaseous form of ventilation with a liquid. Instilling fluid into the lung results in liquid filled alveoli that have a much diminished air–liquid interface and reduced surface tension forces, in much the same way as surfactant. In addition, liquid spreads in a more uniform distribution within the lung compared to gas itself. Attempts at liquid ventilation by instillation of water or electrolyte solutions into the lung were ineffective due to the fact that the solubility of gas within them was low and their high viscosity and density led to increased respiratory work. Liquid ventilation with hyperbarically oxygenated fluid as a survival technique for astronauts and divers was briefly explored in the 1960s but was defeated by the high kinetic viscosity of saline making adequate alveolar ventilation impossible.

The discovery of a new class of compounds known as flurocarbons has overcome most, if not all, of the disadvantages previously associated with the use of liquid as a ventilation medium. These compounds have all the desirable properties for a gas exchanging vehicle that other liquids lack. Perflurocarbon, the one being used in experimental and clinical studies, is a fascinating chemical with a greater solubility for respiratory gases than blood. It has a low surface tension (25% of saline), is twice the density of water and has a low vapour pressure. In addition, it is biologically inert and chemically non-reactive. When instilled into the lung, it is not absorbed into the circulation and, being a hydrocarbon, is eliminated by vaporisation. At present, medically approved usage of perflurocarbon is as a contrast agent in radiological investigations but the discovery of its gas solubility properties has led to preliminary trials of its use in ARF.

Two methods for the application of perflurocarbon assisted ventilation have been investigated. The first, total liquid ventilation (TLV), consists of filling the lung to FRC with perflurocarbon and gas exchanging with an extracorporeal perflurocarbon circuit. The initial studies were performed on either surfactant deficient lambs or those with meconium aspiration. These reported excellent gas exchange while on TLV, which was sustained on return to conventional gas exchange ventilation. In addition, improved lung compliance and lower peak airway pressures were noted, a fact that was ascribed to recruitment of atelectatic lung and more homogeneous lung expansion. However, because of its kinetic viscosity it has to be driven in and out of the lung, purged of CO_2 and recharged with oxygen, resulting in very complex circuitry. The somewhat cumbersome equipment required for TLV has led to investigations into the use of partial liquid ventilation with a mechanical ventilator at conventional settings with the same volume of perflurocarbon instilled to fill the lung to FRC. Fuhrman[51] reported excellent gas exchange in experimental animals with normal lungs when warmed, preoxygenated perflurocarbon was instilled into the lungs up to the volume of FRC with conventional gas ventilation superimposed. This was achieved at low PIP (22 cmH$_2$O). Given the high density of the liquid, the beneficial effects on pulmonary function and gas exchange have been offset to some extent by concerns about adverse effects on cardiac output by physical properties of the liquid in the lung compressing the intra-alveolar vessels and resulting in an increase in PVR and a decrease in venous return. Despite this, surprisingly little effect on cardiac output has been demonstrated.

Since these initial studies a number of controlled studies have been published in either pulmonary lavage induced injury or the prematurity model of induced surfactant deficiency, comparing PLV to gas ventilation. These have demonstrated excellent gas exchange, reduced histological evidence of alveolar damage and improved lung compliance in the perflurocarbon group. There is also the suggestion of a dose response curve for perflurocarbon based on studies that show an increase in PaO$_2$ up to a maximum at 15 ml/kg which is approximately the FRC of the lung. The same relationship does not seem to hold true for the improvement in lung compliance which increased at the lowest dose but showed no further rise with increased volumes instilled into the lung.[52] This observation has led to speculation that the improvement in oxygenation is due to the expansion of alveoli and prevention of their collapse by the perflurocarbon while the increase in compliance is due to the effect on decreasing surface tension. There is also the additional advantage to the use of PLV in ARDS where most of the disease process is in the dependent lung regions which, because of the mechanics of the diaphragm, are difficult to expand and ventilate. Perflurocarbon, because of its density, will preferentially fill these dependent regions and act as a liquid stent – it has been described as "bottled PEEP".

These intriguing experimental findings have lead to preliminary clinical studies of the use of liquid breathing in a small number of neonates with IRDS, initially using a short period of TLV followed by a return to gas ventilation.[53] The results showed the similar improvements in oxygenation and compliance seen in the experimental studies. The technique has also been used in adults with ARDS who were being supported with ECMO therapy. The results from the animal models of lung injury and the human studies have been sufficiently impressive to justify a randomised controlled trial of PLV compared with conventional ventilation in paediatric ARDS which is currently in progress. Children outside the newborn period with a primary diagnosis of ARDS who require FiO_2 ≥ 0.5 and PEEP $\geq 6\,cmH_2O$ for more than 12 hours are eligible for randomisation. Perflurocarbon is instilled into the lung until a meniscus appears in the endotracheal tube (fig 3.10). Liquid ventilation

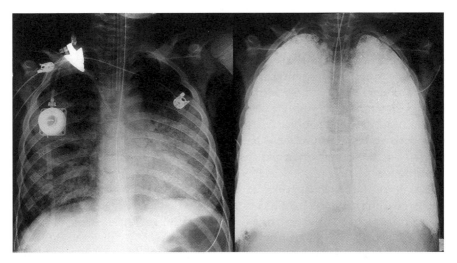

FIGURE 3.10—*Chest x ray before and after installation of perflurocarbon into the lungs of a child with severe ARDS*

is continued for five days. The primary outcome measure is the number of ventilator free days. The appropriate ventilator strategy to be used in terms of tidal volume and PEEP still remains to be determined, particularly as the very large volumes of perflurocarbon that are recommended must cause some lung distortion. In addition, the large tidal volumes are in marked contrast to those currently recommended in other non-conventional ventilator strategies.

Inhaled nitric oxide (iNO)

Few therapies in critical care medicine in the past 20 years have generated the interest and enthusiasm surrounding the medical use of inhaled nitric oxide. Since the first experiments in the 1970s which described the vital role played by the intact endothelium in inducing vascular dilation and the subsequent identification of NO as endothelial derived relaxing factor, there has been rapid progression through experimental studies which have demonstrated that inhaled NO (iNO) is a highly selective pulmonary vasodilator to its introduction into clinical medicine.

It has now become evident that nitric oxide is a biologically important compound with ubiquitous actions that involve multiple organ systems. Nitric oxide is synthetised from L-arginine by the enzyme nitric oxide synthetase (NOS). NO is then diffused rapidly from the endothelial cell into the vascular smooth muscle where it stimulates guanylate cyclase to produce cyclic guanosine monophosphate (CGMP), a potent vasodilator substance. The systemic nitrodilators currently in clinical use work by a similar mechanism but their pulmonary vasodilator effects cannot be separated from the systemic. In the case of iNO the vasodilator effects cannot be confined to the pulmonary circulation because the marked affinity of NO for the haem moiety of haemoglobin results in its rapid binding and inactivation as soon as it crosses the alveolar capillary membrane. Nitric oxide is a very unstable molecule which reacts with oxygen to form higher oxides of nitrogen, the most toxic of which is nitrogen dioxide. The speed of this reaction is proportional to both the concentration of oxygen and the duration of exposure and is greatly enhanced by high inspired oxygen concentrations.

The initial animal experiments on NO demonstrated its remarkable ability to selectively dilate the pulmonary vascular bed after pulmonary vasoconstriction had been induced by either inhalation of a hypoxic gas mixture or the infusion of the potent vasoconstrictor thromboxane. In these studies there seemed to be a dose dependent vasodilator effect as the inhaled concentration was increased from 10 up to 80 ppm.

Perhaps the greatest area of interest of the effects of iNO has been in the control of pulmonary vascular resistance in the transitional period between the adaptation from the foetal to the neonatal circulation and the implications this has for the treatment of persistent pulmonary hypertension of the newborn (PPHN). Studies have shown that endogenous NO modulates the basal pulmonary vascular tone in the late gestation foetus and that blockade of NO inhibits the endothelial dependent pulmonary vasodilation and increased pulmonary blood flow that follows immediately after birth. The pulmonary vasodilation produced by oxygen, as well as that which occurs with lung expansion in the immediate newborn period, have also been shown to be secondary to endogenous NO production. The vasodilator response was preserved in situations where structural abnormalities of the pulmonary vascular bed were induced by compression or ligation of the ductus arteriosus in an attempt to mimic the changes seen in PPHN. In these experiments the vasodilator response to acetylcholine was blunted while that to iNO was preserved, indicating that the NO induced dilation is endothelial independent.

There are now several published studies of iNO in PPHN where the gas has been used as a rescue therapy in newborn infants with severe hypoxaemia despite maximum conventional ventilator therapy where the only other option was ECMO therapy.[54] These have shown that in a significant number of patients iNO in doses of 6–80 ppm resulted in improved postductal PO_2 values, implying a reversal in ductal shunting due to a fall in pulmonary artery pressure. In addition, PaO_2 increased in some infants where there was no ductal shunting, indicating that pulmonary vasodilation produced an improvement in ventilation perfusion matching in the lung. Unlike the animal studies, there seems to be no dose-response relationship between the level of iNO and the increase in PaO_2[55] and there is little rationale in using iNO in concentrations greater than 20 ppm.

All the human newborn studies published to date have used iNO in uncontrolled clinical trials with the gas being delivered by either conventional ventilation, HFOV or while the patient was on ECMO in order to speed the weaning process from extracorporeal support. So far no adverse effects have been reported despite prolonged exposures up to 30 days. Although the response to iNO in ARF in the newborn may be very dramatic, by no means all infants respond. This may reflect the fact that respiratory failure in this group of patients is far from being a single disease entity and individual responses will vary according to the underlying pulmonary pathophysiology. Those infants with pure right to left ductal shunting and little parenchymal lung disease would be expected to respond best while the infant with extensive pulmonary parenchymal disease as a cause of their hypoxaemia (e.g. meconium aspiration) may have little response. There are at present at least three randomised controlled blinded clinical trials in progress of iNO or iNO with HFOV in PPHN. The first of these has shown a significant reduction in the need for ECMO in infants receiving iNO.[56]

There has also been increasing experience in the use of iNO as part of the ventilatory management of both paediatric and adult patients with ARDS. In this situation pulmonary hypertension is secondary to the inflammatory mediated release of pulmonary vasoconstrictors, the development of pulmonary microthrombi and areas of local ventilation perfusion mismatch, rather than being the primary pathophysiological disturbance. Again, the published studies represent experience of its use as rescue therapy in non-controlled clinical trials, often as an adjunct to other alternative ventilation therapies. Most of these show a pulmonary vasodilator effect with a fall in PVR in the range of 20–30% and an improvement in oxygenation secondary to improvement in ventilation perfusion matching.[57,58] These studies suggest that the dose response for iNO is different for enhanced ventilation perfusion compared with reduced PAP. In the former, an effect has been seen at doses of parts per billion while a reduction in PVR requires concentrations of parts per million.

Although the introduction of iNO frequently allows for adjustment of ventilator settings to levels of airway pressure and inspired oxygen less associated with secondary lung injury, it remains to be seen whether there will be a reduction in mortality in this syndrome that is associated with multiple organ failure and where hypoxaemia is frequently not the mode of death.[59] There are also concerns about the safety of adding iNO in situations where sepsis is frequently the underlying aetiology, given the fact that septic shock has been shown to be associated with the overproduction of endogenous NO. The conversion of nitric oxide to peroxynitrite, which has been shown to damage type 2 alveolar epithelial cells, is also potentially hazardous in the already injured lung.[60] These questions can only be resolved by a randomised controlled clinical trial, several of which are presently in progress. The preliminary results from the single published North American randomised controlled blinded trial of iNO in ARDS patients without sepsis has shown no difference in outcome.[61]

Extracorporeal membrane oxygenation

The first experience in the use of extracorporeal membrane oxygenation (ECMO) in the treatment of ARF was published in 1972. In the succeeding five years approximately 120 patients were treated with ECMO therapy with outcomes favourable enough to warrant a multicentre trial. Such a study was conducted in the 1970s where a total of 90 patients were enrolled and the survival in both arms was less than 10%.[62] Not surprisingly, ECMO was largely abandoned as an alternative ventilation strategy, although it continued to be used in Europe. However, the validity of this study by 1990 standards is questionable principally because the PEEP level at the point of randomisation was only 5 cmH$_2$O.

In 1977, Bartlett reported the first successful use of ECMO therapy in the term newborn with acute respiratory failure. Since then over 10 000 newborns with a predicted mortality of greater than 80% have been treated with this therapy with an overall survival of 83%. Since the predicted mortality was based on historical controls, attempts were made to answer the question of whether ECMO was superior to conventional ventilation by undertaking a randomised controlled trial. Two such studies have been completed which have shown improved survival with ECMO but in neither was strict randomisation carried out.[63,64] The outcome from both these studies has also been judged in the light of the fact that there was no standardised protocol used for mechanical ventilation which recognised the fact that oxygenation failure is due, at least in part, to the injury from positive pressure. The importance of taking this into account has been highlighted by studies showing improved survival in PPHN where ventilation with high peak inspiratory pressures was avoided and that by not using aggressive hyperventilation, the survival in PPHN is as good as with ECMO.[65,66] There are also studies which have shown that substantial numbers of infants may be rescued with HFOV prior to ECMO although they have met eligibility criteria.[34,35] At the time of writing, another randomised controlled trial of neonatal ECMO has just been completed in the United Kingdom which fulfilled strict randomisation criteria but did not include a defined protocol for conventional ventilator management and therefore failed to address a fundamentally important issue. Nevertheless, the results have shown improved survival in patients randomised to ECMO treatment.[67]

Outside the newborn period, the issue of whether ECMO is of benefit in the older child with oxygenation failure is even more open to question. The ELSO Registry figures suggest an overall survival of around 40% with a single institution recently publishing a survival of over 80%.[68] The problem with interpreting these figures is the lack of any reliable criteria for predicting mortality in ARF. ECMO will certainly prevent death from hypoxia ARDS, at least temporarily, but when PIPs of 50–60 cmH$_2$O are being used in this situation, it makes one wonder whether the patient is being rescued from the disease or the therapy. In fact, we lack accurate figures for the true mortality.

The issue of adult ECMO has recently been revisited by Morris[69] in the form of a randomised controlled trial of ECMO in ARDS. This compared conventional (volume controlled) mechanical ventilation with a "new therapy" defined as ventilation protocol using PC-IRV followed by low frequency positive pressure ventilation with extracorporeal CO$_2$ removal (LFPPV-ECCO$_2$R) if the PaO$_2$ was <50 mmHg on three consecutive measurements. Forty patients were randomised and there was no statistical difference in survival between the two patient groups (42% vs 33%). Bleeding was a major complication of the ECMO treated group. What is worthy of further comment, however, was that overall survival in both arms (38%) was four times higher than reported survival in the previous ARDS multicentre randomised trial in the 1970s. Several different and somewhat contradictory conclusions can be drawn from this study. The first would be that the comparison of a new therapy with historical controls is not valid, especially when the interval between the two is 20 years and the ventilation protocols were very different (the PEEP level for entry in the previous ARDS trial was only 5 cmH$_2$O). The second would be that the survival with PC-IRV is at least as good if not better than published outcomes using conventional volume controlled ventilation.

Outcome studies in ARF

One of the obstacles to the evaluation of new therapies used in the management of ARF is that we lack good outcome markers. ARDS is a syndrome with many different aetiologies and the outcome will be greatly influenced by the underlying cause. For instance, the mortality in ARDS associated with sepsis is higher than that associated with trauma or patients with single system lung disease without other organ dysfunction. In a published series of adult patients with ARDS, hypoxia was the primary mode of death in only 16% of patients, the rest being due to sepsis and multiorgan failure.[59] Therefore the ability to demonstrate improved oxygenation alone using a non-conventional approach would be unlikey to have a significant impact on outcome unless it could be shown that it either decreases the amount of lung injury or shortens the duration of ventilator support. There is now experimental data which shows that lung overdistension results in the release of cytokines which may be responsible for multiorgan injury and dysfunction. This provides a further rationale for the use of ventilator strategies which prevent this happening.

Attempts have been made in the paediatric literature to define the severity of lung disease and predict a high risk of mortality based on a combination of ventilation settings and blood gases. These are summarised in table 3.3. Most of these are small series which show published mortality rates for ARDS in children which vary from 40% to 70%. The most recent was a multicentre prospective series which evaluated predictors of survival in over 400 patients with ARF (cardiac disease excluded), collected over a one year period, who required the combination of FiO$_2$ ≥ 0.5 and PEEP ≥ 6 cmH$_2$O for more than 12 hours. The overall mortality in this study was 43% with a combination of the OI and PRISM score being the best predictor of death.[26]

Summary

This discussion of non-conventional methods of ventilation has reviewed the current techniques available to oxygenate patients with ARF where

TABLE 3.3—*Predictors of outcome in ARF*

	Study duration	Study design	Inclusion criteria	Patient numbers	Mortality	Predictive of death
Rivera[1]	2.9 years	R	FiO_2 0.9 PIP >25 cmH$_2$O	42	55%	PIP >40 cmH$_2$O A-aDO$_2$ >580 mmHg
Timmons[2]	3 years	R	FiO_2 0.5 PEEP >6 cmH$_2$O	44	75%	A-aDO$_2$ >470 mmHg
Tamburro[3]	4 years	R & P	FiO_2 0.6 PaO$_2$ <60 mmHg	37	46%	A-aDO$_2$ >450 mmHg
Davis[4]	2 years	P	Lung injury score >2.5	60	60%	A-aDO$_2$ >420 mmHg
Timmons[5]	1 year	R (MI)	FiO_2 >0.5 PEEP >6 cmH$_2$O	470	43%	PIP, PEEP, RR, FiO$_2$ PaO$_2$, PaCO$_2$, age, PRISM, postop status

[1] *Anaesth Intens Care* 1990;**18**:385
[2] *J Pediatr* 1991;**119**:896
[3] *J Pediatr* 1991;**119**:935
[4] *J Pediatr* 1993;**123**:35
[5] *Chest* 1995;**108**:789

standard ventilator management has proved inadequate to reverse the hypoxaemia. It has as its premise the frequently overlooked fact that ventilators don't cure lung disease – in fact, they do the opposite. For too long mechanical ventilation has been guided by normal lung physiology with escalations in volume and pressure to achieve "normal" blood gases. We must now recognise that this approach is inherently harmful and that the ventilator strategy in these patients must be adapted to match the underlying pathophysiology of the lung. Limitation of airway pressure and allowing some degree of hypercarbia is already paying dividends in improved survival in the management of status asthmaticus where mortality rates in the 1970s were 25–50% in patients requiring ventilation. In ARDS the "open lung" strategy with prevention of overdistention would seem to have the most to offer. This is particularly true in HFOV where the early application of an aggressive volume recruitment strategy followed by a reduction of mean airway pressure can be highly effective.

Determining improvement in outcome with changing ventilation practice will prove more difficult as it is a syndrome with a multiplicity of causes rather than a single disease entity. Non-conventional ventilation techniques probably have the most to offer patients with hypoxia due to single system pulmonary failure whilst those with immunosuppression and multiple organ dysfunction would be expected to benefit least. Given the multiplicity of therapies now available, there is a pressing need for large, well designed multicentre studies to determine which are truly effective and at what stage in the disease process they should be introduced.

1 Lassen HCA. A preliminary report on the 1952 epidemic of poliomyelitis in Copenhagen with special reference to the treatment of acute respiratory insufficiency. *Lancet* 1953;1: 37–41.
2 Bernard GR, Artigas A, Brigham KL, *et al*. The American–European Consensus Conference on ARDS. *Am J Respir Crit Care Med* 1994;149:818–24.
3 Nash G, Bowen JA, Langlinais PC. "Respirator lung" a misnomer. *Arch Pathol* 1971;21: 234–40.
4 Bendixen HH, Hedle-Whyte J, Laver MB. Impaired oxygenation in surgical patients during general anaesthesia with controlled ventilation. *N Engl J Med* 1963;269:991–6.
5 Froese A, Bryan AC. Effects of anaesthesia and paralysis on diaphragmatic mechanics in man. *Anesthesiology* 1974;41:242–55.
6 Ashbaugh DG, Bigelow DB, Petty TL, Levine BE. Acute respiratory distress in adults. *Lancet* 1967;2:319–23.
7 Gregory GA, Kitterman JA, Phibbs RH, Tooley WH, Hamilton WK. Treatment of the idiopathic respiratory-distress syndrome with continuous positive airway pressure. *N Engl J Med* 1971;284:1333–9.
8 Suter PM, Fairley HB, Isenberg MD. Optimum end expiratory airway pressure in patients with acute pulmonary failure. *M Engl J Med* 1975;292:284.
9 Webb HH, Tierney DF. Experimental pulmonary edema due to intermittent positive pressure ventilation with high inflation pressures. Protection by positive end-expiratory pressure. *Am Rev Respir Dis* 1974;110:556–65.
10 Dreyfuss D, Basset G, Soler P, Saumon G. Intermittent positive pressure hyperventilation with high inflation pressures produces pulmonary microvascular injury in rats. *Am Rev Respir Dis* 1985;132:880–4.

11 Kolobow T, Moretti MP, Fumagalli R, *et al.* Severe impairment in lung function induced by high peak airway pressure during mechanical ventilation. *Am Rev Respir Dis* 1987; **135**: 312–31.

12 Tsuno K, Prato P, Kolobow T. Acute lung injury from mechanical ventilation at moderately high airway pressures. *J Appl Physiol* 1990;**69**:956–61.

13 Dreyfuss D, Soler P, Basset G, Saumon G. High inflation pulmonary edema: effects of high airway pressure, high tidal volume and positive end-expiratory pressure. *Am Rev Respir Dis* 1988;**137**:1159–64.

14 Hernandez LA, Coker PJ, May S, Thompson AL, Parker JC. Mechanical ventilation increases microvascular permeability in oleic acid-injured lungs. *J Appl Phsiol* 1990;**69**: 2057–61.

15 Hernandez LA, Peevy KJ, Moise AA, Parker JC. Chest wall restriction limits high airway pressure-induced lung injury in young rabbits. *J App Physiol* 1989;**66**:2364–8.

16 Corbridge TC, Wood LDH, Crawford GP, Chudoba MJ, Yanos J, Sznajder JI. Adverse effects of large tidal volume and low PEEP in canine acid aspiration. *Am Rev Resper Dis* 1990;**142**:311–15.

17 Sandhar BK, Niblett DJ, Argiras EP, Dunnill MS, Sykes MK. Effects of positive end-expiratory pressure on hyaline membrane formation in a rabbit model of the neonatal respiratory distress syndrome. *Intensive Care Med* 1988;**14**:538–46.

18 Muscedere JG, Mullen JBM, Gan K, Slutksy AS. Tidal ventilation at low airway pressures can augment lung injury. *Am J Respir Crit Care Med* 1994;**149**:1327–34.

19 Reynolds EOR. Effect of alterations in mechanical ventilator settings on pulmonary gas exchange in hyaline membrane disease. *Arch Dis Child* 1971;**46**:152–9.

20 Rappaport SH, Shpiner R, Yoshihara G, Wright J, Chang P, Abraham E. Randomized, prospective trial of pressure-limited versus volume controlled ventilation in severe respiratory failure. *Crit Care Med* 1994;**22**:22–32.

21 Lessard MR, Guerot E, Lorino H, Lemaire F, Brochard L. Effects of pressure-controlled ventilation with different I:E ratios versus volume-controlled ventilation on respiratory mechanics, gas exchange, and hemodynamics in patients with adult respiratory distress syndrome. *Anesthesiology* 1994;**80**:983–91.

22 Darioli R, Perret C. Mechanical controlled hypoventilation in status asthmaticus. *Am Rev Respir Dis* 1984;**129**:385–7.

23 Hickling KG, Henderson SJ, Jackson R. Low mortality associated with low volume pressure limited ventilation with permissive hypercapnia in severe adult respiratory distress syndrome. *Intensive Care Med* 1990;**16**:372–7.

24 Goldstein B, Shannon DC, Todres ID. Supercarbia in children: clinical course and outcome. *Crit Care Med* 1990;**18**:166–8.

25 Amato MBP, Barbas CSV, Medeiros DM, *et al.* Beneficial effects of the "open lung approach" with low distending pressures in acute respiratory distress syndrome. A prospective randomised study on mechanical ventilation. *Am J Respir Crit Care Med* 1995; **152**:1835–46.

26 Timmons OD, Havens PL, Fackler JC. Predicting death in pediatric patients with acute respiratory failure. *Chest* 1995;**108**:789–97.

27 Hamilton PP, Onayemi A, Smyth JA, *et al.* Comparison of conventional and high-frequency ventilation: oxygenation and lung pathology. *J Appl Physiol* 1983;**55**:131–8.

28 DeLemos RA, Coalson JJ, Gerstmann DR, *et al.* Ventilatory management of infant baboons with hyaline membrane disease: the use of high frequency ventilation. *Pediatr Res* 1987; **21**:594–602.

29 McCulloch PR, Forkert PG, Froese AB. Lung volume maintenance during HFO in surfactant deficient rabbits. *Am Rev Respir Dis* 1988;**137**:1185–92.

30 HiFi Study Group. High-frequency oscillatory ventilation compared with conventional mechanical ventilation in the treatment of respiratory failure in preterm infants. *N Engl J Med* 1989;**320**:88–93.

31 Ogawa Y, Miyasaka K, Kawano T, *et al.* A multicentre randomised trial of high frequency oscillatory ventilation as compared with conventional ventilation in preterm infants with respiratory failure. *Early Human Dev* 1993;**32**:1–10.

32 Clark RH, Yoder BA, Sell MS. Prospective, randomised comparison of high-frequency oscillation and conventional ventilation in candidates for extracorporeal membrane oxygenation. *J Pediatr* 1994;**124**:447–54.

33 Clark RH, Gerstmann DR, Null DM, DeLemos RA. Prospective randomised comparison of high-frequency oscillatory and conventional ventilation in respiratory distress syndrome. *Pediatrics* 1992;**89**:5–12.

34 Carter JM, Gerstmann DR, Clark RH, *et al*. High-frequency oscillatory ventilation and extracorporeal membrane oxygenation for the treatment of acute neonatal respiratory failure. *Paediatrics* 1990;**85**:159–64.

35 DeLemos RA, Yoder B, McCurnin D, Kinsella J, Clark R, Null D. The use of high-frequency oscillatory ventilation (HFOV) and extracorporeal membrane oxygenation (ECMO) in the management of the term/near term infant with respiratory failure. *Early Human Dev* 1992;**29**:299–303.

36 HiFO Study Group. Randomised study of high-frequency oscillatory ventilation in infants with severe respiratory distress syndrome. *J Pediatr* 1993;**122**:609–19.

37 Arnold JH, Hanson JH, Toro-Figuero LO, Gutierrez J, Berens RJ, Anglin DL. Prospective, randomised comparison of high-frequency oscillatory ventilation in pediatric respiratory failure. *Crit Care Med* 1994;**22**:1530–9.

38 Carlon GC, Howland WS, Ray C, Miodownik S, Griffin JP, Groeger JS. High frequency jet ventilation. A prospective randomized evaluation. *Chest* 1983;**84**:551–9.

39 Smith DW, Frankel LR, Derish MT, *et al*. High-frequency jet ventilation in children with the adult respiratory distress syndrome complicated by pulmonary barotrauma. *Pediatr Pulm* 1993;**15**:279–86.

40 Keszler M, Donn SM, Bucciarelli RL, *et al*. Multi-center controlled trial comparing high-frequency jet ventilation and conventional ventilation in newborn infants with pulmonary interstitial emphysema. *J Pediatr* 1991;**119**:85–93.

41 Kolobow T, Powers T, Mandava S, *et al*. Intratracheal pulmonary ventilation (ITPV): control of positive end-expiratory pressure at the level of the carina through the use of a novel ITPV catheter design. *Anesth Analg* 1994;**78**:455–61.

42 Ravenscraft SA, Burke WC, Nahum A, *et al*. Tracheal gas insufflation augments CO_2 clearance during mechanical ventilation. *Am Rev Respir Dis* 1993;**148**:345–451.

43 Downs JB, Stock MC. Airway pressure release ventilation: a new concept in ventilatory support. *Crit Care Med* 1987;**15**:459–61.

44 Sydow M, Burchardi H, Ephraim E, Zielmann S, Crozier TA. Long-term effects of two different ventilatory modes on oxygenation in acute lung injury. Comparison of airway pressure release ventilation and volume-controlled inverse ratio ventilation. *Am J Respir Crit Care Med* 1994;**149**:1550–6.

45 Bradley TD, Holloway RM, McLaughlin PR, Ross BL, Walters J, Liu PP. Cardiac output response to continuous positive airway pressure in congestive heart failure. *Am Rev Respir Dis* 1992;**145**:377–82.

46 Bott J, Carroll M, Conway JH, *et al*. Randomised controlled trial of nasal ventilation in acute ventilatory failure due to chronic obstructive airways disease. *Lancet* 1993;**341**:1555–7.

47 Brochard L, Mancebo J, Wysocki M, *et al*. Noninvasive ventilation for acute exacerbations of chronic obstructive pulmonary disease. *N Engl J Med* 1995;**333**:817–22.

48 Albert RK, Leasa D, Sanderson M, Robertson HT, Hlastala MP. The prone position improves arterial oxyenation and reduces shunt in oleic-acid-induced acute lung injury. *Am Rev Respir Dis* 1987;**135**:628–33.

49 Jobe A. Pulmonary surfactant therapy. *N Engl J Med* 1993;**328**:861–8.

50 Anzueto A, Baughman RP, Guntupalli KK, *et al*. Aerosolised surfactant in adults with sepsis induced acute respiratory distress syndrome. *N Engl J Med* 1996;**334**:1417–21.

51 Fuhrman BP, Paczan PR, DeFrancisis M. Perflurocarbon-associated gas exchange. *Crit Care Med* 1991;**19**:712–22.

52 Tutuncu AS, Faithfull NS, Lachmann B. Intratracheal perfluorocarbon administration combined with mechanical ventilation in experimental respiratory distress syndrome: dose-dependent improvement of gas exchange. *Crit Care Med* 1993;**21**:962–9.

53 Greenspan JS, Wolfson MR, Rubenstein D, Shaffer TH. Liquid ventilation of human preterm neonates. *J Pediatr* 1990;**117**:106–11.

54 Kinsella JP, Neish SR, Dunbar D, Shaffer E, Abman SH. Clinical responses to prolonged treatment of persistent pulmonary hypertension of the newborn with low doses of inhaled nitric oxide. *J Pediatr* 1993;**123**:103–8.

55 Finer BR, Etches PC, Kamstra B, Tierney AJ, Peliowski A, Ryan CA. Inhaled nitric oxide in infants referred for extracorporeal oxygenation: dose response. *J Pediatr* 1994;**124**: 302–8.

56 Neonatal Inhaled Nitric Oxide Study Group. Inhaled nitric oxide in full-term and near full-term infants with hypoxic respiratory failure. *N Engl J Med* 1997;**336**:597–604.

57 Rossaint R, Falke K, Lopez F, *et al.* Inhaled nitric oxide for the adult respiratory distress syndrome. *N Engl J Med* 1993;**328**:399–405.

58 Abman SH, Griebel JL, Parker DK. Acute effects of inhaled nitric oxide in children with severe hypoxic respiratory failure. *J Pediatr* 1994;**124**:881–8.

59 Montgomery AB, Stage MA, Carrico CJ, Hudson LD. Causes of mortality in patients with the adult respiratory distress syndrome. *Am Rev Respir Dis* 1985;**132**:485–9.

60 Haddad IY, Gyorgy P, Hu P, Galliani C, Beckman JS, Matalon S. Quantification of nitrotyrosine levels in lung sections of patients and animals with acute lung injury. *J Clin Invest* 1994;**94**:2407–13.

61 Dellinger RP, Zimmermann JL, Hyes TM, *et al.* Inhaled nitric oxide in ARDS: preliminary results of a multicenter clinical trial. *Crit Care Med* 1996;**24**:A29.

62 Zapol WM, Snider MT, Hill JD, *et al.* Extracorporeal membrane oxygenation in severe acute respiratory failure. A randomized prospective study. *JAMA* 1979;**242**:2193–6.

63 O'Rourke PP, Crone RK, Vacanti JP, *et al.* Extracorporeal membrane oxygenation and conventional medical therapy in neonates with persistent pulmonary hypertension of the newborn: a prospective randomized study. *Pediatrics* 1989;**84**:957–63.

64 Bartlett RH, Roloff DW, Cornell RG, Andrews AF, Dillon PW, Zwischenberger JB. Extracorporeal circulation in neonatal respiratory failure: a prospective randomised study. *Pediatrics* 1985;**76**:479–87.

65 Wung JT, James LS, Kilchewskey E, James E. Management of infants with severe respiratory failure and persistence of the foetal circulation without hyperventilation. *Paediatrics* 1985;**76**:488–94.

66 Dworetz AR, Moya FR, Sabo B, Gladstone I, Gross I. Survival of infants with persistent pulmonary hypertension without extracorporeal membrane oxygenation. *Pediatrics* 1989; **84**:1–6.

67 UK Collaborative ECMO Trial Group. UK collaborative randomised trial of neonatal extracorporeal membrane oxygenation. *Lancet* 1996;**348**:75–82.

68 Moler FW, Custer JR, Bartlett RH, *et al.* Extracorporeal life support for severe pediatric respiratory failure: an updated experience 1991–1993. *J Pediatr* 1994;**124**:875–80.

69 Morris AH, Wallace CJ, Menlove RL, *et al.* Randomized clinical trial of pressure-controlled inverse ratio ventilation and extracorporeal CO_2 removal for adult respiratory distress syndrome. *Am J Respir Crit Care Med* 1994;**149**:295–305.

4: Home ventilation: indications, ethics, and practicalities

JONATHAN GILLIS, PAUL HUTCHINS

The ability to ventilate children artificially at home has been shown on many occasions and in many countries to be both technically and practically feasible.[1-14] The technology dependent child presents a significant challenge to child health[15] and to medical ethics.[16] As many as one in 1000 school children has some needs[17] which can be defined as technology dependent.[14] For the patient and family, home care provides the most appropriate environment for the child, gives the family control and removes the emotional, financial, energy, and time burdens of hospital visiting.[18] For the hospital, home care reduces nosocomial complications and the pressures on the resources of intensive care. The decision on whether to ventilate a child at home usually arises in an intensive care unit and has therefore become an issue for paediatric intensivists and a subject for chapters in books on paediatric intensive care. A good argument can be made that this location is an inappropriate domain for this subject and this will be one of the main themes of this chapter.

Intensive care units are not commonly confronted with a decision on whether to ventilate a child at home, but when such a consideration does occur, it consumes a great deal of time, emotional effort, and resources and has a major impact on the functioning of the intensive care unit. The child and the family become an integral part of the life of the unit and staff develop a highly ambivalent attitude ranging from possessive devotion to the irritating awareness that a valuable acute bed is being occupied. Ward rounds are interminably prolonged with wide ranging discussions on the child's and family's emotional and psychological needs. There are frequently divergent opinions amongst staff about whether the treatment should be continued, with vastly different attitudes and levels of knowledge about the quality and cost of prolonged ventilator living. Intensive care units and those that work within them are geared to the acute, the great miracle or the noble failure, a world of action and instant gratification. This is not a world attuned to the problems of chronic disability and the slow but steady rehabilitation needed for the chronically ventilated child. Since, of necessity, these children originate in the paediatric intensive care unit, it is necessary for those working in the area to be familiar with the issues involved.

The main themes of this chapter will be as follows.

- Home ventilation for children is possible, practical and advantageous compared with institution living.
- Home ventilation should always be supported by a comprehensive, coordinated and continuous management programme.
- The main problems are not technical. The main issues are the emotional and practical demands on the family and the provision of appropriate support.
- Issues for the child and family and the resources required differ greatly, depending on associated disabilities and whether ventilation is required full time or only at night.

Our approach derives from an examination of the medical and nursing literature, liaison with colleagues from other parts of the world and the experience of our own designated home ventilation programme.[4,71] Established in 1989, our programme currently supports 12 individuals ventilated at home; this is 40% of the total Australian experience in children and young adults recently reviewed by the National Health and Medical Research Council.[5] This review emphasised the issues and costs of long term ventilation, rather than the specifics of daily care. It reported 26 children who were ventilated, 20 wholly or partially at home. British experience until 1990 reported a similar number of ventilator dependent children.[11] A further 20 adults under 40 years of age were reported in the Australian review, though this is probably an underestimate. Later that year, a survey by the Australian Quadriplegic Association[20] in New South Wales alone identified 99 cases of all ages, most with partial and non-invasive ventilation. A South Australian survey[21] estimated that 42 children and adults would require home ventilation support in 1995 in that state.

This chapter will endeavour to answer the following questions.

- Who are the children who might be candidates for home ventilation?
- What are the practical considerations for the intensive care unit?
- What are the essentials of a programme to support such children?
- What is the future of home ventilation?

Which children?

Children who may be considered for ventilation at home are those who are either fully or partially ventilator dependent and are in a relatively stable state. Diseases that result in such a state are either neuromuscular or pulmonary. Neuromuscular conditions include cervical spinal cord injuries, neuromuscular diseases and congenital central hypoventilation ("Ondine's curse"); pulmonary conditions include bronchopulmonary dysplasia and congenital airway anomalies. Support is required for an increasing number of children with disordered sleep physiology impairing daytime function. It may also be requested for those awaiting lung transplantation, as in cystic fibrosis.

Presentation is acute in cervical cord injury or in congenital central hypoventilation from birth; an acute presentation may also be precipitated by an intercurrent illness in those with neuromuscular or chronic lung parenchymal disorders. Such children often "creep up on" the intensive care unit. We have coined the phrase "the phenomenon of entrapment" to describe this situation.[4,22] The child requires urgent ventilator support for acute respiratory failure. The processes of resuscitation and intensive care take their inexorable course because of the immediate need to stabilise the situation. One can never be sure initially that there is not a possibility of recovery to the point of being independent of ventilation. In those children with preexisting neuromuscular disease there is always the chance that there has been an acute reversible insult such as a viral illness. No matter how well they have been prepared in previous discussions about progressive diseases, patient and family still face a crisis.[23,24,25] The uncertainty of outcome compels treatment to be continued. By the time ventilator dependence is apparent, the child is alert and sometimes, particularly in neuromuscular disease, in better health than before. As we have previously pointed out: "Whilst the concept of entrapment is not new and must be very familiar to all intensivists, it requires greater consideration. The entrapped person is the most affected, but he or she is not the only one entrapped. So are the family, involved professionals and the facilities and resources which might produce far greater benefits for others".[22]

Some question whether patients should be allowed to refuse life support early in the intensive care phase of treatment when outcome is uncertain, sometimes leading to heated debate.[26-30] Others follow a presumption by medical care providers that they could not live with such disability.

Categories of home ventilation children

Children who require long term artificial ventilation are a heterogeneous population. The complex considerations are not uniform and differ according to eventual prognosis. They must take into account quality of life, family disruption, and logistical considerations. Such considerations involve:

- whether nocturnal or full ventilation is required;
- whether there is a need for tracheostomy or whether mask ventilation or negative pressure ventilation can be used;
- whether the child is predicted to eventually resume spontaneous ventilation;
- whether there are major associated handicaps, for example, quadriplegia or cognitive handicaps;
- whether the underlying disease is non-progressive or progressive, as in muscular dystrophy.

Children who require nocturnal ventilation and have no other handicaps, as in congenital central hypoventilation, can often lead a normal life by day with their only handicap being a tracheostomy.[31,32] It is probable that in time such children may be able to be ventilated by face mask or cuirass ventilator with even less disruption to everyday life. In neuromuscular diseases, nocturnal ventilation may significantly improve daytime activity, cognitive, and social function and can be commenced with non-invasive techniques. In some myopathic disorders, weaning may be possible; in others the progress is inexorable, in spite of ventilation. Children who require full ventilation for bronchopulmonary dysplasia are ventilated with the expectation that they will eventually be able to resume normal ventilation. This is possible because of continued growth and development of the lung parenchyma; numbers of alveoli increase until 8 years of age. The move from neonatal to "older" paediatric intensive care facilities highlights practical and ethical decisions about their management and ongoing ventilation. Home ventilation is offered to this group much less in Australia than in North America, where it provides the predominant experience of home ventilation.[7]

Children with cervical spinal cord damage, however, are in a position of extreme handicap and dependence, in which the practicalities of ventilation may present as the prime problems but pale beside the disability and care needed for high cervical quadriplegia.[33,34] They present the greatest practical and ethical challenge and sharpest example of "entrapment". The die is often cast at the scene of the trauma when resuscitation is initiated.

95

Deciding to continue ventilation

The purpose of long term ventilation is to prolong life in an individual who desires it, to relieve the discomfort of respiratory failure, and to improve outcome. Home ventilation aims to prolong life in an environment which will enhance individual potential. For a child, the essence is growth and care within the family, peers and social world. Physical well being and growth are important. Though ethical issues seem paramount in the well equipped intensive care unit, the bigger hurdle is the long term adequacy of professional caregivers, equipment and funding to support the family's burden.[35-37]

Criteria for selection

Patient selection criteria must be established by the professionals responsible for coordinating the home ventilation programme. The essential criterion is that the family must be willing and have the ability to undertake long term home management. They must be helped to understand the demands involved and give informed consent to proceed with this course; this includes an acceptance of the true nature of the child's disability and prognosis. All parties must be clear about the level of routine and emergency home care required and what services are realistically available to support it. This often necessitates a compromise between family commitment, optimum management, and actual resources.

Medical criteria include a stable clinical state with a reliable airway, low (if any) oxygen dependence, and steady standard ventilator settings without the need for end expiratory pressure. In general, the child should have a non-progressive condition without other major disabilities, e.g. severe cognitive impairment, which preclude an acceptable quality of life. There is a stark spectrum between the normality of daytime function with congenital central hypoventilation and the profound disability of ventilator dependent quadriplegia.

The participation of an adolescent in decisions to initiate or discontinue treatment is particularly poignant, as discussed in two thoughtful papers[39,40] and the Australian overview.[5,28,41] The position of "mature minors", younger than the statutory 16 years yet able to understand the nature and risks of the proposed treatment, must be considered. Notwithstanding official admission age policies, older adolescents and even young adults may present to the paediatric intensive care unit, particularly in children's hospitals which have provided care for the underlying condition for many years.

96

Adolescent consultation and counselling are particularly relevant in neuromuscular disorders, such as muscular dystrophy. Decisions in this group compound the complexity of the "non-progressive" criterion. Ventilation will not slow progression of the disease, but well being can be improved by non-invasive ventilation, particularly if introduced early. Patients' and families' attitudes and decisions and retrospective reviews of life before and after home ventilation indicate that half may elect for ventilation, others are undecided and a minority decline; those who have continued believe that their decision was correct.[23] All views emphasise the need for early, repeated, detailed explanations and the opportunity to meet others experiencing home ventilation.[24,25] There will be a growing number of conditions and children who will be considered for assisted ventilation, perhaps after a period on supplemental oxygen. Examples include lower cervical quadriplegia, brainstem anomalies, as in neural tube defects, connective tissue dysplasia with brainstem compression, as in achondroplasia, and lung impairment from scoliosis.

Such emotional and ethical decisions cannot be taken rapidly and the involvement of health care professionals who will manage home support is essential. They can share the burden with intensive care staff, can guide the family and patient with knowledge of other families' experience and set the base of continuing care. Indeed, a speedy discharge will be unlikely, with a minimum of several months needed to acquire equipment, engage and train family and carers and, if compensatable, acquire funding from the complex legal and insurance procedures.[35-37]

Life expectancy depends greatly on the primary diagnosis, associated problems, and the potential for further growth and development. Combined with the hoped-for miraculous cure, it is not surprising that long term survival does not feature heavily in immediate decision making about whether to continue. Published survival figures may be inflated by the inclusion of patients with bronchopulmonary dysplasia who eventually wean. In cervical cord injury, survival statistics into adulthood are derived from cohorts who became ventilator dependent two or three decades ago. Morbidity and mortality, prevalence according to diagnostic group, and length of stay have undoubtedly changed greatly due to advances in care.[42]

Funding

When home ventilation is deemed appropriate, society should provide the resources that an individual family needs, although this rarely occurs.[5] The decision to ventilate must be taken on clinical grounds. The possibility of discharge from intensive care either within or outside the hospital, however, is often complicated by arguments about cost as well as the vagaries of the legal and compensation systems. Different countries and localities have different funding systems and finite budgets.[5,6,10,14] Our own experience mirrors that elsewhere, i.e. that the costs of 24 hour nursing care are similar in hospital and home; the main gain, therefore, is humanitarian in that the child is at home. The Australian Association of Paediatric Teaching Centres[38] explored the costs of technology dependent care in 1991 and assessed annual costs of full time ventilator dependence to be at least AUD 250 000. A South Australian study[21] examined costs of cervical cord injury in three patients, two with electrophrenic pacing and one mechanically ventilated, and found that nursing costs were AUD 600 per day. In 1988 a United States Task Force suggested annual costs of home ventilation of about US$80 000, with the greatest saving for children with bronchopulmonary dysplasia who would often have a substantial part of their care undertaken by parents.[14] The Health Care Committee of the National Health and Medical Research Council summarised the Australian situation as it existed in 1993.[5]

Practical considerations for the intensive care unit

For the professional working in paediatric intensive care, such patients affect unit function in a number of ways:

- the adaptation of the unit's processes to a problem involving chronic rehabilitation rather than acute resuscitation;
- the establishment of a programme leading to home ventilation;
- the pressure of other acute admissions.

Adaptation of the intensive care unit

The reprocessing of intensive care to cope with a chronic patient with rehabilitation needs often presents a major difficulty for intensive care units. Considerations regarding home ventilation should only be an issue for intensive care in the very early phases. Once the decision has been made to continue ventilation, a coordinated, comprehensive home ventilation programme should immediately be instituted with the aim of discharging the patient from the intensive care to a general ward and eventually home. Our own experience[4] and other position statements[5,6,8,14,18] attest that management is best organised by a rehabilitation team in association with respiratory physicians and should be regionalised so that expertise is maintained.[5,37] In some hospitals there will be no choice but for the child to remain in the ICU, ideally in a single room, allowing normalisation of daily routines and insulation from some of the daily trauma and tragedy.

Establishment of a programme leading to home ventilation

In establishing long term ventilation, steps for the intensive care unit should include the following.

Respiratory care

The establishment of a stable, secure airway is of paramount importance. For most acute patients this requires endotracheal intubation followed by early tracheostomy. Tracheostomy is needed for infants, many children under 8–10 years, those requiring extended daily ventilation and those with poor cough and bulbar function. Tubes should be uncuffed and small enough to allow an air leak with positive pressure which facilitates speech. Non-invasive ventilation by nasal masks or mouthpiece or by negative pressure may be considered, particularly in neuromuscular diseases.[43-45] Mask ventilation in young children requires very special expertise that is available in few locations.

Stable ventilation parameters should be established as soon as possible. Ventilation rates are likely to be lower than expected due to lower metabolic demand. Hypocapnia may be difficult to readjust if children become accustomed to the comfort and sensation of low PCO_2. Ventilation demands and techniques will differ greatly according to the diagnosis and age of the child.

Ventilators used in these situations should be electronically driven, reliable, light and portable; they must incorporate alarms and backup battery power.[46,47] Larger tidal volumes with a leak around the tracheostomy are used to facilitate talking. A speaking valve can be added and most children learn to talk during the inspiratory phase of the ventilator. The Life Care PLV and LP series are examples of such ventilators. Disconnection and high pressure alarms are mandatory. It is also essential to have a self-inflating resuscitator available for emergency ventilation and portable suction apparatus. We have not used positive end expiratory pressure in these patients.

Other needs include humidification, replacement tracheostomy tubes and suction catheters. For humidification, heat and moisture exchangers are usually adequate and aid mobility.[13] If oxygen is required (usually for intercurrent illness) an oxygen concentrator is best.[48,49] The equipment required for home care should be established and acquired early, even while in the intensive care unit. Different setups can be trialled and stable ventilation established on a portable ventilator with satisfactory sleep physiology studies before moving to the ward. A backup ventilator must be available to cover servicing or malfunction.

Electrophrenic pacing has been used in few Australian patients. Experience over 30 years and current indications have been recently reviewed by Fodstad.[50] It is most effective for disorders of respiratory control or cervical medical lesions above the phrenic nerve cell bodies. It is not appropriate in respiratory muscle paralysis or secondary phrenic nerve damage. Even though the absence of a ventilator may improve body image, pacing requires the same care and supervision as mechanical ventilation. It costs about AUD 50 000 and is no cheaper than two ventilators. Pacing does not usually allow closure of the tracheostomy, as there is poor coordination between the paced diaphragm and upper thoracic muscles; decannulation in high quadriplegia is rarely successful.[51] It may allow greater mobility for children needing some ventilatory support during the day, e.g. those with congenital central hypoventilation.[31] If pacing is to be used, conditioning the diaphragm can occur within weeks if the diaphragm is still active. It may take more than a year to condition diaphragm muscles which have not been used, e.g. after long term mechanical ventilation.

Establishment of discharge focused rehabilitation

1. A primary nurse should be appointed within the ICU staff as the main coordinator of management. This provides continuity in communication with child, family, and ICU staff and with the home ventilation programme.
2. Early attempts should be made to normalise as many activities and routines as possible. Early involvement of occupational therapists,[52] ward teachers, play therapists, and volunteers, e.g. "ward grannies", can establish a daily routine into which the nursing care and monitoring should fit. A portable ventilator should be acquired as soon as possible so that the child can leave the ICU for short periods. Strenuous efforts should be made to allow the child to attend the hospital child care centre, preschool or school.
3. In order to "deintensify" the care of the child, laboratory or radiological investigations should be minimised as well as monitoring and observations. Invasive blood gas monitoring is not needed; end tidal CO_2 and pulse oximetry measurements and an apnoea alarm in younger children are adequate once stability is achieved. The scaling down of monitoring may cause some ICU staff philosophical difficulties.
4. Equipment acquisition is one of the barriers to the achievement and the speed of discharge to the "step down" ward. Spinal injury has extensive

nursing and resource demands, including the need to purchase a wheelchair capable of accommodating a portable ventilator.[33,34,53] Funding for compensatable injury must be sought early. Non-funded patients impose a major burden on hospital budgets or community schemes. Administrators and lawyers must be invited to an early case conference to discuss requirements and funding. These needs, although uncommon, are predictable and past experience should avoid the tendency to "reinvent the wheel". In individual cases, local ingenuity and collaboration are beneficial.[12] Consultation with regional, national or international home ventilation programmes is advisable. Home management will require a local discharge liaison coordinator, home nursing and respite services. Paediatric home care programmes exist in a few centres.[54] Coordination will use local rehabilitation, respiratory and spinal units, biomedical, orthotic, and computer engineers. Other patient support organisations may also be able to provide invaluable experience, information, and resources.

5. It is crucial to encourage early involvement of parents and other home carers. Regular case conferences are essential and should include parents, the child's general paediatrician, and family doctor.[27] Parents and carers should be encouraged to be actively involved in all aspects of the child's care. Training in respiratory care, including suction and tracheostomy tube change, should be provided.

6. Active planning for a move to a ward or to another step down facility in preparation for home care occurs as soon as the need for long term ventilation is confirmed. The child is essentially not ill and requires normal family interaction and physical and psychological development opportunities as soon as possible in an environment very similar to that which will be present at home.

7. Consultation with experienced home ventilation programmes and one or two visits by them to consult with family and staff may be invaluable to confirm that their experiences are "usual" and that the care is appropriate.

Pressure of acute admissions

By 1980, in one paediatric intensive care unit in the United States, 50% of the beds were occupied by patients who were receiving long term ventilator support.[7] This has important resource implications where there is a high demand for acute intensive care beds. It also highlights that the intensive care unit is not the ideal environment for the child with a chronic condition. Parents witness that once the acute phase is over, all the action and "fuss" is around high priority acute admissions. Other children come and go while their child stays; some children die. The unit's activity continues while their child may appear to lose status and priority. The emphasis should therefore be on early discharge to a ward as a step to home.

Essentials of a home programme

Discharge from the intensive care unit

The ideal transfer from the intensive care unit depends on commitment from the receiving ward, explicit and detailed planning with sensitive and thorough handover of nursing care. There is seldom a tailormade step down ward or other acute rehabilitation service in a hospital which can cope with ventilation. A finite date for transfer should be set, resisting the urgency created by acute pressure on beds. The ventilated patient has no alternative to intensive care until the patient, family, and ward are appropriately prepared and must not have "second class priority" for an ICU bed. Staff from the receiving ward, particularly a new primary nurse, should work in the ICU to establish a relationship with the child and family and become familiar with care procedures and equipment. Even though hospital policies for ventilator care may demand 1:1 staffing, in this context it is not essential or practical. Ventilator dependent spinal cord injury is the most nurse dependent diagnostic group, greater than almost all other patients with similar length of stay.[55]

The child should also be prepared by visiting the ward and, if possible, by attending the hospital child care centre, preschool or school. Staffing and lines of responsibility must be clarified to guarantee that the child is safely transferred between the ward and school. In young children, needing ventilation when asleep, the usual daytime sleep must be arranged and supervised.

Definitive preparation of carers

The techniques of care are readily learned by ward staff and parents and other carers. Two family members living with the child must become competent in care. By the time discharge is looming, the parents will, and should, be more expert than many of the nurses. Indeed, frustration with rotating and relieving nurses who are not familiar with the child, but who find it hard to surrender authority and decisions to a parent, is a source of stress for the family. Nurses who are to be involved in home care should be engaged, trained, and provide care in hospital prior to discharge. This is easier with insurance compensation as a private nursing agency can be contracted. A coordinating nurse should be elected. As such children are relatively uncommon, agencies experienced in home ventilation should be given preference as they have the advantages of continuing staff education, coordination, and a pool of experienced nurses. There should be regular meetings for the home nurses (whose shifts do not overlap) and occasional reviews with the home ventilation team. This may require strong representation to insurers who may wish to engage a cheaper but less experienced agency; in our experience they do not last the course.

The debate and decision about whether nurses or trained carers should be engaged wholly or partly are the source of much emotion, professional competition, and costly court decisions. Nurses are extensively trained in specific and general needs of paediatric patients and are professionally accredited, accountable, and indemnified. As parents will provide some (or most) of the care, other "lay" carers can be trained to do the same. However, if lay carers are used they must be thoroughly trained, skills must be maintained, and they themselves must have good practical and emotional support. In our estimation, attendant care is only half the cost of that provided by full time registered nurses.[5]

Though all funding systems try to argue against expensive nurse care, there are no "controlled trials" of care and it must be evaluated for each patient and family. Some literature[3] suggests that care of ventilated children by lay carers may be equal or superior to nurses only when they are relatives or close friends of the child and family, presumably with added commitment and understanding. Not all families want full time nursing, even in ventilator dependent quadriplegia. Most want some relief from the invasion of privacy. If nurses are employed, hours of nurse care may diminish over time, though this may need to increase at times of intercurrent illness to avoid readmission.[56] Family stress is less if nurses rather than lay carers provide care.[57] Whoever provides care, there must be flexibility in staffing and funding to allow additional support during family illness and other life disruptions.

Discharge to home

Before discharge, the parents and nurses must have experienced totally independent care, mirroring the home situation as far as possible.[33] They must demonstrate that they can care for the child, never leaving the child unattended, that all routine and emergency care is given effectively, and that they are familiar with all the technology used. They must respond appropriately to emergencies, including "planned sabotage", and demonstrate that they can follow telephone instructions.[58] Individual knowledge and instruction programmes can be evaluated before discharge.[59] Close observation in the hospital setting then leads into day passes and overnight stays at home, initially accompanied by one of the discharge team and home nurses, extending the number of nights until the child and family are ready to go home. Appropriate community agencies and services must be prepared and the family must be guaranteed 24 hour telephone advice and readmission for review or respite.

Technical support is essential in evaluating, servicing, and checking the safety of equipment in the home, especially electrical and oxygen safety.[60] Backup equipment must be obtained for home and for school, particularly suction and hand ventilation apparatus.

Coordinating community supports

During these home trials, probably over a week or two, a case conference should be held (possibly at home) with all the relevant community support agencies, especially the family doctor, local paediatrician, home nursing staff, respite care staff, and school staff.[56] It is particularly important to engage the child in specialised or regular day care, preschool or school and to prepare, equip, and support those settings adequately.[61-63] It is our experience that most ventilator dependent children can attend mainstream school with appropriate nursing and care support. This may necessitate building modifications to facilitate access.

Community agencies must be informed; power and telephone utilities need to be unequivocally committed to maintaining support in emergencies, correcting problems urgently and, hopefully, rebating costs of services. The family and all involved must have comprehensive, updated lists of personnel, agencies involved, their roles, and how they can be contacted. Current information about the child's clinical status and care needs and about home ventilation in general should be available to the nurses and all other groups involved.

Resuscitation

The excitement and fulfilment of going home feels such a victory that it is difficult to discuss attitudes to and procedures for future resuscitation. In our experience, even years later, this discussion is painful for families, reminding them of the acute decisions when long term ventilation was first decided upon. However, this is essential for the family, carers, and all agencies in routine contact with the child and particularly for unfamiliar clinicians with whom the family may have to deal at times, such as holidays, staying with relatives, and school camps. These issues should be discussed before discharge and perhaps one or two specifically planned. For camps and holidays, local medical care, e.g. paediatricians and hospitals, should be alerted and given a clinical summary, including instructions regarding resuscitation.

Long term follow up

Ideal management involves the home ventilation team in regular home visits in the first instance and comprehensive annual reviews. Once routines of care are established, parents need easy contact for advice, with visits on request rather than at fixed intervals. Frequency of visits for equipment support, e.g. circuit changes, depends on family competence and preference. There should be at least an annual reassessment of the patient involving multispecialty clinical review, revision of care techniques and equipment, review of family and carer stress, and support and inservice training for carers and nurses. Adolescents need to become responsible for directing their own care and aware of the implications of their disability. Transfer to adult care is a particular challenge for individuals who do not receive compensation and where there is a lack of coordinated home support programmes.

Ventilator dependent individuals, clinicians, equipment suppliers, and support organisations meet at international conferences on home ventilation, held every two years in Denver, Colorado, or Lyons, France.

The future

Short term mortality and morbidity

If the child is clinically stable and well on discharge, the risk of short term major complications or of death is low. Most at risk are infants with bronchopulmonary dysplasia, particularly during infections such as pertussis and influenza. Children with high cervical cord injury who lack any life sustaining respiratory effort, e.g. accessory muscle ventilation, are also at higher risk. Pooled statistics over two decades for all ages suggest 40% mortality (usually due to respiratory infection) for ventilated spinal cord injury victims in the first year. Children probably fare much better.[64,65] Readmission is uncommon except for about one admission a year for reassessment, such as sleep studies; half may have no admissions.[67,71] A home care team, particularly those using registered nurses, can usually manage the child through intercurrent infections, thereby avoiding admission.

Effects on family

Home ventilation is an enormous and unique challenge. The effects in any one family are not predictable. All parents are assumed to be totally committed to their child, but must be allowed to decide for themselves if they can face the demands of home care. All parents and patients continue in one way or another to hope for a miracle. Reports of surgical and medical research to correct cervical cord injury continue to raise hopes. There are a few questionnaire studies of family realities but none of direct observation. In a survey of children in our programme, parents nearly all felt pleased their child was at home and maintained directly by their efforts.[71]

Families say that the main burden of home ventilation is the precision, meticulous detail, and constancy of care.[25] Some see family coping declining with time, "purchasing" stability at the expense of the primary carers. Family costs include personal demands, anxiety, financial burdens of equipment, and restrictions on employment and promotion. Families' perceptions of stress and their general coping skills are major determinants of stress, rather than the severity or prognosis or hours on the ventilator.[69] In 48 families, 25% of whom were on ventilation, Patterson[70] found that protection against family stress included more structure and control of family functioning and more community supports. There was less family strain if carers were professional nurses rather than parents or lay home carers.

Parental illness increased with added financial burden, less care hours from nurses, and degree of technology dependence. Families all have concerns about "problems with the system" providing the what, who, and when of their needs. Uncertainty about the continuity of support is strong, particularly with respect to public health services. There are also concerns about compensation and legal systems changing rules and procedures and that lump sums granted may not last throughout the patient's life. In one study,[19] 40% of families discharged on ventilation (most having bronchopulmonary dysplasia) had no case manager, 20% depended on their physician, and only 20% had some arranged psychosocial support.

Parents' main concerns for the child are maintenance of good health, developmental outcomes, and lifetime financial support. Home care involves invasion of privacy, with some tension regarding the competence and authority of the parents and the carers. Parents may exhibit frustration with the health professionals' apparent lack of expertise with their child and lack of continuity. Care becomes very mundane and long term continuity of care demands special commitment to the child and family. The intimacy, chronicity and routines of care may put some pressure on professional attitudes, with a real or perceived conflict between carers as professional partners or "multiple mothers". The authority and culture of the family must be respected, the child's developmental needs and progress must be acknowledged, and increasing autonomy encouraged through adolescence. Many of these issues need regular discussion and urgent action on problems; they benefit from long term social work support and other guidance, e.g. from adolescent workers. Transfer to adult care usually involves the loss of intimate, intense collaboration between child, family, and paediatric home care team. Adult support services may not have equivalent coordinated programmes, ethos and funding.

Judgment of quality of life

Assessments by the family and patient of their life situation are usually more optimistic than the professionals would suspect. We and others show that ratings of functional status and personal adjustment are often close to normal range.[19,71,72,73,75] Studies are usually retrospective and of small numbers, though Fleming[74] interviewed 91 ventilated individuals aged less than 19 years among 848 cervical cord injury victims.

Long term survival

Long term outcome depends more on associated disabilities than the need for ventilation, which is relatively straightforward. Estimates of longevity are crucial in compensation settlements, such as cervical cord injury.[64,65,66] There is a risk of unexplained sudden death,[3] a small risk of accidental disconnection, and well publicised but uncommon cases of suicide. Estimates for quadriplegia not requiring ventilation suggest a loss of life expectancy of 10–20%. Statistics from North America suggest that after a 25% first year mortality, survival in ventilator dependent quadriplegia is up to 20 years.[65] For children now entering a life of long term ventilation, improving techniques of care, personal vocational and social opportunity, and fulfilment may extend these estimates.

107

Ethics

Ethical perspectives on home ventilation pervade every action and decision in management[72,73] and are discussed throughout this chapter. Choices about available resources and cost benefit to the individual and society will become sharper as technology gives children and young adults increasing access to recreational activities and employment, with promise of a fulfilling life within the limits of their disability. Increased survival and costs of technology and labour and general pressures on health funding are on a collision course. Any decision as to whether to continue long term ventilation should acknowledge the phenomenon of "entrapment". Decisions should not be driven by the relentless processes of resuscitation and intensive care. Control has to be regained by the child, the relatives, and the health professions involved. "It requires courage to admit futility and to realise that just because the treatment has started and is 'working' it does not of necessity have to be continued."[22]

If a decision is made to initiate longer term ventilation, the essential issue is that a society that actively supports (and sometimes enforces) such decisions must then provide adequate, flexible and reliable funding and resources to maximise quality of outcome.

Summary

Long term home ventilation demands an approach to optimum care which is creative, constructive, persistent, and optimistic. Practical, personal, professional, and ethical challenges are complex and demand some compromise. Safe and effective care demands proper patient selection and exemplary preparation of, and collaboration between, parents and all others caring for the child. Experience clearly demonstrates that children and adolescents should be discharged as soon as possible from the acute care setting into an active rehabilitation programme where families can achieve home support and community living.

Acknowledgments

We are grateful to the staff of the home ventilation programme for their help in the preparation of this review, particularly Catherine Lockwood, Roger Hall and their predecessors, and to our secretaries, Marina Giokas and Chris Fuller. Above all, we acknowledge the children and parents who have taught us so much about humanity, dignity, resourcefulness, and heroism.

1 Burr BH, Guyer B, Todres ID, *et al.* Home care for children on respirators. *N Engl J Med* 1983;**309**:1319–23.
2 Goldberg AI, Faure EA, Vaughn CJ, *et al.* Home care for life-supported persons: an approach to program development. *J Pediatr* 1984;**104**:785–95.
3 Frates RC, Splaingard ML, Smith EO, Harrison GM. Outcome of home mechanical ventilation in children. *J Pediatr* 1985;**106**:850–6.
4 Gillis J, Tibballs J, McEniery J, *et al.* Ventilator-dependent children. *Med J Aust* 1989; **150**:10–14.
5 Health Care Committee. *Home mechanical ventilation for children and young adults.* Canberra: National Health and Medical Research Council, 1994.
6 European Respiratory Society Executive Committee. Recommendations for home mechanical ventilation. *Eur Resp Rev* 1992;**2**:303–442.
7 Schreiner MS, Donar ME, Kettrick RG. Pediatric home mechanical ventilation. *Pediatr Clin North Am* 1987;**34**:47–60.
8 Eigen H, Zander J. Home mechanical ventilation of pediatric patients. *Am Rev Resp Dis* 1990;**141**:258–9.
9 Howard P. Home mechanical ventilation and respiratory care in the United Kingdom. *Eur Resp Rev* 1992;**10**:416–7.
10 Goldberg AI. Home mechanical ventilation – the free market system (USA). *Eur Resp Rev* 1992;**10**:422–5.
11 Keens TG, Davidson Ward SL. Ventilatory treatment at home. In: Beckerman RC, Brouillette RT, Hunt CE, eds, *Respiratory control disorders in infants and children.* Baltimore: Williams and Wilkins, 1982:371–85.
12 Robinson RO. Ventilator dependency in the United Kingdom. *Arch Dis Child* 1990;**65**: 1235–6.
13 Kinnear WJM. *Assisted ventilation at home. A practical guide.* Oxford: Oxford University Press, 1994.
14 Task Force on Long-term Health Care Policy. Report to Congress and the Secretary by the task force on technology dependent children. Washington: Government Printing Office, 1988.
15 Oates RK. Challenge for child health in Australia. *Arch Dis Child* 1992;**67**:1406–9.
16 Health Care Committee. Ethics of limiting life-sustaining treatment. Canberra: National Health and Medical Research Council, 1988.
17 Palfrey JS, Walker DK, Haynie M, *et al.* Technology's children: report of a statewide census of children dependent on medical supports. *Paediatrics* 1991;**87**:611–8.
18 Ad Hoc Task Forces on Home Care of Chronically Ill Infants and Children, American Academy of Pediatrics guidelines for home care of infants, children and adolescents *Paediatrics* 1984;**74**:434–6.
19 Aday LA, Wegener DH, Andersen R, *et al.* Home care for ventilator assisted children. *Health Affairs* 1989;**8**:137–47.
20 Australian Quadriplegic Association. Survey of home ventilation needs in New South Wales and ACT. Sydney: AQA, 1993.
21 Springgay, M. *Draft report: coordination of services to longterm ventilation dependent patients.* South Australian Health Commission Statewide Services Division, 1990.
22 Gillis J, Kilham H. Entrapment. *Crit Care Med* 1990;**18**:897.
23 Gilgoff I, Prentice W, Baydur A, *et al.* Patient and family participation in the management of respiratory failure in Duchenne's muscular dystrophy. *Chest* 1989;**95**:519–24.
24 Miller JR, Colbert AP, Schock NC. Ventilator use in progressive muscular diseases: impact on patients and their families. *Dev Med Child Neurol* 1988;**30**:200–7.
25 Miller JR, Colbert AP, Osberg JS. Ventilator dependency: decision making, daily functioning and quality of life for patients with Duchenne muscular dystrophy. *Dev Med Child Neurol* 1990;**32**:1078–86.
26 Patterson DR, Miller-Perrin C, McCormick TR, *et al.* When life support is questioned early in the care of patients with cervical-level quadriplegia. *N Engl J Med* 1993;**328**: 506–9. (Reply by Ross LF *et al.* **329**:663–4.)
27 Frader J. Perilous life-sustaining therapy and the primary care physician: should the buck stop here? *Clin Pediatr* 1994;**33**:185–188.

109

28 Torda TA, Gerber P. To resuscitate or not, that is the question. *Med J Aust* 1989;**151**: 243–5.

29 Gardner BP, Theocleous F, Watt JWH, *et al*. Ventilation or dignified death for patients with high tetraplegia. *Br Med J* 1985;**291**:1620–2.

30 Purtillo RB. Ethical issues in the treatment of chronic ventilator dependent patients. *Arch Phys Med Rehab* 1986;**67**:718–21.

31 Weese-Mayer DE, Brouillette RT, Hunt CE *et al*. Pediatric diaphragm pacing in infants and children. *J Pediatr* 1992;**120**:1–8.

32 Marcus CI, Jansen MI, Poulsen MD, *et al*. Medical and psychosocial outcome of children with congenital central hypoventilation syndrome. *J Pediatr* 1991;**119**:888–95.

33 Miller MD, Steele NF, Nadell JM, *et al*. Ventilator assisted youth: appraisal and nursing care. *J Neurosci Nurs* 1993;**25**:287–95.

34 Stern LM, Campbell DA, Hartley EM *et al*. High cervical cord injury: medical, nursing and psychosocial aspects of rehabilitation. *J Paediatr Child Health* 1992;**28**:244–8.

35 Plummer AL, O'Donohue WJ, Petty TL. Consensus conference on problems in home mechanical ventilation. *Am Rev Respir Dis* 1989;**140**:555–60.

36 DeWitt PK, Jansen MT, Davidson Ward SL, Keens TG. Obstacles to discharge of ventilator assisted children from the hospital to home. *Chest* 1993;**103**:1560–5.

37 Goldberg AI. Home health care for children assisted by mechanical ventilation: the physician's perspective. *J Pediatr* 1989;**117**:378–83.

38 Australian Association of Paediatric Teaching Centres. *Technology dependent children: a discussion paper*. AAPTC, 1991.

39 King NMP, Cross AW. Children as decision makers; guidelines for pediatricians. *J Pediatr* 1989;**115**:10–16.

40 Leikin S. A proposal concerning decisions to forgo life-sustaining treatment for young people. *J Pediatr* 1989;**115**:17–22.

41 Newton-John H. Longterm mechanical ventilation of patients in Australia. *Med J Aust* 1989;**150**:3–6.

42 Simson Nelson V, Carrol JC, Hurvitz, EA. Home mechanical ventilation in children: parameters of change in 15 years of experience. *Dev Med Child Neurol* 1994;**36**:supplement 70.

43 Bach JR, Saporito LR. Indications and criteria for decannulation and transition from invasive to non-invasive long-term ventilatory support. *Resp Care* 1994;**39**:515–31.

44 Piper AJ, Parker S, Torzillo PJ, *et al*. Nocturnal nasal patients with cystic fibrosis and hypercapnic respiratory failure. *Chest* 1992;**102**:846–50.

45 Heckmatt JZ, Loh L, Dubowitz V. Nocturnal hypoventilation in children with nonprogressive neuromuscular disease. *Paediatrics* 1989;**83**:250–5.

46 Muir JF. Home mechanical ventilation. *Eur Respir Buyers* 1995;**1**:7–12.

47 Muir JF. Home mechanical ventilation. *Thorax* 1993;**48**:1264–73.

48 Fauroux B, Desguerre I. Home oxygen therapy equipment and mechanical ventilators for children. *Eur Respir Buyers* 1995;**1**:13–19.

49 Masters IB, Asher MI. Domiciliary oxygen therapy in children: position paper of Thoracic Society of Australia and New Zealand. *J Paediatr Child Health* 1993;**29**:259–62.

50 Fodstad, H. Phrenico-diaphragmatic pacing. In: Roussos C, Clenfant C, eds, *The thorax*. New York: Dekker, 1995:2597–617.

51 Carter RE. Experience with ventilator dependent patients. *Paraplegia* 1993;**31**:150–3.

52 Young H, Cocks N. The ventilator dependent spinal injured child; a new challenge for occupational therapists. *Aust Occup Ther* 1991;**38**:101–3.

53 Flett PJ. The rehabilitation of children with spinal cord injury. *J Paediatr Child Health* 1992;**28**:141–6.

54 Tatman MA, Woodroffe C. Paediatric home care in the United Kingdom. *Arch Dis Child* 1993;**69**:677–80.

55 Richmond TS, Metcalf J, Daly M. Requirements for nursing care services and associated costs in acute spinal cord injury. *J Neurosci Nurs* 1995;**27**:47–52.

56 Fields M, Rosenblatt A, Pollack M, *et al*. Home care cost effectiveness for respiratory technology dependent children. *Am J Dis Child* 1991;**145**:729–33.

57 Wegener DH, Aday LA. Home care for ventilator-assisted children: predicting family stress. *Pediatr Nurs* 1989;**15**:371–6.
58 Steele NF, Morgan J. Emergency preparations for technology assisted children. *J Pediatr Nurs* 1989;**4**:81–7.
59 Burke SA, Zarafu I, Santos AM. Family education and teaching program: transitioning care from hospital to home for technology dependent children. *Dev Med Child Neurol* 1995;**37**: supplement 73, 4556.
60 Goldberg AI. Technology assessment and support of life-sustaining devices in home care. The home care physician's perspective. *Chest* 1994;**105**:1448–53.
61 Stutts AL. Selected outcomes of technology dependent children receiving home care and prescribed child care services. *Pediatr Nurs* 1994;**20**:501–6.
62 Delaney N , Zolondick K. Day care for technology dependent infants and children: a new alternative. *J Perinatal Neonat Nurs* 1991;**5**:80–5.
63 Walker P. Where there is a way, there is not always a will: technology, public policy and the school integration of children who are technology assisted. *Child Health Care* 1991; **20**:68–74.
64 DeVivo MJ, Stover SL. Longterm survival and causes of death in spinal cord injury. In: Stover SL, DeLisa JA, Whiteneck GG, eds, *Clinical outcomes from model systems*. Maryland: Aspen, 1995.
65 DeVivo MJ, Ivie CS. Life expectancy of ventilator dependent persons with spinal cord injury. *Chest* 1995;**108**:226–32.
66 Sneddon DG, Bedbrook G. Survival following traumatic tetraplegia 1982. *Paraplegia* 1982;**20**:201–7.
67 Canlas Yamsuan M, Sanchez I, Kesselman M, *et al.* Morbidity and mortality patterns of ventilator dependent children in a home care program. *Clin Pediatr* 1993;**32**:706–13.
68 Quint RD, Chesterman E, Crain LS, *et al.* Home care for ventilator dependent children. *Am J Dis Child* 1990;**144**:1238–41.
69 Keens SE, Jansen MT, Lipsker LE, *et al.* Coping resources to combat stress in parents caring for a ventilator assisted child at home. *Pediatr Res* 1990;**27**(4):11A.
70 Patterson JM, Leonard BJ, Titis JC. Home care for medically fragile children: impact on family health and wellbeing. *J Dev Behav Pediatr* 1992;**13**:248–55.
71 Fonseca K, Lockwood C, Hutchins P. Quality of outcome in home ventilated children and young adults. *J Paediatr Child Health* 1996;**32**(3):A27.
72 Orlowski JP. Ethical and quality of life issues in ventilator dependent children. *Clin Pediatr* 1993;**32**:714–7.
73 Farrel PM, Frost NC. Long-term mechanical ventilation in pediatric respiratory failure: medical and ethical considerations. *Am Rev Resp Dis* 1989;**140**:S36–40.
74 Fleming J, Challela M, Eland J, *et al.* Impact on the family of children who are technology dependent and cared for in the home. *Pediatr Nurs* 1994;**20**:379–88.
75 Baldwin-Myers AS, Oppenheimer EA. Quality of life and quality of care data from a 7-year pilot project for home ventilator patients. *J Ambulatory Care Manage* 1996;**19**(1): 46–59.

Useful Internet sites for professionals and patients

http:/www.eskimo.com/ ~ jlubin/disabled/vent/
http://www.theshop.net/kkulhman/resp.htm
http://www.aarc.org/cpgs/othefcpg.html

5: Management of paediatric trauma

NEIL T MATTHEWS

Care of the injured child requires an organised and coordinated approach by a team familiar with the management of this age group. Trauma clinicians need to appreciate the anatomical and physiological differences that predispose children to patterns of injury which differ from adults and be aware of paediatric pathophysiology that results from trauma.

Epidemiology and prevention strategies

Trauma is the leading cause of death in children, accounting for 50% of deaths from 1 to 14 years in the USA.[1] Because behaviour patterns are age related, causes of injury are most commonly falls, assaults, and foreign body aspirations in the younger age group and motor vehicle, pedestrian, and bicycle accidents in older children. These causes mainly lead to blunt injury of the central nervous system, thorax, abdomen, and/or musculoskeletal system, with head injuries accounting for 30% of fatalities.[2] Penetrating injury is uncommon.

In the past, little effort, money or research was directed at paediatric trauma. However, new emphasis has seen the development of prevention strategies, including:

- injury surveillance, prevention research, legislation, and public safety campaigns;
- education programmes directed at caregivers (Advanced Trauma Life Support, American College of Surgeons);
- nationally coordinated approaches to trauma care.

The importance of these initiatives has been demonstrated in Sweden where a significant reduction was achieved in childhood injury fatalities[3] by a long term approach over 25 years, involving research into injury surveillance and prevention, a broad based safety education campaign, and the production of safer environments through legislation and regulation. Reduction in mortality can be achieved by mandatory use of seat belt restraints in vehicles and wearing of helmets by cyclists.[4] Prevention strategies against common paediatric injuries are listed in table 5.1.

TABLE 5.1—*Prevention strategies*[38]

Paediatric injuries	Prevention strategies
MVA – occupant	Child car seat
	Seat belt restraint
MVA – pedestrian	Safety programmes in schools
Bicycle	Helmet
Drowning	Pool fencing
Burns	Smoke detectors
	Water tap regulator
	Flammable fabric legislation
Poisoning	Preventive packaging
Violence	Handgun legislation
	Crisis resolution counselling

Initial approach to management of the traumatised child

As with adults, there is a trimodal distribution of mortality in children.

1. Immediate death at the accident scene is due to airway obstruction, haemorrhage, and head or spinal injury. The majority of these patients are beyond salvage.
2. During the first hour or hours (the so-called "golden hour") at the time of stabilisation and transport, mortality and morbidity are caused by airway obstruction, aspiration, haemorrhage, and head injury. Appropriate care at this time may have a significant impact on outcome, especially with regard to airway and haemorrhage control in major head, chest, abdominal, and bony injury.
3. Mortality days to weeks later results from intensive care related complications such as respiratory distress syndrome, sepsis, and multisystem organ failure. Effective resuscitation in the early stages of injury may influence these delayed complications.

As mentioned previously, resuscitation requires an organised, coordinated, and informed team effort. Initially, the approach requires accurate appraisal of the patient's history, consideration of the events resulting in the injury, and rapid, repeated clinical assessment and management. It is important to understand that these steps must be

113

accomplished simultaneously and that responses should be quickly prioritised, with immediate attention to life threatening injuries. The Advanced Trauma Life Support (ATLS) programme of the American College of Surgeons[5] advocates a systematic approach to initial management based on five phases:

1. rapid primary evaluation (primary survey or ABCs);
2. resuscitation of vital functions;
3. a detailed secondary evaluation (secondary survey);
4. institution of definitive care;
5. triage.

Primary survey

The approach to initial care in the primary survey recognises the ABCs of resuscitation together with cervical spine stabilisation, haemorrhage control, neurological assessment, and complete examination of the patient by exposure. The aim of the primary survey is to identify life threatening injuries within minutes.

Airway

Airway maintenance and intubation require a special approach in children due to differences in anatomy. Children have:

- a relatively larger head with a prominent occiput;
- more pharyngeal soft tissue and a relatively larger tongue;
- a shorter neck with a larynx that is more superior and anterior;
- an epiglottis that is relatively large and has less cartilage;
- a subglottis that is the narrowest part of the airway (as opposed to the vocal cords in adults);
- a shorter trachea and smaller airways.

These differences are most marked in neonates and infants and make it more difficult to position the head, maintain the airway, visualise the larynx, and intubate. Children beyond the age of 4–5 years are usually easy to intubate. The structural differences described disappear by approximately 12 years of age.

Due to the risk of cervical spine injury, it must be assumed that the cervical spine is injured until proved otherwise and the head kept at all times in an in-line neutral position without traction. The airway should be first maintained by simple manoeuvres such as chin lift, jaw thrust and suction but if these fail, insertion of an oral or nasal airway or intubation may

114

be required. Surgical airways such as needle cricothyroidotomy, incisional cricothyroidotomy and tracheostomy are more difficult in children and are rarely indicated. Oxygen should be administered immediately in high concentration and later adjusted following pulse oximetry and/or blood gas analysis.

Breathing

Ventilation is assisted where necessary using a bag and mask device followed by intubation. In these situations, gastric distention is common and should be relieved as soon as possible with a gastric tube to minimise regurgitation and allow for easier ventilation. Indications for intubation in trauma are:

- Glasgow Coma Score less than 8;
- failure to maintain an airway, including facial injuries and burns;
- the need for airway protection from gastric contents or blood;
- ventilatory assistance which is required in the presence of hypoxaemia, central hypoventilation, treatment of raised intracranial pressure, seizures, and where anaesthesia is required for investigations (e.g. CT scan) or surgery;
- airway protection during transport.

Intubation is performed with the head maintained in a neutral position without traction by an assistant, using an endotracheal tube of size appropriate for age. It is easier with a straightbladed laryngoscope and a rapid sequence induction should be performed using a muscle relaxant and sedative. A common pitfall in children is incorrect placement of the endotracheal tube tip, either not being in far enough, leading to spontaneous extubation, or in too far with endobronchial intubation. Care must be taken by noting measured insertion of the tube at the lips or nose and confirming tip placement by x ray. The tube should be well secured to avoid accidental extubation.

Circulation

Haemorrhage is the commonest cause of shock in children. Circulation is assessed clinically by observation of:

- heart rate;
- blood pressure;

- respiratory rate (increased when compensating for metabolic acidosis);
- capillary refill (normal less than two seconds);
- conscious state;
- urine output (normal 1–2 ml/kg/h).

The initial response to hypovolaemia is tachycardia and blood pressure is well maintained until 25% of the circulating blood volume is lost. It is important to remember that heart rate, blood pressure, and respiratory rate vary normally with age and this should be taken into account during

TABLE 5.2—*Differences in heart rate (HR), systolic blood pressure (Sys BP), and respiratory rate (RR) with age*

Age	HR	Sys BP	RR
1 month	140	80	30
2 years	120	90	20
10 years	100	100	15

assessment (table 5.2). Obvious haemorrhage should be looked for and controlled, while volume loss is replaced with crystalloid, colloid and/or blood (depending on availability). Children lose large volumes from scalp lacerations and hidden losses occur in the chest, abdomen, pelvis, and retroperitoneum. Hypotension should be treated as hypovolaemia until proved otherwise – hypovolaemia is the cause of death in 30% of trauma patients.[6]

Access to the vascular space can be difficult in children, the options being percutaneous peripheral IV line, IV cutdown, central venous line, and intraosseous needle. Choice depends on the clinical state of the patient, equipment available, and expertise of the clinician. As soon as vascular access is achieved, blood must be taken for crossmatch. The intraosseous needle should not be underestimated as a method of fluid and drug administration and is the method of choice where peripheral access cannot be achieved within 90 s[7] (depending upon urgency). It provides easy vascular access and requires little expertise. The needle is best inserted on the flat medial aspect of the upper tibia 2 cm below the tibial tuberosity. Complications are few, but include compartment syndrome from inadvertent extraosseous tissue placement of the needle, osteomyelitis, cellulitis, and disruption of the tibial growth plate. The volume administered and rate of infusion depend on the degree of hypovolaemia (table 5.3). Hypovolaemia is initially treated with 20 ml/kg of fluid and repeated as necessary. Response to fluid is carefully monitored by frequent reassessment of vital signs. If the patient remains unstable, sites of ongoing haemorrhage should be sought.

116

TABLE 5.3—*Blood loss and clinical diagnosis of shock*

| | Blood volume loss | | |
	<25%	25–40%	>40%
Cardiac	Tachycardia	Tachycardia	Hypotension and bradycardia when terminal
Central nervous system	Lethargy, irritability, confusion, aggression	Reduced level of consciousness and response to pain	Comatose
Skin	Cool peripheries	Cyanosis, reduced capillary refill	Pale, cold
Renal	Reduced urine output	Low urine output	No urine output

Neurological deficit

Repeated neurological assessment is necessary to allow for early recognition of cardiovascular or intracranial pathology. Assessment of the central nervous system using the Glasgow Coma Scale can be difficult and intimidating to those not using it on a regular basis. A more simple approach from the ATLS, American College of Surgeons, relies on observing the pupil's responses to light and assessing the patient's level of consciousness using the AVPU mnemonic to grade response as (a) *a*lert, (b) responding to *v*ocal stimuli, (c) responding to *p*ainful stimuli or (d) *u*nresponsive.

Application of an ECG monitor is helpful but pulse oximetry and end tidal CO_2 (in the intubated patient) are more useful where available. Gastric distention is common in children and gastric decompression with a gastric tube aids ventilation while minimising aspiration of gastric contents. Nasal tubes, whether endotracheal or gastric, are contraindicated in the presence of basal skull fractures which should be suspected in the presence of CSF rhinorrhoea or otorrhoea, orbital haematomas, mastoid haematomas or blood in the external auditory meatus. Urinary catheters assist the assessment of urinary output but should not be passed via the urethra when urethral injury is suspected. Thermoregulation is important because children have a greater body surface area to weight ratio and have a tendency to hypothermia from heat loss, which is best avoided by warming IV fluids and using a warming blanket.

Secondary survey

The secondary survey comprises a thorough head to toe evaluation as soon as life threatening problems have been controlled and involves examination of the head, neck, chest, abdomen, and extremities. Radiology of the chest, abdomen and pelvis are best performed at this stage, while accurate documentation should be commenced as soon as possible. Following stabilisation, a more comprehensive management plan can be instituted, with consideration of the need for operative procedures, fracture stabilisation, analgesia, and referral to a tertiary institution.

Head injury

At least 80% of children dying from multiple trauma have significant head injuries, compared with 50% for adults.[8] The more compliant cranial vault is less protective and there is a larger head to body size ratio, providing more momentum and likelihood of injury.

Signs and symptoms of raised ICP in children are:

● depressed level of consciousness;
● changes in respiratory pattern, blood pressure, and pulse rate;
● full or bulging fontanelle (less than 18 months old);
● motor weakness;
● cranial nerve palsies;
● decorticate or decerebrate posturing;
● convulsions;
● vomiting;
● headache;
● increased head circumference (less than 18 months old);
● papilloedema.

As mentioned previously, assessment of neurological status using the Glasgow Coma Scale (GCS) can be difficult and this is especially the case for children, where scores tend to be more subjective. When using the original scale described for adults, children score differently because under 5 years of age they are unable to score normally for verbal and motor responses. Normal aggregate Glasgow Coma Scores for age are 9 at 6 months, 11 at 12 months, and 13–14 at 5 years. This has led to attempts to modify the scale by either changing the scoring assessment signs and maintaining the same potential score or reducing the total score by elimination of some response categories.[9] These methods have not been validated and do not allow for comparison of outcome data. An example of a commonly used scale which has been simply modified for infants is shown in table 5.4.

TABLE 5.4—*Glasgow Coma Scale*

Glasgow Coma Scale			Glasgow Coma Scale modified for infants		
Activity	Best response	Scale	Activity	Best response	Scale
Eye opening	Spontaneous	4	Eye opening	Spontaneous	4
	To speech	3		To speech	3
	To pain	2		To pain	2
	None	1		None	1
Verbal	Orientated	5	Verbal	Coos, babbles	5
	Confused	4		Irritable cries	4
	Inappropriate words	3		Cries to pain	3
	Non-specific sounds	2		Moans to pain	2
	None	1		None	1
Motor	Obeys commands	6	Motor	Spontaneous activity	6
	Localises pain	5		Withdraws to touch	5
	Withdraws to pain	4		Withdraws to pain	4
	Abnormal flexion	3		Flexion to pain	3
	Extensor response	2		Extension to pain	2
	None	1		None	1

Management of head injury

The aim of management is to maintain adequate cerebral blood flow, while preventing secondary ischaemic injury and herniation from raised intracranial pressure. Deterioration in level of consciousness and the appearance of signs of herniation must be rapidly recognised by continual and repeated reassessment. Attention to the ABCs of resuscitation, as previously described, is important. Hypotension is most likely due to blood loss (especially from scalp lacerations) and not brain injury. Hyperthermia should be avoided with the use of a servo controlled cooling blanket, while mild hypothermia (to 35°C) reduces cerebral oxygen consumption and may provide cerebral protection. Cerebral venous return should be optimised by neutral head positioning to prevent venous obstruction.

Posttraumatic seizures are more common under 2 years of age.[10] Seizures are treated initially with diazepam (0.2 mg/kg), followed by phenytoin (20 mg/kg IV) which causes less CNS depression than barbiturate or repeated benzodiazepine therapy and allows for continued neurological assessment. Seizures result in increased cerebral blood flow, but are difficult to monitor in the paralysed patient because systems for continuous

119

electroencephalographic monitoring are too complex to interpret at the bedside and provide limited information. Jugular venous oxygen saturation (SjO$_2$) can be continuously monitored via fibreoptic reflection oximetry and allows for identification of global cerebral hypoperfusion and ischaemia.[11] Technical difficulties, probably related to catheter position against venous endothelium, limit its use in paediatrics at the present time.

A cranial CT scan should be performed when the GCS is less than 13 and helps to:

- exclude surgically treatable lesions;
- assess the size of CSF spaces including the basal cisterns;
- detect herniation and shift;
- show the presence of hyperaemia, oedema, intracerebral haematomas, contusion, and fractures.

However, a normal CT scan does not exclude raised ICP and the following are poor signs:

- ablated basal cisterns and midline shift;
- reversal of grey/white differentiation;
- subdural haemorrhage (an indication of significant damage to underlying brain tissue).

Cranial ultrasound, where the fontanelle is open (i.e. the patient is less than 18 months old) is useful for serial assessment of ventricular size in the unstable patient.

Intracranial pressure (ICP)

The causes of raised ICP in childhood trauma are:

1. increased intracranial blood volume:
   - intracranial bleeding;
   - cerebral hyperaemia in the first 1–2 days post injury;[12]
   - increased cerebral blood flow from increased PaCO$_2$, decreased PaO$_2$ or convulsions;
2. cerebral oedema after day 2;[13]
3. hydrocephalus from subarachnoid haemorrhage.

The concern of persistently raised and uncompensated ICP is cerebral ischaemia and herniation which both result in neuronal death. Herniation can be cingulate, uncal (temporal lobe), cerebellar tonsillar, upward cerebellar (posterior fossa hypertension) or transcalvarian (through vault defects).

Measurement of ICP is indicated where intracranial hypertension has or is likely to develop (GCS 8 or less) or where signs are hidden by anaesthesia. There are several approaches to measuring ICP in children. Subdural catheters and intracranial transducers are widely used but require expertise for careful placement and interpretation. Subarachnoid bolts, such as the Richmond screw, fail at high pressures and need special threads to maintain stability in thin cranial vaults, which makes them difficult to insert under 12 months of age. Ventricular catheters allow estimation of compliance and removal of CSF to reduce ICP, but are difficult to insert when ventricles are small due to raised ICP and readings are difficult to interpret when ventricles collapse against the catheter lumen. Non-invasive applanation devices over the anterior fontanelle allow trending of pressure in neonates[14] but have not been well accepted. New strain gauge technology being developed will allow easier intracranial (including intracerebral) pressure measurement via thin, flexible probes.

The significance of elevated ICP is that outcome is poor when it remains above 40 mmHg.[15] However, it must be remembered that measured ICP does not reflect regional pressure and perfusion and maintenance of a normal ICP does not ensure a good outcome. Several mechanisms allow physiological compensation for increased intracranial contents in children:

- displacement of cerebrospinal fluid (CSF) to distensible spinal subarachnoid spaces;
- compression of the intracranial veins;
- increased CSF readsorption;
- reduced CSF production;
- stretching of dura, unfused skull bones, and skin when cranial sutures are not yet fused (i.e. less than 18 months old).

In the child under 18 months of age, gradual increase in intracranial volume is achieved without elevation of intracranial pressure by an increase in head circumference. Thus, measurement of head circumference is an important clinical sign, especially in the chronic evolution of subdural haemorrhage, because this compensation can delay recognition of clinical signs and diagnosis in the face of emerging pathology.

Reduction of raised ICP

Specific measures to reduce raised ICP include hyperventilation, osmotic and diuretic agents, sedation, muscle relaxation, meticulous nursing, controlled hypothermia (to 35°C), and surgical decompression in selected cases.

Hyperventilation lowers raised ICP acutely but when overdone, may result in cerebral ischaemia and $PaCO_2$ should be maintained between 35 and 40 mmHg. Care must be taken when weaning from hyperventilation to minimise rebound rises in ICP when $PaCO_2$ is allowed to return to normal.[16] Fluid restriction helps alleviate raised ICP provided circulating blood volume is maintained. Mannitol (0.25–0.5 g/kg IV over 20–30 min) reduces raised ICP by increasing the osmotic gradient across the intact blood–brain barrier and reducing cerebral oedema.[17] Its effects may also be due to reduced blood viscosity and induced cerebral vasoconstriction. Maintain serum osmolality below 315 mosm/l and the osmolar gap (the difference between measured osmolarity and calculated osmolality) at less than 20 mosm to avoid hyperosmolar states. Frusemide (1 mg/kg) reduces cerebral water and CSF production and can also be helpful. However, excessive diuretic therapy reduces circulating blood volume and compromises oxygen delivery. Initial results of surgical decompression and removal of brain tissue as a method of treating unremitting cerebral oedema from head trauma were not encouraging, but recent studies have shown improved results where the oedema is focal.[18]

There are implications for the maintenance of cerebral perfusion pressure (CPP) in children, which depends on the difference between mean arterial pressure and ICP when ICP is higher than central venous pressure (CVP). However, values vary with age and dependence on blood pressure is more important in the younger age group, because physiological systolic pressures are lower, being 85 mmHg at 6 months, 95 mmHg at 2 years, and 100 mmHg at 7 years.[19] In addition, normal ICP is lower in the younger age group,[20] being up to 5 mmHg at 2 years and up to 10 mmHg at 5 years. In the younger age groups relative hypotension can have a profound effect on CPP and outcome[21] and hypotension significantly affects cerebral blood flow. CPP should be maintained above 60 mmHg[22] with maintenance of an adequate blood volume and normal blood pressure with pressor agents if required.

Outcome of head injury

Despite comments that recovery of children is better than that of adults, outcome data are inconsistent and more information is required. Outcome has been shown to be better than for adults,[23] worse for those under 2 years of age,[24] and no different when comparing adults and children in blunt trauma.[25] During the acute phase of injury, it can be difficult to predict short and long term outcome. The presence or absence of somatosensory evoked potentials is a promising reliable predictor of outcome in children.[26]

122

With regard to brain death, criteria for its diagnosis in the Australian and New Zealand Intensive Care Society statement on brain death are the same for adults and children.[27] However, the report recommends children under 2 months of age be given longer observation times, although the length of time is not stipulated. With any dying child, relatives must be allowed time to come to terms with the diagnosis and it is often helpful to have relatives watch the physical examination required for brain death. Clinicians have a responsibility to consider the possibility of organ donation whenever brain death criteria are met.

Thoracic trauma

Treatment of chest injuries is aimed at stabilising respiratory and cardiac function, remembering that hypoxia is the main threat to initial survival. In children, thoracic injuries are most commonly due to blunt trauma as opposed to penetrating trauma. Although the incidence is low in children the mortality is high[28] due to the association with high speed accidents and multiorgan injury. Because of the child's small size and more elastic chest wall, there is more transmission of kinetic energy to intrathoracic structures and a high incidence of pulmonary contusion without rib fractures or flail chest.

Life threatening injuries require immediate intervention. Upper airway obstruction results from loss of consciousness, blood, gastric contents, and direct airway trauma. Airway management as described above is extremely important. Tension pneumothorax is also life threatening and is clinically recognised by difficulty in oxygenation and ventilation, hypotension, and deviation of the trachea away from the affected side, with hyperinflation, hyperresonance, decreased chest movement, and reduced breath sounds on the same side. Treatment is commenced as soon as clinically recognised, by needle aspiration without waiting for radiological confirmation, and then insertion of an intercostal catheter or drain in the mid or anterior axillary line at the fifth intercostal space. Open pneumothorax occurs in the presence of any "sucking" chest wound, which should be sealed with an airtight dressing to minimise lung collapse. Flail chest is demonstrated by paradoxical chest wall movement and signifies severe underlying lung contusion; the need for intubation and ventilation should be anticipated. Pericardial tamponade results in hypotension, distended neck veins, and muffled heart sounds (Beck's triad) but needs to be differentiated from hypotension due to blood loss and tension pneumothorax before needle pericardiocentesis is performed. The pericardium can be decompressed by inserting a long needle from the xiphisternum angled to the tip of the left scapula and into the pericardial sac. Massive haemothorax causes hypotension, dullness to percussion, and decreased breath sounds and requires blood replacement and insertion of a chest drain. Should large blood losses from the chest drain continue (more than 40 ml/kg), surgical consultation and thoracostomy are necessary.

Potentially life threatening injuries are airway disruption, pulmonary contusion, ruptured aorta, diaphragmatic rupture, oesophageal perforation, and blunt cardiac injury. Airway disruption should be considered in the presence of extensive surgical emphysema and will be apparent when air continues to escape from a chest drain inserted for tension pneumothorax. Urgent bronchoscopy and surgical intervention are required in these situations. Pulmonary contusion causes difficulty in oxygenation and ventilation, while radiological changes may not be apparent for several hours and are indistinguishable from aspiration pneumonitis. Aortic rupture requires a high index of suspicion following any high speed accident and is suggested if chest radiology shows a widened mediastinum, fractures of the first and second ribs, left pleural cap, deviation of the trachea to the right, and obliteration of the aortic knuckle. It is important to avoid hypertension in these patients and aortography continues to be the investigation of choice for aortic rupture in children.[29]

Abdominal trauma

Abdominal trauma is usually due to blunt trauma in children and injuries are predominantly to liver and spleen. The abdominal wall and thoracic cage are more compliant and provide less protection to intraabdominal organs. Also, the liver and spleen are relatively large and more exposed below the rib cage and thus forces do not need to be excessive to cause rupture of either organ. Massive peritoneal or retroperitoneal haemorrhage, hollow viscus perforation, and renal tract injury also need to be recognised.

Abdominal trauma is more often managed conservatively in children,[30] especially with improvements in radiological imaging techniques. A conservative approach requires appropriate monitoring and supervision in a paediatric setting, with an awareness of the need for urgent surgical intervention and laparotomy. Indications for laparotomy are profound hypovolaemia, persistent haemorrhage (more than 40 ml/kg), penetrating injury, gastrointestinal perforation, signs of peritonism, increased intraabdominal pressure over 20 mmHg with renal impairment, and pancreatic injury. An abdominal CT scan with intraluminal and intravenous contrast aids this non-operative approach and allows for examination of solid organs and renal tract function and detection of intraperitoneal blood, free air, and pancreatic injury. Diagnostic peritoneal lavage is rarely indicated in children. It is performed when the source of apparent blood loss is undetermined or where a prolonged procedure or observation period is anticipated in a setting without CT scan assessment being available.

Spinal cord injury

The paediatric spine is more mobile and subject to stress. The cervical spine under 8 years of age has less muscular support, its ligaments and joint capsules are more flexible, and its facet joints more horizontal. The relatively large head mass increases momentum, with the fulcrum of mobility at C2–C3 as opposed to C4–C5 in the adult; thus paediatric cervical spine injuries tend to be above C4. However, the use of lap seat belts has led to an increase in lumbar spinal cord injury[31] with cord transection.

Clinical assessment of neurological deficits is difficult in the young child and requires careful observation. Interpretation of radiological investigations is complex because growth plates can mimic fractures, a degree of subluxation is normal, and spinal cord injury without obvious radiological abnormality (SCIWORA) is a recognised entity in children.[32] A high index of suspicion should be maintained at all times. Detection of abnormalities is improved when both plain radiological and CT scan examination are combined.[33] Sensory evoked potentials can also help diagnosis.

From the time of injury, the spine should be assumed to be unstable until proved otherwise and immobilised. High likelihood of spinal injury is suggested by the presence of:

- signs or symptoms suggesting neurological spinal deficit;
- a history of loss of consciousness;
- altered mental status;
- a history of a high speed accident or significant fall;
- significant head or chest trauma.

Spinal cord injury can then only be dismissed after repeated clinical and radiological assessment, which may include magnetic resonance imaging in the non-acute setting. However, delayed onset of spinal neurological signs has been reported in children[34] following initial normal examination.

Additional difficulty comes when deciding to which tertiary institute to transfer the child with a spinal injury, that is, to a paediatric intensive care unit or a specialised spinal unit. This decision ultimately will be determined by the age of the child and the stability of the spine. Infants should not be cared for in adult spinal units, whereas for older children expertise in spinal care may be more important. In the acute setting, a team approach is required between intensive care and spinal injury clinicians. Once spinal column stability and surgical fixation have been achieved, children with spinal cord injury are best cared for in paediatric intensive care facilities. Ongoing care is complex and requires a long term multidisciplinary approach.

Non-accidental injury

A high index of suspicion is needed to diagnose non-accidental injuries and abuse, which include physical assault, sexual abuse, emotional abuse, and neglect. From the history, suspicion should be raised when:

- the cause of the injury cannot be satisfactorily explained by the caregivers;
- there is discrepancy between the volunteered history and the sustained injury;
- there is a history of repeated injuries;
- it is alleged that the injury is self-sustained;
- there is a prolonged delay in seeking care.

Physical examination needs to be thorough with careful documentation. Patterns of injury from abuse include multiple bruises in differing stages of development and burns from forced immersion in hot water, with sparing of the groin area, and from cigarettes. Suspicion should be raised where head trauma is associated with retinal haemorrhages, subdural haematomas or skull fractures. Retinal haemorrhages are typical of head shaking, but may also be caused by cardiopulmonary resuscitation.[35] Whole body x ray screening and bone scan are required to detect multiple fractures in different stages of healing.

Non-accidental injury in children must be referred to a multidisciplinary team used to the diagnosis and care of these patients. An approach is required by a specialised child protection unit to deal with the medical and legal issues and the counselling of the family unit. Care and safety of other siblings and family members should be urgently evaluated.

Transport

Prehospital stabilisation and transport are best provided by teams based in tertiary paediatric intensive care units and staffed by medical and nursing staff who are subspecialists in paediatric critical care medicine.[36] Secondary insults occur more frequently when paediatric personnel are not used for transport.[37] However, both the referring and receiving clinicians share responsibility for patient transfer and telephone communication and advice are important components of patient stabilisation before the transport team arrives. In addition, local health care providers have a responsibility to maintain sufficient skills to adequately stabilise critically ill children. The paediatric retrieval service works best when regular educational outreach services provide close links between the tertiary centre and outlying hospitals.

Summary

Treatment of the injured child begins by recognising the differences required for management as compared to the adult. Caring for the critically ill traumatised paediatric patient requires unique expertise and can be a difficult and emotional experience. This is especially so when parents and/ or other siblings have been killed or severely injured in the same accident and cannot be with the child for support. In addition, a team approach with emotional support and counselling for health care professionals is an important component of care for the child.

1 Peclet MH, Newman KD, Eichelberger MR. Patterns of injury in children. *J Pediatr Surg* 1990;**25**:85–91.
2 Centers for Disease Control, Division of Injury Control, Center for Environmental Health and Injury Control. Childhood injuries in the United States. *Am J Dis Child* 1990;**144**: 627–46.
3 Bergman AB, Rivara FP. Sweden's experience in reducing childhood injuries. *Paediatrics* 1991;**88**:69–74.
4 MacKellar A. Deaths from injury in childhood in Western Australia, 1983–1992. *Med J Aust* 1995;**162**:238–42.
5 American College of Surgeons. *Advanced trauma life support program*. Chicago: American College of Surgeons, 1988.
6 Baker CC, Oppenheimer L, Stephens B. Epidemiology of trauma deaths. *Am J Surg* 1980;**140**:144.
7 Inaba AS, Seward PN. An approach to pediatric trauma. *Emerg Med Clin North Am* 1991; **9**:523–47.
8 Kissoon N, Dreyer J, Walia M. Pediatric trauma: differences in pathophysiology, injury patterns and treatment compared with adult trauma. *Can Med J* 1990;**142**:27–34.
9 Simpson D, Reilly P. Paediatric coma scale (letter). *Lancet* 1982;**2**:450.
10 Hahn YS, Chyung C, Barthel MJ, Bailes J, Flannery AM, McLone DG. Head injuries in children under 36 months of age. Demography and outcome. *Child's Nerv Syst* 1988;**4**: 34–40.
11 Dearden NM, Midgley S. Technical considerations in continuous jugular venous oxygen saturation measurement. *Acta Neurochir Suppl Wien* 1993;**59**:91–7.
12 Bruce DA, Alavi A, Bilaniuk L, Dolinskas C, Obrist W, Uzzell B. Diffuse cerebral swelling following head injuries in children: the syndrome of "malignant brain edema". *J Neurosurg* 1981;**54**:170–8.
13 Snoek JW, Minderhoud JM, Wilmink JT. Delayed deterioration following mild head injury in children. *Brain* 1984;**107**:15–36.
14 Colditz PB, Williams GL, Berry AB, Symonds PJ. Fontanelle pressure and cerebral perfusion pressure: continuous measurement in neonates. *Crit Care Med* 1988;**16**:876–9.
15 Longfitt TW, Gennarelli TA. Can the outcome from head injury be improved? *J Neurosurg* 1982;**56**:19–25.

16 Havill JH. Prolonged hyperventilation and intracranial pressure. *Crit Care Med* 1984;**12**: 72–4.
17 Stephenson HE, Safar P, Arfors KE, *et al.* Treatment potentials for reversing clinical death. *Crit Care Med* 1988;**16**:1034–42.
18 Katayama Y, Tsubokawa S, Miyazaki T, Kawamata T, Yoshino A. Oedema fluid formation within contused brain tissue as a cause of medically uncontrollable elevation of intracranial pressure: the role of surgical therapy. *Acta Neurochir Suppl* 1990;**51**:308–10.
19 Horan MJ. Report of the second task force on blood pressure in children. *Paediatrics* 1987;**79**:1–25.
20 Welch K. The intracranial pressure in infants. *J Neurosurg* 1980;**52**:693–9.
21 Raju TN, Vidyasagar D, Papazafiratou C. Cerebral perfusion pressure and abnormal intracranial waveforms: their relation to outcome in birth asphyxia. *Crit Care Med* 1981; **9**:449–53.
22 Chan KH, Dearden NM, Miller JD, Andrews PJ, Midgley S. Multimodality monitoring as a guide to treatment of intracranial hypertension after severe brain injury. *Neurosurgery* 1993;**32**:547–52.
23 Bruce DA, Raphaely RC, Goldberg AI, *et al.* Pathophysiology, treatment and outcome following severe head injury in children. *Child's Brain* 1979;**5**:174–91.
24 Mahoney WJ, D'Souza BJ, Haller JA, Rogers MC, Epstein MH, Freeman JM. Long-term outcome of children with severe head trauma and prolonged coma. *Paediatrics* 1983; **71**:756–62.
25 Eichelberger MR, Mangubat EA, Sacco WS, Bowman LM, Lowenstein AD. Comparative outcomes of children and adults suffering blunt trauma. *J Trauma* 1993;**28**:430–4.
26 Taylor MJ, Farell EJ. Comparison of the prognostic utility of VEPs and SEPs in comatose children. *Pediatr Neurol* 1989;**5**:145–50.
27 Australian and New Zealand Intensive Care Society. *Statement and guidelines on brain death and organ donation – 1993.* Melbourne: ANZICS, 1993.
28 Peclet MH, Newman KD, Eichelberger MR, *et al.* Thoracic trauma in children: an indicator of increased mortality. *J Pediatr Surg* 1990;**25**:961–6.
29 Spouge PE, Armstrong D. Traumatic aortic rupture in the pediatric population: role of plain films, CT and angiography in the diagnosis. *Pediatr Radiol* 1991;**21**:324–8.
30 Erin S, Shandling B, Simpson J, Stephens C. Nonoperative management of traumatised spleen in children. *J Pediatr Surg* 1978;**13**:117–9.
31 Newman KD, Bowman LM, Eichelberger MR. The lap belt complex: intestinal and lumbar spine injury in children. *J Trauma* 1990;**30**:1133–40.
32 Dickman CA, Rekate HL, Sonntag VKH, Zabramski JM. Pediatric spinal trauma: vertebral column and spinal cord injuries in children. *Pediatr Neurosci* 1989;**15**:237–56.
33 Borock EC, Gabram SGA, Jacobs LM, *et al.* A prospective analysis of a two-year experience using computed tomography as an adjunct for cervical spine clearance. *J Trauma* 1991; **31**:1001–6.
34 Pang D, Wilberger JE. Spinal cord injury without radiological abnormalities in children. *J Neurosurg* 1982;**57**:114–29.
35 Goetting MG, Sowa B. Retinal haemorrhage after cardiopulmonary resuscitation in children: an etiological re-evaluation. *Paediatrics* 1990;**89**:585–8.
36 Johnson CM, Gonyea MT. Transport of the critically ill child. *Mayo Clin Proc* 1993;**68**: 982–7.
37 McNab JM. Optimal escort for interhospital transport of pediatric emergencies. *J Trauma* 1991;**31**:205–9.
38 Stylianos S, Eichelberger MR. Pediatric trauma prevention strategies. *Pediatr Clin North Am* 1993;**40**:1359–68.

6: Acute brain insults in infants and children: management and outcome prediction

GEOFF KNIGHT, PAUL SWAN

Overview

Acute cerebral injuries are the major cause of death and disability in infants and children in Western societies. The effect of a child's death is devastating, not only to its family, but also to the community as a whole. Similarly, survival of a child with severe neurological handicap may be disastrous, as considerable emotional and financial burden is placed on both the family and the community to provide the required long term care. The challenge to the paediatric intensive care practitioner is, therefore, not only to develop therapies which improve the chances of survival and recovery to the preinjury state but also to minimise the risk of producing a severely brain damaged survivor who would otherwise have died. There is great interest in the development of treatments aimed at improving outcome from acute brain injury and in monitoring techniques that more accurately predict poor prognosis. Reliable prognostic tools may guide subsequent withdrawal of therapy.

The most common causes of acute cerebral insults can be prevented by appropriate public health measures in diverse areas. These measures include motor vehicle and road safety programmes, construction of swimming pool enclosures, and vaccination against some causes of meningitis. They involve community resources, education, appropriate legislation, and other public health initiatives. The major causes of acute brain insults in paediatric

TABLE 6.1—*Major causes of acute brain insults in infants and children*

1. Traumatic cerebral insults
   Concussive blunt trauma
   Penetrating injuries
   Crush injuries
   Non-accidental (child abuse)

2. Cerebrovascular insults
   Vascular malformations with spontaneous haemorrhage
   Thromboembolic events

3. Metabolic cerebral insults
   Hypoxic-ischaemic injury
      cardiac arrest
      immersion incidents
      near miss sudden infant death syndrome
      suffocation
      iatrogenic misadventure (e.g. accidental ventilator disconnection)
   Infection
      meningitis, encephalitis
      cerebral abscess
      cerebral effects of generalised sepsis
   Metabolic injury
      hypoglycaemia
      hypernatraemia
      hyponatraemia
      hyperosmolar states
      hypothermia
      hepatic encephalopathy
      Reye's syndrome
      haemolytic uraemic syndrome
      drug intoxication
      poisoning
      inborn errors of metabolism
   Status epilepticus

practice are shown in table 6.1. Near miss sudden infant death syndrome and non-accidental injury (child abuse) are the commonest causes in the first year, after the neonatal period. Immersion in swimming pools is the major cause of death in preschool infants in some warm climate countries. In general, however, traumatic injuries due to falls and motor vehicle, pedestrian or bicycle accidents are the most common cause of acute brain insults in children. In the following discussion of acute cerebral insults in children, the pathophysiology and intensive care management of traumatic brain injury will be dealt with in detail. The significant differences in those patients with other causes of brain insults will be highlighted.

Pathophysiology

A logical approach to the treatment of acute brain insults requires an understanding of the pathophysiology involved. The brain is a delicate organ which depends on structural integrity and precise metabolic control to maintain its complex voluntary and involuntary functions. Lost neurones are not replaced. Further, the paediatric brain is developing and any injury may interrupt this process and prevent milestones being reached at the anticipated age.

The injurious event may be regarded as causing the "primary injury". Subsequently, the brain may respond in a variety of ways leading to either recovery or amplification of the primary injury. This amplification process, the "secondary injury", may worsen outcome. It is extremely important to understand the nature of this secondary injury as it represents a potential opportunity for intervention. Such intervention would hopefully result in improved outcome.

Primary injury

Traumatic

Traumatic cerebral insults produce a variable combination of pathological events. The physical application of force is somewhat dissipated through the skull bone which protects the underlying brain. Whilst the thin, more cartilaginous skull of children under the age of 2 years may not fracture, it does provide less protection than the thicker skull of older children and adults. The injurious force causes sudden acceleration, then deceleration, of the soft brain, accompanied by shear stresses. This causes the physical disruption of neurones, supporting cells and cerebral vessels producing contusions, petechial haemorrhages and/or haemorrhagic collections in or around the brain. Neuronal tissue may be damaged immediately below the point of impact, along the path of the shear stresses, producing diffuse axonal injury, or on the opposite side of the head; this results in the so-called contre coup injury caused by the soft brain suddenly decelerating against the skull.

Following severe head injury, intracranial bleeding occurs in 20–25% of children. This incidence is low compared to the 40–50% incidence seen in adults. Subdural haematomas are most common and are generally associated with severe brain injury. Extradural haematomas and intracerebral collections are less common. Bleeding may produce an expanding mass causing progressive cortical, and ultimately brainstem, compression. Unless diagnosis and surgical evacuation are performed expeditiously death may result.

Metabolic

The brain is an obligate aerobic organ. It depends on a continuous supply of oxygenated blood and glucose to generate adenosine triphosphate (ATP) via glycolysis and the citric acid cycle. In health ATP is consumed in almost equal proportions by the processes that maintain cellular integrity and those that generate neuronal electrical signals. There are minimal brain stores of oxygen, glucose or ATP. Interruption of their supply therefore causes rapid development of lactic acidosis, accumulation of intracellular toxic metabolites, and failure of membrane pumps responsible for the maintenance of cellular integrity. This results in cell swelling and, ultimately, neuronal death. Metabolic insults are the end result of either failure of substrate delivery or failure of normal cellular activity. Examples of failed substrate delivery include arterial hypoxaemia, global or focal ischaemia, and hypoglycaemia. Cellular activity may fail because of the toxic effects of drugs, poisons, infection or other systemic metabolic diseases.

The underlying causes of metabolic injuries are listed in table 6.1. In addition to encephalopathies secondary to liver failure and deficiencies of substrate delivery, such as hypoxaemia and hypoglycaemia, there are also a number of primary metabolic disorders which can have a neurological presentation in childhood. Presenting problems include lethargy, vomiting, and acutely altered conscious state. Reye's syndrome is a rare disorder characterised by an acute encephalopathy following a short vomiting illness with associated abnormalities of liver function, hyperammonaemia, and often hypoglycaemia. The associated marked cerebral oedema can be life threatening. Many of the inherited disorders of metabolism, such as urea cycle defects and organic acidurias, can be suspected when encephalopathy is accompanied by hypoglycaemia, lactic acidosis or hyperammonaemia.

Hypoxic ischaemic encephalopathy

Profound hypoxic events in children are often due to immersion but can also occur secondary to head trauma or strangulation, during either an assault or a suicide attempt. Hypoxia interrupts the normal aerobic metabolic pathway to production of ATP. As has been discussed, ATP is essential for the maintenance of cellular membrane functions and much less is produced via anaerobic metabolism. Ischaemia adds to the cellular insult by further decreasing substrate delivery and allowing accumulation of cellular waste products such as lactic acid.

Secondary injury

There are a number of pathological changes which develop in the brain following the primary injury. These include altered cerebral metabolism and blood flow, cerebral oedema, and raised intracranial pressure. Each of these events may add a further hypoxic and/or ischaemic insult. Areas of marginal viability are then at risk of cell death or irreversible dysfunction.

Hypotension and hypoxaemia

Hypotension is very common following trauma (table 6.2), and may also occur in patients with bacterial meningitis associated with septic shock. It

TABLE 6.2—*Causes of hypotension following traumatic brain insults*

Hypovolaemia
    large bone fractures(femur/pelvis/tibia/humerus)
    liver/spleen/kidney laceration
    haemothorax
    lacerations, particularly scalp
    intracranial collection in infants
Pericardial tamponade
Tension pneumothorax
Myocardial injury
Loss of sympathetic tone (e.g. spinal cord or brainstem injury)
Acute gastric dilation

reduces cerebral perfusion pressure and is an extremely potent cause of further ischaemic injury. Raised intracranial pressure, when associated with hypotension, is more difficult to control than it is when the patient is normotensive. The presence of either hypoxaemia or hypotension at the time of admission increases the risk of death 2–3 times.

Altered coupling of cerebral metabolism and blood flow

The brain weighs 2–3% of body mass in the adult, yet it receives 15% of the cardiac output and accounts for 20% of total oxygen consumption and 25% of total resting glucose consumption. In the newborn, the brain weighs 10–12% of body weight and thus, at this age, consumes an even higher percentage of resting energy demands. Although the global oxygen consumption of the brain varies little in health, there are fluctuations in regional cerebral blood flow during changes in cerebral activity.

The normal cerebral metabolic rate of oxygen ($CMRO_2$) is 3.5 ml/min/100 g. However, this represents the "average" consumption by the brain. The $CMRO_2$ of grey matter areas, including the cortex and deep nuclei, is 50–100% higher, whilst white matter has a lower metabolic rate. $CMRO_2$

increases by 200% or more during seizures and by 10–13% per °C temperature rise in core body temperature. Hypothermia, on the other hand, reduces the rate 7% per °C. Following brain injury, the $CMRO_2$ falls roughly in proportion to the degree of coma; in deep coma and under barbiturate anaesthesia it reaches a nadir of approximately 50% of normal, equivalent to the energy requirements for basic cellular integrity. Cerebral blood flow (CBF) is governed according to Poiseuille's law:

$$CBF = (k \times CPP \times r^4)/8\,hl$$

where CPP is cerebral perfusion pressure (mean arterial pressure minus intracranial pressure), r is vessel radius, h is blood viscosity and l is vessel length. As can be seen, the vessel diameter is a major determinant of cerebral blood flow. In the healthy brain, fluctuations in CPP and/or viscosity are countered by alterations in vessel diameter at the arteriolar level. This process, termed autoregulation, allows a constant CBF to be maintained over a wide range of CPP. In health cerebral blood flow is tightly coupled to the brain's metabolic needs. Fluctuations in local metabolic requirements cause local vasodilation and increased regional cerebral blood flow. The factors which control this response are unclear but may involve release of adenosine, carbon dioxide or nitric oxide from metabolically active tissue. Following any acute brain injury, the above control mechanisms may be impaired or lost. Without autoregulation, cerebral blood flow becomes pressure dependent and may therefore fall to ischaemic levels even with mild hypotension. Conversely, hypertension may cause hyperaemia and increase the risk of oedema formation. As will be seen, various interventions utilised in the management of brain injury act by altering parameters of the above equation, in particular cerebral perfusion pressure, blood viscosity, and vessel diameter.

At a microscopic level, focal disturbances may occur after temporary interruption of blood flow. There may be occlusion of arterioles and venules by spasm or thrombus formation, endothelial swelling secondary to release of vasoactive substances including the products of arachidonic acid metabolism (leukotrienes, thromboxane) and/or impaired local nitric oxide production. This may result in occlusion of capillaries causing the "no reflow" phenomenon; ischaemia is subsequently perpetuated.

Cerebral oedema

Under normal conditions, intracellular water balance depends on maintenance of active transport membrane pumps. These force sodium and water out of the cell and balance the opposite tendency to follow concentration gradients into the cell. The extracellular interstitial space is controlled largely by the blood–brain barrier. This is created by tight junctions between blood vessel capillary endothelial cells. Lipid soluble molecules pass this barrier easily and large molecules, such as plasma proteins, do not enter the interstitial space. As there is no lymphatic system in the brain, interstitial fluid drains along the planes of white matter into the cerebral ventricles and returns to the circulation, along with cerebrospinal fluid, via the arachnoid granulations and the cerebral venous sinuses.

Three forms of cerebral oedema can develop:

1. Vasogenic oedema occurs secondary to disruption of the blood–brain barrier, allowing leakage of water soluble molecules and plasma protein into the interstitial space. This form of oedema is worsened by systemic hypertension and by conditions or drugs, in particular ketamine, which increase cerebral blood flow. Vasogenic oedema occurs in head trauma, following prolonged ischaemia, in acute central nervous system infections, and around certain inflammatory tumours. It can occur within hours of the primary injury.
2. Cytotoxic oedema occurs secondary to cellular metabolic failure. As membrane pumps fail, sodium and water pass down their concentration gradients and the cells swell. Cytotoxic oedema results from hypoxia and ischaemia and is often delayed in onset for 2–3 days. It also occurs in metabolic brain disease, especially hepatic coma, and may rapidly develop in severe hyponatraemia.
3. Interstitial oedema is caused by any condition which interferes with cerebrospinal fluid drainage such as communicating or obstructive hydrocephalus.

Intracranial hypertension

The cranial contents are enclosed in a rigid, semi-closed box (the skull with its foramina). There are three incompressible elements: brain tissue, blood, and cerebrospinal fluid. The Monroe–Kelly doctrine, which is central to understanding the process and management of intracranial hypertension, states that unless an increase in the volume of one intracranial component is matched by a reduction in the others, the intracranial pressure will rise. One component of the intracranial contents increases acutely in cases of haemorrhage, cerebral oedema or acute obstructive hydrocephalus, and raised intracranial pressure results. If the volume change occurs over a long period, as occurs with tumours and abscesses, the intracranial pressure does not rise rapidly; this adaptation occurs because the surrounding cerebral tissue shrinks to some degree. In addition, if the lesion is slowly growing the head may increase in size. The shape of the pressure–volume

135

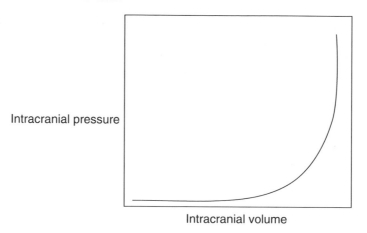

Intracranial pressure

Intracranial volume

FIGURE 6.1—*Intracranial compliance curve*

curve reflects the compensating events as volume is added acutely inside the cranial cavity (fig 6.1). Initially, cerebrospinal fluid in the cerebral ventricles and basal cisterns is displaced out of the head into the spinal subarachnoid space. The cerebral blood volume is also reduced by cerebral venous compression. During this phase intracranial pressure increases minimally. However, as the compensation mechanisms are quite limited, further increases in intracranial volume cause progressively greater increases in intracranial pressure. The infant skull responds somewhat differently; the sutures are not fused and this allows some degree of expansion of the cranial vault.

There are two major complications of intracranial hypertension: cerebral ischaemia and herniation. As intracranial pressure rises, cerebral perfusion pressure falls unless there is an equal rise in blood pressure. The reduction in cerebral perfusion pressure adds further ischaemic injury to areas with marginal perfusion and in those areas with impaired autoregulation. Ultimately, when cerebral perfusion pressure equals mean arterial pressure, cerebral perfusion pressure falls to zero and brain death results.

The cranial cavity is partly divided into compartments by the horizontal tentorium cerebri and the vertical falx cerebri. These tough fibrous septa help stabilise the brain during head movement. The second major complication of intracranial hypertension results when swelling in one large compartment causes a pressure gradient which pushes the brain towards another compartment. This typically produces downward herniation across the tentorium. The uncal gyrus of the temporal lobe presses medially onto the brainstem, initially stimulating, then terminally depressing, the respiratory and cardiac centres. This process is almost always accompanied by dysfunction of oculomotor tone, resulting in pupillary constriction and then dilation. Rarely, tentorial herniation occurs in an upward direction from an expanding mass in the posterior fossa. Herniation may occur at an intracranial pressure less than that required for global cerebral ischaemia. Conversely, cerebral perfusion pressure may fall to zero well before herniation occurs, particularly in the face of systemic hypotension. Occasionally, the two events coincide.

Pathophysiology of non-traumatic brain insults

It is not difficult to delineate the primary insult from the secondary in conditions such as trauma and acute anoxia. Cerebral insults that are infectious in origin or secondary to generalised illnesses are more difficult to characterise.

Bacterial meningitis and viral meningoencephalitis

Infection of the central nervous system occurs locally in the form of meningitis, encephalitis or abscess. In addition, infection in non-cerebral sites may cause brain dysfunction, the so-called "septic encephalopathy".

Bacterial meningitis generally occurs secondary to bacteraemia. Children at high risk include those with impaired immune function, those with foreign bodies such as a ventriculoperitoneal shunt in place, and those in whom there is a breach of the meninges, as occurs with an open skull fracture and neural tube defects. Inflammation occurs in the subarachnoid space and around blood vessels and the inflammatory process may involve the brain tissue itself, resulting in cerebritis. Vasculitis can lead to infarction. There are, in addition, several potential secondary insults associated with meningitis. Increased cerebral blood flow can contribute to an increase in intracranial pressure. Hypotension, secondary to septic shock, and cerebral oedema, secondary to inappropriate antidiuretic hormone secretion and hyponatraemia, may add to the primary brain insult. The organisms responsible for bacterial meningitis vary with age. Neonatal meningitis is usually due to Gram negative organisms, Group B streptococci or *Listeria monocytogenes*. In young children meningitis is caused by *Neisseria meningitidis*, *Streptococcus pneumoniae* or *Haemophilus influenzae* type b. Immunisation has markedly reduced the incidence of the previously common Haemophilus meningitis. Subdural effusions and hydrocephalus are recognised complications and are particularly seen following pneumococcal infection.

Other bacterial infections of the central nervous system include brain abscess and subdural empyema. Abscesses may arise due to contiguous spread from middle ear disease. They are also seen in patients with cyanotic

137

congenital heart disease or endocarditis. Subdural empyema arises from extension of sinus or middle ear disease. The common presenting symptoms of both problems are headache, seizures, and focal neurological signs.

Viral infections of the central nervous system may be limited to meningitis or involve the brain itself in the process of encephalitis. The common causes include enteroviruses, herpes simplex, arboviruses, mumps, and measles. Herpes encephalitis can present in many ways but should always be suspected in patients who present with encephalopathy and seizures, in whom there is no history of trauma.

Status epilepticus

Status epilepticus in children may occur as the presenting episode of epilepsy, as a febrile seizure or when a known epileptic patient undergoes a change in therapy. Physiological changes include increased systemic blood pressure and increased cerebral blood flow. The neurological insult in status epilepticus may be secondary to one or a combination of three factors:

1. the effects of the original disorder precipitating the seizures;
2. any secondary insult occurring during the seizure such as hypoxia, ischaemia, hypoglycaemia and hyperpyrexia;
3. the direct effect of the seizure on the brain.

The increased metabolic requirements of the brain appear to be matched by increased cerebral blood flow in most cases, provided oxygenation is not impaired. The incidence of long term morbidity following status is lower in children than adults. Although it is recognised that permanent sequelae may follow seizures of greater than 60 min duration, an underlying neurological disorder is the major determinant of sequelae.[1]

Primary intracranial haemorrhage

In contrast to adults, the most common origin of primary intracranial haemorrhage in children is an arteriovenous malformation; aneurysms are uncommon. The presenting symptoms of both problems are similar, however. Headache, altered conscious state, and seizures are most common. The cerebral insult occurs for a variety of reasons including the effects of the actual haemorrhage and subsequent vascular disruption, secondary vasospasm, and raised intracranial pressure. The intracranial hypertension may be due to mass effect of a haematoma, oedema or obstructive hydrocephalus.

Clinical management

When an infant or child presents with an acute cerebral disorder, there must be a rapid yet orderly response leading to resuscitation, diagnosis, and subsequent management. It is important to note that much of the current "standard" therapy is based on clinical experience as opposed to carefully evaluated scientific evidence. Standard neurological care has changed over the past few years and it is now recognised that certain treatment options, in particular hyperventilation, may actually worsen the outcome in some cases. It has been established that a severe secondary brain injury can be caused by postinsult hypoxia and hypotension. Patients who develop intracranial hypertension in any cerebral disorder are also more likely to have a poor outcome. These factors should be borne in mind throughout all stages of management in order to minimise secondary insult.

TABLE 6.3—*Management approach in acute brain insults*

1. Basic resuscitation: airway, breathing, circulation, protect cervical spine.
2. Assess the nature and extent of cerebral injury or pathology.
3. Rapid assessment for injury or dysfunction in other organ systems.
4. Subsequent management.
5. Institute specific monitoring and therapy.
6. Perform prognostic tests.
7. Progress to rehabilitation following the acute phase.

Table 6.3 summarises the basic steps in management of any acute cerebral disorder. Each step will be discussed in detail, initially reviewing current standard therapy, followed by new directions in management.

Initial management

The resuscitation phase is a dynamic period. As unexpected deterioration may rapidly develop, the child must be constantly monitored and the response to every intervention carefully reviewed. Although the causes of acute cerebral injuries are diverse, the basic approach should be similar. The aim is always to firstly restore the delivery of oxygenated blood to all regions of the brain as soon as possible, followed by assessment of the likely cause of the problem and the degree of neurological injury. The final step is institution of specific therapy. The initial management covers the first three points of table 6.3.

Basic resuscitation

The first priority is to assess the airway, breathing, and circulation. Oxygen should be given to all patients and oxygen saturation measured by pulse oximeter. Apnoea or hypoventilation must be immediately treated with assisted ventilation via bag and mask. This manoeuvre should precede any attempt at intubation. A large bore peripheral intravenous cannula should be rapidly inserted. If venous access cannot be achieved, an intraosseous needle should be placed; the proximal tibia is the most suitable site. Insertion of central venous lines should not be attempted in unstable hypovolaemic children as the procedure may be difficult, time consuming and be complicated by pneumothorax, haemothorax or arterial puncture. In addition, a deterioration in haemodynamic, respiratory or neurological status may occur during this time and not be recognised. If central venous access is subsequently required, the procedure should be performed, following resuscitation, by an experienced clinician in a carefully monitored environment. All trauma patients should have cervical stabilisation until cervical spine *x* rays are reviewed by an experienced paediatric radiologist or neurosurgeon. This stabilisation can be achieved using a collar, sandbags or even rolled towels.

Tracheal intubation should be performed in comatose children if the airway cannot be maintained, oxygen saturation is less than 94%, shock is present or there is hypoventilation, detected either by clinical examination or a measured $PaCO_2$ greater than 45 mmHg (6 kPa). Successful atraumatic intubation requires preparation. All the necessary equipment, including drugs, suction and alternative endotracheal tubes, must be at hand and it should be assumed that all patients have a full stomach. Preoxygenation and cricoid pressure should be applied prior to orotracheal intubation. Unresponsive, areflexic patients will usually not need anaesthetic drugs to provide good intubating conditions. Comatose patients who have some reflex motor activity are best managed with paralysis induced by succinylcholine 1.5–2 mg/kg intravenously. Atropine (0.02 mg/kg) should be given if bradycardia occurs or is likely to occur.

The use of anaesthetic drugs to attenuate the hypertensive response to intubation is appropriate depending on the degree of haemodynamic stability. Although thiopentone (2–5 mg/kg) or propofol (0.5–2 mg/kg) are excellent agents, they should only be used if the patient is normovolaemic and not hypotensive. Narcotic opioids (for example, fentanyl 1–4 µg/kg) in combination with short acting benzodiazepines (for example, midazolam 0.05–0.15 mg/kg) are useful alternatives in the haemodynamically unstable patient. It is better to err on the side of "light anaesthesia" than to cause hypotension and risk worsening the cerebral injury. Ketamine should never be used as it increases cerebral metabolic rate and cerebral blood flow; it may therefore worsen intracranial hypertension and brain injury.

Concern about cervical injury should not lead to delay in performing tracheal intubation in hypoxic or hypoventilating patients. Although unstable cervical spine injury occurs in children, it is rare and delay in securing the airway is likely to result in secondary hypoxic cerebral damage. If intubation is required in a child with a cervical injury, careful manual inline stabilisation (not traction) should be performed by an assistant, to minimise neck movement. The intubation itself should be performed by the most skilled person available. The appropriate sized endotracheal tube, once placed, should be fixed and air entry to both lung fields repeatedly checked. The pulse oximeter should confirm a sustained oxygen saturation of over 95%. Problems following intubation include right endobronchial intubation and rapid enlargement of a previously undetected pneumothorax. Ventilation should deliver a tidal volume of approximately 12 ml/kg at 12–20 breaths per minute, depending on age. Normocapnia should be the aim as hyperventilation may reduce cerebral oxygen delivery by causing excessive cerebral vasoconstriction.

Failure to detect hypoventilation by clinical evaluation frequently occurs and a blood gas analysis is an important investigation but it should not delay implementation of interventions such as intubation. Other initial investigations should include measurement of haemoglobin, platelet count, blood glucose, sodium, potassium, creatinine, and urea levels. In cases of trauma blood should be crossmatched. A gastric tube should be inserted in all children with acute neurological insults. Acute gastric dilation is very common and causes diaphragmatic embarrassment and increases the risk of aspiration. An orogastric tube should be used in head trauma as there may be an unrecognised basal skull fracture and a nasogastric tube may enter the cranial cavity. A nasogastric tube may be used in all other cases.

Hypotension is a late sign of hypovolaemia in children but is common following trauma (table 6.2). Tachycardia, pallor, and slow capillary refill are important early signs of reduced cardiac output. Blood loss may have occurred from wounds, especially of the scalp, or be concealed in the chest, abdomen, pelvis, long bones or skull. A number of relatively minor injuries may contribute to major volume loss and subsequent shock. A large scalp laceration and one major bone fracture, each resulting in a 150 ml haemorrhage, could account for the loss of 30% of a 10 kg child's circulating blood volume. Although hypotension also occurs secondary to systemic sepsis associated with bacterial meningitis, with drugs and poisons which depress cardiac output and/or vasomotor tone, and for non-hypovolaemic reasons in trauma patients, it is important to remember that hypovolaemia is the major cause of hypotension. Plasma volume expansion should be achieved using a non-dextrose containing isotonic crystalloid solution (Ringer's lactate or 0.9% sodium chloride 20–30 ml/kg), or a colloid solution (albumin 5% in saline 10–20 ml/kg). The response, in terms of blood

141

pressure, heart rate, and neck vein filling, should be reviewed and the dose repeated at least once if there is persistent hypotension.

The patient must be continuously monitored during resuscitation. If volume expansion beyond 30 ml/kg of colloid is required, in the absence of external blood loss, a source of uncontrolled concealed haemorrhage must be sought. This may be intrathoracic, intraperitoneal, retroperitoneal or from major long bone or pelvic fractures. The use of ongoing volume expansion makes serial measurement of haemoglobin mandatory. An early chest x ray will diagnose or exclude intrathoracic blood loss. Persistent hypotension needs careful clinical evaluation for other evolving problems. Distention of neck veins suggests pneumothorax, cardiac tamponade or myocardial failure. Blood pressure usually normalises rapidly after drainage of the affected pleural space or pericardium. Hypotension with inappropriate bradycardia and cutaneous vasodilation is strongly suggestive of a high spinal cord lesion, particularly if accompanied by priapism. The functional sympathectomy which occurs secondary to such a lesion makes the patient extremely sensitive to hypovolaemia. If hypotension persists despite aggressive volume expansion, and exclusion of the other problems listed above an infusion of a vasoactive drug should be administered (dopamine 5–15 µg/kg/min; or noradrenalin 0.1–0.5 µg/kg/min). The dose needs to be titrated until the blood pressure is normal for age.

There is experimental evidence that hypertonic fluids may be superior to the standard intravenous fluids in haemodynamic resuscitation and could perhaps improve outcome. Haemodynamic stability can be achieved quickly using hypertonic saline (7.5%, 2400 mOsm/l) in hypovolaemic subjects using a much smaller volume (4 ml/kg) than is required when using isotonic solutions. This fluid regime is most useful during initial resuscitation and in situations of controlled haemorrhage.[2] There is evidence that, in patients with combined hypovolemic and brain injury, hypertonic fluid resuscitation improves cerebral circulation and, by inducing vasoconstriction, leads to a reduction in intracranial pressure.[3,4]

Initial assessment of neurological injury

During the resuscitation phase, there should be a rapid neurological evaluation to determine the depth of coma and the presence of localising neurological signs. This assessment should include examination of the posture, muscle tone in each limb, movement in response to command, and tendon reflexes. In comatose patients, the response to pain in each extremity and in the trigeminal nerve distribution must be assessed. Detailed examination of the cranial nerves and retinoscopy should not be performed at this stage, but ocular examination is mandatory. Gaze palsies, pupil size, and response to light should be recorded. The oculocephalic, or doll's eye,

142

reflex must not be checked until the cervical spine has been radiologically cleared. In addition, the pattern of breathing should be noted. The Cheyne–Stokes pattern or hypoventilation is seen in patients who have brainstem compression, are postictal or are affected by depressant drugs such as opioids or benzodiazepines. Hypoventilation is also seen in spinal cord injury. Spontaneous hyperventilation occurs with pontine haemorrhage, in metabolic acidosis, and after ingestion of stimulatory drugs, in particular aspirin.

The Glasgow Coma Scale (GCS) score permits serial assessment of coma depth and the score at six and 72 hours also has a limited degree of prognostic value. A modified paediatric score has been produced and is

TABLE 6.4—*Modified Glasgow Coma Scale*

Motor	Eye opening	Voice (child)
1. Flaccid	1. Nil	1. Nil
2. Decerebrate/abnormal extension	2. To pain	2. Moans/cries
3. Decorticate/abnormal flexion	3. To command	3. Unintelligible words
4. Withdrawal	4. Spontaneous	4. Confused speech
5. Localises pain		5. Normal
6. Obeys commands		
	Total score: 3–15	

used widely (table 6.4). Scoring should be performed after resuscitation and reversal of central nervous system depressant drugs. The best response in each category should be the one recorded. It is notable that seizures are common in the prehospital phase of many acute neurological insults. Both the ictal and postictal state will worsen the GCS score and possibly lead to an overestimate of the severity of injury.

Unilateral pupillary dilation at presentation may be a sign of injury to the globe or its oculomotor pathways as far back as the brainstem. However, progressive dilation in a previously normal sized pupil indicates possible brainstem compression and impending death, particularly if the contralateral pupil subsequently dilates. This is classically accompanied by bradycardia, hypertension, and unilateral hypertonia. The hypertension and corticospinal signs may not occur in some patients and hence bradycardia is an ominous sign. It should also be kept in mind that seizures may result in bilaterally, and occasionally unilaterally, dilated pupils.

A unique aspect of acute brain trauma in children is that of non-accidental injury or child abuse. This diagnosis should be considered when the injuries sustained are inconsistent with the reported history. Physical signs such as bruising and skin markings in unusual patterns or injuries to the mouth or genitalia may indicate abuse. As bilateral retinal haemorrhages resulting from violent shaking are very suggestive signs, a thorough ophthalmological examination should be undertaken whenever there are suspicions. A skeletal survey can also be useful in making the diagnosis in small children by detecting clinically silent fractures of ribs and long bones. Fractures of different ages may be documented by this survey and this may help clarify the clinical picture. The unreliable history makes neurological assessment very difficult because the injury may have occurred days prior to presentation, hypoxia may have subsequently occurred and there may have been previous non-accidental brain insults.

Injury or dysfunction in other organ systems

Although the presence of organ failure or injury will often become apparent during the initial resuscitation phase, it is easy to miss other injuries unless a systematic examination is made and repeated subsequently. It is mandatory to perform a head to toe examination, including visualisation of the back. Diagnosis of spinal cord injury may be difficult in comatose patients. The incidence of cervical spinal cord injury approaches 100% in those children who are apnoeic at the accident site and who subsequently require cardiopulmonary resuscitation in the prehospital phase. Absence of limb movements combined with priapism, areflexia, paradoxical movement of the chest and abdomen or rhythmic flaring of the alae nasi (Duncan's sign) is suggestive of a high spinal lesion. A cervical spine x ray series should be obtained in all trauma victims to look for bony or ligamentous disruption. In contrast to adults, in whom unstable fracture dislocations of the lower cervical spine are common, children tend to suffer injuries of the upper cervical spine. This is probably because of the relatively large heavy head. Such high injuries often result in disruption of the upper spinal cord or cervicomedullary junction and lead to immediate cardiorespiratory failure and death. It is only the administration of immediate expert resuscitation that allows such patients to reach emergency departments alive.

Early in the resuscitation process a urine catheter should be inserted. The urine should be analysed for macroscopic or microscopic haematuria. A chest x ray should be performed in all cases to diagnose or exclude lung injury, pulmonary aspiration, pleural collections, and mediastinal collections. Although rare in children, aortic dissection can occur and is suggested by a widened upper mediastinum, accompanied by pleural capping, haemothorax, and lateral displacement of the orogastric tube. These signs should lead to a contrast computed tomographic (CT) scan of the chest, supplemented by transoesophageal echo or aortic angiography. The presence of intraabdominal trauma in children is best addressed by abdominal CT scan. Intraabdominal injury should be suspected when there is distention, localised bruising or requirement for volume replacement that cannot be explained otherwise. Undisplaced fractures of long bones are often missed, though they retain less priority in the sedated ventilated patient.

Subsequent management

After the initial assessment and resuscitation, the need for mechanical ventilation, mannitol, cranial CT scan, and neurosurgery must be considered.

Mechanical ventilation

Even if the criteria for intubation were not met in the initial resuscitation phase, mechanical ventilation should be instituted in those patients with a GCS of eight or less, rapidly worsening coma, coma with localising signs or accompanied by bradycardia and hypertension. The technique of intubation has been described. Once the endotracheal tube has been secured, non-depolarising muscle relaxants should be given (for example, pancuronium 0.1 mg/kg intravenously) as required to facilitate ventilation and prevent straining, at least until after the CT scan has been reviewed. Sedation with opioids supplemented by benzodiazepines should be given to prevent hypertension but administered with caution if hypotension persists despite resuscitation.

Mannitol

Mannitol (0.25 g/kg intravenously) is indicated in patients with signs of severe raised intracranial pressure. As will be discussed it is a useful alternative to cerebrospinal fluid drainage and hyperventilation during the subsequent course as well. A urethral catheter should be in place to monitor urine output.

Computed tomography (CT)

A cranial CT scan should be performed in patients with a GCS of less than 10, in those with focal neurological deficits, and in patients with undiagnosed coma. The aim of CT is to diagnose:

145

1. surgically treatable mass lesions;
2. brain swelling due to hyperaemia or oedema which may benefit from specific therapy in the ICU;
3. skull fractures.

A CT scan should be considered, even in cases of less severe head trauma, prior to anaesthesia for major orthopaedic, thoracic or abdominal surgery. The CT examination may extend to the spine, as well as to the chest and abdomen in a search for solid organ injuries. Spinal cord injury without radiological abnormality (SCIWORA) is a well recognised entity in children and at least 50% of children with clinical evidence of spinal cord injury will have no bony damage visible on plain x rays. This group will need subsequent myelography with CT and/or magnetic resonance imaging 24–48 h after stabilisation has taken place in the intensive care unit.

Neurosurgery

In most centres, management of paediatric head trauma is jointly coordinated by neurosurgeons and intensive care specialists. Urgent surgery to remove extradural or subdural collections associated with any midline shift or significant brain compression should be performed as soon as possible. If surgery is delayed, lethal intracranial hypertension and transtentorial herniation may rapidly develop. Small collections may be treated conservatively but CT scans must be repeated immediately if the neurological status deteriorates. Surgery may also be required for acute hydrocephalus or a depressed skull fracture.

The intracranial pressure should be monitored in all children with a modified GCS of less than eight, if significant cerebral swelling is present on CT examination, and postoperatively following drainage of an intracranial haematoma. Intracranial pressure monitors may be placed in the extradural or subdural spaces, in either lateral ventricle or directly into the cerebral tissue. Pressure is usually monitored through a soft catheter placed in the lateral ventricle or subdural space. These are connected to an external transducer. The advantages of external transducers include the option to re-zero as required, less baseline drift and lower cost. However, there must be careful positioning of the transducer relative to the brain; it is usually aligned to the external auditory meatus. Other systems in use include a fibreoptic catheter placed in the extradural space and a microtransducer placed directly into the cerebral tissue or ventricle. The advantage of transducer tipped devices is that intracranial pressure measurement is not influenced by a change in patient position. Baseline drift and inability to re-zero following insertion are potential problems with this technology.

Although there has been controversy about the best means of monitoring intracranial pressure, there is good evidence that an intraventricular catheter offers two significant advantages. Firstly, this technique is more accurate than subdural and extradural methods which frequently underestimate intracranial pressure, particularly when it is elevated. Secondly, the ventricular catheter also has a therapeutic role as it permits cerebrospinal fluid drainage which leads to a reduction in intracranial pressure. The major disadvantage of intraventricular catheters is the risk of infection and ventriculitis. The risk is lessened by strict asepsis in handling the catheter and by having the catheter inserted through a subcutaneous tunnel. Placement within the ventricle may be limited by the size of the ventricles at the time of surgery. If the patient does not need to be transferred to the operating room for a craniotomy for haematoma evacuation, the intracranial pressure monitor can be inserted in the intensive care unit. This avoids the problems inherent in intrahospital transport, especially alterations in the pattern of ventilation and level of monitoring which may worsen control of cerebral perfusion. Suitable facilities, including adequate lighting, are of course a prerequisite to this approach.

Monitoring and therapy: intensive care management

The intensive care of a patient with any acute cerebral insult requires constant careful observation of the general and neurological status. The primary aim is to maintain cerebral oxygen delivery, give specific therapy for the primary problem, and prevent secondary cerebral insults. Specific neurological monitoring must be utilised to detect any deterioration, in the hope of optimising outcome.

General care

The function of each organ system should be carefully assessed. Monitoring of respiratory pattern and depth, blood pressure, neurological status, and oxygenation are essential when the patient is breathing spontaneously. The GCS score and pupillary size and reaction should be recorded each hour. Controlled ventilation may be facilitated by administration of long acting muscle relaxants and/or sedatives. Sedation helps limit the increase in blood pressure and oxygen consumption seen with coughing and straining. Morphine (30–50 µg/kg/h) with midazolam (50–100 µg/kg/h) is a suitable regime. Additional sedation may be required to prevent increased intracranial pressure during endotracheal suction, physiotherapy or painful procedures. An intraarterial catheter is useful for continuous measurement of blood pressure and sampling of arterial blood.

147

Efficacy of ventilation is monitored by continuous pulse oximetry and, if there is no significant alveolar–arterial CO_2 gradient, capnography. The PaO_2 should be over 100 mmHg (13.3 kPa) and $PaCO_2$ 35 mmHg (4.7 kPa). Blood pressure should be maintained in the normal range for age. Surface cooling should be used if the core temperature exceeds 38°C, as hyperpyrexia can have a detrimental effect on the injured brain.

Seizure prophylaxis

Seizures following head injury are common and can add to any secondary injury by increasing metabolic requirements and intracranial pressure and by impairing oxygen delivery. Seizures are most common after penetrating trauma, depressed skull fracture, and with focal collections. In addition to the above high risk groups, all paralysed patients and patients who have already suffered a seizure should receive anticonvulsant therapy. Phenytoin (20 mg/kg) is suitable initially; it is efficacious and does not significantly depress the conscious state. There is evidence that anticonvulsant therapy is effective at preventing early posttraumatic seizures but such treatment is only effective in the first week.[5] Phenytoin may also impair cognitive function and should therefore be continued only in the high risk groups and for a short period.[6] In practice many patients receive an effective anticonvulsant, through the benzodiazepine infusion given as sedation.

Management of intracranial hypertension

Management of cerebral perfusion pressure is, by definition, intimately linked with the control of systemic blood pressure and intracranial pressure. It is generally accepted that maintenance of an adequate cerebral perfusion pressure is desirable, although there is no strong evidence that this is associated with improved outcome. In adult patients a cerebral perfusion pressure greater than 70 mmHg is the aim.[7] In children, an adequate cerebral perfusion pressure is more difficult to define because of the variation in normal blood pressure with age; most accept a minimum cerebral perfusion pressure of 50 mmHg in young infants. A critical pathway for the management of established intracranial hypertension has been produced.[7] Though designed for adult patients, its principles are applicable to children.

The desired cerebral perfusion pressure should initially be met by optimising blood pressure. If intracranial hypertension develops and a ventricular drain is *in situ*, cerebrospinal fluid should be drained. If this is unsuccessful or there is no ventricular drain, mannitol (0.25 g/kg) should be given. This can be repeated at intervals provided it does not induce hypovolaemia and the osmolality remains less than 315 mOsm/l. Barbiturate therapy, moderate hypothermia, and hyperventilation could subsequently be considered. Suboptimal cerebral perfusion pressure can also be addressed by raising the mean arterial pressure. This can be done by modest expansion of the intravascular compartment and via inotropic agents, such as dopamine, or vasoconstrictors, such as phenylephrine.

Fluid management in the acutely brain injured patient should be based on optimising intravascular volume initially and subsequently minimising the possibility of accumulation of excess interstitial and intracellular fluid. Normovolaemia is a minimum requirement in the equation of cerebral perfusion and blood pressure. In some cases of raised intracranial pressure, expanding the intravascular space to promote cerebral perfusion may be useful. A hypoosmolar state should be avoided as this can lead to an increase in brain oedema. Subsequent to the resuscitation phase intravenous crystalloid solutions should be limited to 50% of usual daily requirements. This may in fact be greater than many patients require because of the minimisation of losses in the intensive care environment. The fluid should provide a minimum of 3 mmol/kg of sodium per day and any decrease in serum osmolality should be countered by further reduction in administered fluid. There is a trend in some areas to actively raise the serum osmolality in the hope that this will limit oedema formation. Although theoretically sound, there is little evidence to support this approach.

Mannitol is effective at reducing intracranial pressure and may also improve cerebral blood flow.[8] Much of its early effect occurs secondary to altered red cell rheology and induction of vasoconstriction. Subsequently the osmotic and then the diuretic action help to reduce brain water. Mannitol is very useful in the patient who develops signs of severe raised intracranial pressure. However, repeated use is limited often by the development of a hyperosmolar state. The intravascular space may be depleted following a mannitol induced diuresis and volume expansion may subsequently be required to maintain optimal cerebral perfusion pressure.

Head posture remains a controversial aspect of the care of the head injured patient. The head should be kept in the midline to optimise venous drainage. The arguments related to head elevation are that, on the one hand, lying flat reduces the potentially beneficial effects of gravity on intracranial pressure and, on the other, that having the patient head up potentially reduces cerebral perfusion pressure. Studies suggest that in the majority of patients head elevation to 30° provides a beneficial effect on intracranial pressure without a reduction in cerebral perfusion pressure or cerebral blood flow.[9,10] It is important to note, however, that individual variation was a feature of the response pattern in the patients in these studies. Therefore, one reasonable approach to this problem is to elevate

149

the head 30° after a period of stabilisation; any subsequent deterioration in cerebral perfusion pressure suggests that the patient should be managed flat.

High dose barbiturate therapy is known to lower intracranial pressure and does so by reducing cerebral metabolism and this in turn may lead to a reduction in cerebral flow. It has no effect in the prophylaxis of intracranial hypertension. However, when used in patients with raised intracranial pressure refractory to conventional therapy, it has been shown to be effective and may contribute to improved outcome.[11] The patients whose intracranial pressure responded to barbiturates had improved mortality outcome compared to those who did not respond. Care must be taken to avoid a reduction in cerebral perfusion pressure secondary to induced hypotension. The aim of therapy is to reduce intracranial pressure or to induce a burst suppression electroencephalographic pattern. A loading dose of 2–5 mg/kg thiopentone and then an infusion of 1–5 mg/kg/h is an approximate guide and pharmacokinetics have been shown to be similar in children and adults.[12] Blood levels can be monitored although there is no clear correlation between therapeutic effect, cardiovascular side effects, and serum levels.

There is renewed interest in the use of moderate hypothermia in the brain injured patient. Marrion et al. have demonstrated improved outcome in adult patients with an initial GCS of 5–7 who were managed with hypothermia to 34°C for 48 h.[13] Significant improvements were seen at six months but not at 12 months. It has also been shown that moderate hypothermia leads to a reduction in cerebral metabolic rate but does not reduce cerebral blood flow.[14] The studies of hypothermia in adults may not be directly applicable to small children but the use of hypothermia should be considered in cases of refractory intracranial hypertension, particularly in adolescents. The potential complications of moderate hypothermia in children include altered platelet function, coagulopathy, impaired leucocyte activity, and reduced cardiac and renal function. The overall clinical state needs to be carefully considered, therefore, prior to initiating hypothermia.

Hyperventilation, by inducing cerebral vasoconstriction, can reduce intracranial pressure. For this reason it had been used in the management of severe head injury, in adults and children, for many years. Children were thought to develop cerebral hyperaemia frequently following traumatic brain injury and might therefore particularly benefit from hyperventilation. It has been shown, however, that a hyperaemic response is uncommon.[15] Although often effective at rapidly lowering intracranial pressure, hyperventilation is not routinely indicated because of the risk of cerebral ischaemia, subsequent to reduced cerebral blood flow. A randomised, controlled study assessing the value of prophylactic hyperventilation in adults demonstrated improved outcome when hyperventilation was not used.[16] Refractory cases of raised intracranial pressure may benefit from hyperventilation and in such cases bedside assessment of cerebral blood flow is useful.

The measurement of jugular venous oxygen saturation ($SjvO_2$), via a catheter placed in the jugular venous bulb, enables indirect monitoring of global cerebral blood flow. The technique of placement in children is as described for adults. In diffuse brain injury it is theoretically best to place the catheter into the dominant jugular vein. The dominant vein can be determined by monitoring the effect on intracranial pressure of manual occlusion of each jugular in turn. If no difference can be detected the right side should be cannulated; it is also technically easier to place the catheter into the right. (A left handed operator may, however, find it easier to place a left sided catheter).

A single episode of desaturation to less than 50% has been associated with a poorer outcome.[17] Despite this, $SjvO_2$ monitoring is not indicated in all severely head injured patients for a number of reasons. Firstly, jugular venous oxygen saturation reflects global cerebral blood flow rather than regional and does not therefore indicate flow to the injured part of the brain. In addition, the systems in current use require frequent calibration which limits the value of continuous monitoring. Finally, $SjvO_2$ monitoring may not provide information that cannot be gleaned from standard monitoring devices. It is of value in the patient whose intracranial pressure is poorly controlled despite standard management, including ventriculostomy drainage and mannitol. In such a circumstance hyperventilation should be considered and $SjvO_2$ monitoring allows assessment of the response to hyperventilation and it may therefore help avoid any degree of ischaemia that results. Raised intracranial pressure with high jugular venous oxygen saturation, indicating luxury perfusion, can be controlled with hyperventilation also. Induced hypocapnia has been found to be the most common cause of desaturation.[18] One further advantage of continuous $SjvO_2$ monitoring lies, therefore, in measurement of the physiological effect of the various necessary interventions in the brain injured patient. Endotracheal suction, hand ventilation, and painful procedures may have effects on $SjvO_2$ prior to any change in intracranial pressure.

Decompressive craniotomy would seem to be a logical method of managing raised intracranial pressure. Although no controlled studies have been published there have been small series reported and these suggest some benefit.[19] The procedure may not have been adequately assessed as it has traditionally been performed after a period of sustained intracranial hypertension, when significant secondary damage may already have occurred. Surgical decompression should certainly be considered in cases of metabolic encephalopathy, such as Reye's syndrome, that are complicated by intracranial hypertension. As neurological sequelae may be entirely due to the secondary insult in these cases, aggressive control of intracranial pressure has the potential to dramatically alter outcome.

Aspects of management of non-traumatic brain insults

The basic management of all patients with an acute brain insult is similar, with emphasis on early restoration of oxygenation and cerebral perfusion. There are specific illnesses that have points worthy of discussion, however.

The aggressive approach to management of intracranial hypertension outlined above is not relevant to all causes of brain injury. In particular, patients who have suffered a primary hypoxic brain insult do not appear to benefit from invasive monitoring and management of raised intracranial pressure.[20] Children who have suffered a severe hypoxic insult will either recover well, die or remain in a persistent vegetative state independent of treatment administered.[21] Such patients should be stabilised haemodynamically and restored to normothermia. If coma persists after 24 h prolonged aggressive treatment will only produce a survivor in a persistent vegetative state and treatment should therefore not be continued.

Status epilepticus is a medical emergency and should be controlled as soon as possible. Benzodiazepines are the most useful initial drugs; diazepam (0.2 mg/kg) or lorazepam (0.05–0.1 mg/kg) administered intravenously is effective. As intermittent frequent seizures are as likely to cause damage as persisting status, a longer acting drug should follow these agents. Either phenytoin (20 mg/kg) or phenobarbitone (20 mg/kg) can be used though phenytoin is less likely to cause respiratory depression and hypotension. If the above measures are ineffective seizures can be controlled by thiopentone (1–5 mg/kg intravenously). As this essentially means induction of anaesthesia artificial ventilation will be required. During the process of stabilisation attention should be paid to control of hyperpyrexia and maintenance of glucose homoeostasis.

Suspected bacterial meningitis is confirmed by analysis of cerebrospinal fluid. The timing of lumbar puncture requires careful consideration. The risks outweigh the benefits in patients who are significantly obtunded, as evidenced by a GCS of less than 8, or those who have recently had a seizure, are shocked or have a marked coagulopathy. In such cases treatment should be empiric and commence with a third generation cephalosporin (cefotaxime 50 mg/kg 6-hourly or ceftriaxone 100 mg/kg daily) and penicillin (60 mg/kg 4-hourly). If a lumbar puncture has been performed antibiotic therapy can be rationalised once sensitivities are known. Steroids appear to improve neurological outcome and should be given in all cases of bacterial meningitis, prior to antibiotic administration if possible.[22]

Dexamethasone 0.4 mg/kg 12-hourly for two days is a suitable regime. Herpes encephalitis has protean modes of presentation and early diagnosis is difficult. As the outcome is improved by the early use of acyclovir, empirical treatment should be considered in cases of encephalopathy of unknown cause, particularly when associated with seizures.

CT is usually sufficient to make the diagnosis of primary intracranial haemorrhage; lumbar puncture is only required when uncertainty remains after CT. Definition of the vascular formation will often require magnetic resonance imaging, magnetic resonance angiography or formal angiography. The basic management is as described for other acute brain insults. Raised intracranial pressure or intracranial collections are managed in the standard manner. Vasospasm complicates aneurysm rupture as in adults, but is not often a problem associated with arteriovenous malformations. Protective agents, such as calcium channel blockers, have been used to manage vasospasm but there is no clear evidence of their benefit. Children are at greater risk of rehaemorrhage than are adults and must be closely observed for several days.

Specific metabolic encephalopathies require management based on the above principles. Additional management in hyperammonaemic states may include limitation of protein intake and enhancing ammonia metabolism using arginine or sodium benzoate.

Prognosis and outcome

The outcome of acute brain insults depends on the factors described in this chapter: the nature and severity of the primary injury and the extent to which the quality of resuscitation and subsequent critical care either prevent or reduce any secondary brain injury.

Outcome can be assessed in two ways. The first method is to characterise any residual focal deficit such as hemiplegia or visual impairment. The second and most important method is the assessment of recovery of higher cerebral functions: intellectual ability, vision, speech, ongoing neurodevelopment, and personality. This has been quantified for the purpose of comparison in the Glasgow Outcome Scale (GOS)[23] (table 6.5).

TABLE 6.5—*Glasgow Outcome Scale*

1. Dead
2. Persistent vegetative state
3. Severe disability – conscious but disabled
4. Moderate recovery – disabled but independent
5. Good recovery

Outcome categories may be alternatively grouped into favourable, which includes good and moderate disability, and unfavourable, including severe disability, persistent vegetative, and death. The two main areas of interest to intensive care practitioners in paediatric brain injury outcome are:

1. prediction of outcome at the time of presentation and throughout the acute phase (early outcome prediction);
2. the subsequent prognosis for further improvement in those children who survive their acute illness with residual deficits.

Information regarding long term outcome is also of great importance to families in order for them to commence any degree of planning for the child's future needs.

Early outcome prediction

A number of tools can be used, alone or in combination, to allow the clinician to make a prediction of outcome at an early stage of management. This process is important to the treating physician who may be disinclined to continue life saving treatment if an accurate early prediction of an unfavourable outcome, particularly death or vegetative states, could be made. In order for these tools to be suitable for guiding therapy in individual patients, they must be proven to be specific, detecting only patients who will do badly and never incorrectly identifying as hopeless a patient who would do well. It is far worse to not treat a patient who would otherwise have done well than it is to continue to treat a patient who eventually has a poor outcome.

Clinical assessment

Clinical prognostic factors include the nature of the primary injury, the initial GCS score, and the severity of subsequent insults such as hypoxia and hypotension. Although often unreliable in predicting outcome from trauma, clinical signs are important in certain situations. Any patient who presents to the emergency department without vital signs is unlikely to survive. If the cause is an acute hypoxic event the chance of survival in the absence of systemic hypothermia is zero. Clinical assessment becomes more accurate with the passage of time. This is particularly true in patients with hypoxic ischaemic insults and some metabolic substrate injuries. Hypoglycaemic coma persisting beyond four hours after appropriate resuscitation is associated with a very high chance of residual neurological deficit. Similarly, failure to recover consciousness within 24 h of a hypoxic ischaemic event is of grave significance. On the other hand, in traumatic

154

head injury there may be eventual complete recovery even in cases where coma persists for more than a week.

The accuracy of the first GCS score is of vital importance and it is possible that the relative failure of the GCS as an outcome predictor is in part due to poor technique. When first assessed in the emergency department, the patient may suffer from a variety of conditions leading to a false overestimation of brain injury severity. Conditions which worsen the apparent clinical state include unrecognised seizures, uncorrected hypoxaemia or hypovolaemia, pain, hypothermia, hypoglycaemia, and action of drugs including sedatives, opioids, and skeletal muscle relaxants. It is therefore important to correct all of these problems prior to assigning the "true" initial GCS. As a generalisation, a lower GCS after appropriate resuscitation is associated with a worse primary injury and higher chance of an unfavourable outcome. Furthermore, the motor component of the GCS is more predictive of the outcome than the total score and it is therefore useful to express the score in categories in the following style: motor 2, eyes 1, vocalisation 1. Beca *et al.* reported a large series of children with severe brain injury from varied causes and showed a 25% unfavourable outcome in children who could localise pain (motor score 6) at presentation and a 47% favourable outcome in children whose best motor response was extensor posturing (motor score 2).[24] Prognosis is, however, more predictable in patients with an initial postresuscitation GCS of 3; absence of motor response in the non-sedated, non-paralysed patient is a specific predictor of unfavourable outcome.[24] In other situations the GCS score allows little confidence in assigning prognosis in individual patients.

It has been shown that hypotension markedly increases morbidity and mortality in patients with traumatic brain injuries but not in traumatised patients without brain injuries. Hypotension, not corrected prior to arrival at the hospital emergency department, indicates a worse prognosis than in those patients where blood pressure is normalised in the prehospital phase. A single event of systolic hypotension below 90 mmHg in adults increases mortality by 150%.[25] In children with severe head injuries, it has been shown that patients who suffered neither hypoxia nor hypotension had a survival rate four times that of children who had suffered either secondary insult.[26] Hypotension was found to be the dominant factor influencing outcome in this study.

Computed tomography

CT has not been shown to be a reliable early predictor of outcome in children. Signs of a shearing injury, evidenced by scattered small intracerebral haemorrhages, the presence of intracerebral and subdural haematomas, and diffuse brain swelling with ablation of the basal cisterns are all poor prognostic features. However, there have been sufficient numbers of patients who have had a good outcome despite having one or all of these features to make CT an unreliable guide for clinical decision making.

Somatosensory evoked potentials and electroencephalography

Somatosensory evoked potentials (SEP) are recorded over the sensory cortex following stimulation of a peripheral nerve and are assessed in terms of delay or absence. Beca et al., in a study of children with a variety of acute brain disorders, found that by excluding patients with a physical barrier to cutaneous reception, SEP measured within four days of injury could accurately predict poor outcome in 100% of patients.[24] Outcome was assessed at a minimum of six months however, and, as will be discussed, progress after traumatic injury commonly continues after this time.

The EEG has not traditionally been used as a prognostic tool in head injured patients as it has not been found to correlate with outcome. Gutling et al. demonstrated, in a series of adult patients, that interpretation of EEG reactivity to external stimuli could predict outcome following head injury. Accurate poor outcome prediction at 18 months was made in 92% of cases.[27] It was a superior method to interpretation of SEP but use of both methods had added specificity. SEP was not as accurate as it has been found to be by Beca and this may, in part, be explained by the longer follow up. EEG reactivity requires interpretation and therefore lacks the precision that may be required for it to become an accepted prognostication method. The use of neurophysiological tools to guide withdrawal of treatment remains an individual decision for clinicians.

Long term outcome

Following acute brain injury children may have deficits in mobility, cognitive skills, language, memory, and social abilities. Following discharge from hospital the likelihood of subsequent further recovery in survivors of severe brain injury is largely related to the nature of the primary injury, residual structural damage, the GOS at the time of discharge, and duration of coma.

As has been discussed, there are several acute brain insults in which the clinical picture correlates poorly with outcome. Children may develop deep coma secondary to hepatic encephalopathy and make a full recovery after successful liver transplantation. The response of the brain to trauma is quite different to all other acute insults. Children who survive a severe head injury generally show continued improvement, sometimes of a remarkable

156

degree, and much of the recovery occurs in the first year. Jaffe *et al.* have documented steady improvement in areas such as intelligence, problem solving, memory, academic and motor performance, and attainment of living skills over the first 12 months after injury.[28] Rates of improvement tend to plateau after this time though further recovery may continue for several years. Most intensive care units have experience of children who, having survived a stormy course of intracranial hypertension and prolonged coma following head trauma, leave the intensive care unit in a severely disabled state and yet make a near full recovery.

The outcome from hypoxic ischaemic insults is much more clear and predictable. Motor and cognitive outcome is closely linked to duration of coma. Patients unconscious for greater than 24 h have a poor prognosis. In a series of 25 children who suffered severe anoxic brain injury and remained comatose 24 h following the insult, 72% were profoundly impaired when assessed at 12 months.[29] Near drowning appears to have specific outcome characteristics that are worse than other anoxic insults. In Kriel's study no survivor of near drowning, who remained unconscious for 24 h, progressed past the smiling stage and none were ambulatory at 12 months and the majority remained in a persistent vegetative state.[29] Although progress from a hypoxic injury related persistent vegetative state does occur up to nine months following the event, very few patients can be expected to become independent subsequently.[30] Patients with bacterial meningitis have a poorer prognosis if there are persisting focal neurological deficits, focal or intractable generalised seizures or coma beyond 2–3 days. In other forms of coma associated with acute disturbances in serum electrolytes, persistence of coma after correction of the metabolic disturbance suggests a poorer outcome.

Structural lesions following traumatic or vascular events are generally defined by CT and occasionally by magnetic resonance imaging. Focal lesions, including subdural, extradural, and intracerebral haemorrhages, are associated with an increased risk of seizures and may correlate with focal neurological deficits such as hemiplegia. The final outcome is also dependent on coexistent diffuse brain injuries. Ross *et al.*, in a study comparing adult head injured patients with and without focal abnormalities on CT, found that those with focal abnormalities had impaired neuropsychological performance in the short term. The two groups performed similarly at 12 months, however.[31] Radiological signs of acute infarction following vascular events also correlate poorly with final neurological outcome as significant clinical improvement is often seen after the acute phase.

Outcome using the GOS is described as good if the patient can return to a full and independent life, despite minimal deficits. Moderate disability includes patients with significant neurological or intellectual impairment but who are still independent. A severely disabled patient has recovery of consciousness but is totally dependent on others for daily activities. A persistent vegetative state is one where the patient has no meaningful interaction with the environment, although there may be some apparent sleep/wake cycles, eye opening, chewing, and swallowing; this patient is totally dependent on full time care. Massagli *et al.* found that good late outcome at 5–7 years after traumatic brain injury in children was best predicted by the early GOS.[32]

The duration of coma also strongly correlates to the degree of final recovery. Of children in a persistent vegetative state 30 days following traumatic injury, Heindl and Laub found 34% had regained some degree of responsiveness by three months; 63% had made the same step by six months and 80% by 12 months. However, very few improved after 12 months and only 15% had become independent in daily life by 19 months following the injury.[30] Of another group of children who were unconscious 90 days after a variety of brain insults, more than 50% remained in a persistent vegetative state or had limited social responsiveness at nine months.[33] Only one patient in this series became independent; this patient suffered a traumatic injury. Following anoxic injury it has been found that children who were eventually able to communicate at 12 months after the insult were conscious within 60 days and all those who were able to walk were conscious within 30 days.[29]

Outcomes assessed as good at discharge or even at several years from injury may not translate to good long term outcome. Massagli identified four of 10 patients discharged with a GOS indicative of good recovery who received a lower score at follow up; this deterioration was due largely to personality and academic problems related to limited concentration.[32] Despite a normal neurological state and near normal intelligence, adults who suffered a brain injury in childhood may still not function in society. It has been found that they can find gaining and maintaining employment difficult because of memory or personality disturbances.[34]

Rehabilitation

The rehabilitation process should commence early so that there is a seamless progression from intensive care to ward based care. The physiotherapist is often involved in the acute management and their role should evolve into dealing with long term issues such as maintenance of joint mobility and appropriate posturing. A rehabilitation physician should direct a coordinated rehabilitation programme for all patients who leave the intensive care unit with residual neurological problems. This will ensure that the programme is optimal and that issues such as seizure control and hypertonia are addressed. The team should consist of physiotherapists, speech, and occupational therapists and have the services of teachers and clinical psychologists.

1 Maytal JS, Moshe SL, Alvarez LA. Low morbidity and mortality of status epilepticus in children. *Pediatrics* 1989;**83**:323–31.
2 Krausz MM. Controversies in shock research: hypertonic resuscitation – pros and cons. *Shock* 1995;**3**:69–72.
3 Sheikk AA, Matsuoka T, Wisner DH. Cerebral effects of resuscitation with hypertonic saline and a new low-sodium hypertonic fluid in haemorrhagic shock and head injury. *Crit Care Med* 1996;**24**:1226–32.
4 Taylor G, Myers S, Kurth CD, *et al*. Hypertonic saline improves brain resuscitation in a paediatric model of head injury and haemorrhagic shock. *J Pediatr Surg* 1996;**31**:65–70.
5 Temkin NR, Dikmen SS, Wilensky AJ *et al*. A randomised, double-blind study for the prevention of post-traumatic seizures. *N Engl J Med* 1990;**323**:497–502.
6 Dikmen SS Temkin NR, Miller B, Machamer J, Winn HR. Neurobehavioural effects of phenytoin prophylaxis of post-traumatic seizures. *JAMA* 1991;**265**:1271–7.
7 Bullock R, *et al*. Guidelines for cerebral perfusion pressure. Brain Trauma Foundation. *J Neurotrauma* 1996;**13**:639–734.
8 Fortune JB, Feustel PJ, Graca L, Hasselbarth J, Keuhler DH. Effect of hyperventilation, mannitol, and ventriculostomy drainage on cerebral blood flow after head injury. *J Trauma* 1995;**39**:1091–7.
9 Feldman Z, Kanter MJ, Robertson CS, *et al*. Effect of head elevation on intracranial pressure, cerebral perfusion pressure, and cerebral blood flow in head-injured patients. *J Neurosurg* 1992;**76**:207–11.
10 Rosner MJ Colwy IB. Cerebral perfusion pressure, intracranial pressure, and head elevation. *J Neurosurg* 1986;**65**:636–41.
11 Eisenberg HM, *et al*. High-dose barbiturate control of elevated intracranial pressure in patients with severe head injury. *J Neurosurg* 1988;**69**:15–23.
12 Russo H, Bressolle F, Duboin MP. Pharmacokinetics of high-dose thiopental in pediatric patients with increased intracranial pressure. *Ther Drug Monit* 1997;**19**:63–70.
13 Marrion DW, Penrod LE, Kelsey SF, *et al*. Treatment of traumatic brain injury with moderate hypothermia. *N Engl J Med* 1997;**336**:540–6.
14 Metz C, Holzschuh M, Bein T, *et al*. Moderate hypothermia in patients with severe head injury: cerebral and extracerebral effects. *J Neurosurg* 1996;**85**:533–41.
15 Sharples PM, Stuart AG, Matthews DS, Aynsley-Green A, Eyre JA. Cerebral blood flow in children with severe head injury. Part 1: relation to age, Glasgow coma score, outcome, intracranial pressure, and time after injury. *J Neurol Neurosurg Psychiatr* 1995;**58**:145–52.
16 Muizelaar JP, Marmarou A, Ward JD, *et al*. Adverse effects of prolonged hyperventilation in patients with severe head injury: a randomized trial. *J Neurosurg* 1991;**75**:731–9
17 Robertson CS, Gopinath SP, Goodman JC, *et al*. SjvO2 monitoring in head-injured patients. *J Neurotrauma* 1995;**12**:891–6.
18 Lewis SB, Myburgh JA, Reilly PL. Detection of cerebral venous desaturation by continuous jugular bulb oximetry following acute neurotrauma. *Anaesth Intens Care* 1995;**23**:307–14.
19 Cho DY, Wang YC, Chi CS. Decompressive craniotomy for acute shaken/impact baby syndrome. *Pediatr Neurosurg* 1995;**23**:192–8.
20 Le Roux PD, Jardine DS, Kanev PM, Loeser JD. Pediatric intracranial pressure monitoring in hypoxic and non-hypoxic brain injury. *Child's Nerv Syst* 1991;**7**:34–9.
21 Biggart MJ, Bohn DJ. Effect of hypothermia and cardiac arrest on outcome of near-drowning accidents in children. *J Pediatr* 1990;**117**:179–83.
22 Schaad UB, Lips U, Gnehm HE, *et al*. Dexamethasone therapy for bacterial meningitis in children. *Lancet* 1993;**342**:457–61.
23 Jennet B, Bond M. Assessment of outcome after severe brain injury: a practical scale. *Lancet* 1975;**1**:480–4.
24 Beca J, Cox PN, Taylor MJ, *et al*. Somatosensory evoked potentials for prediction of outcome in acute severe brain injury. *J Pediatr* 1994;**126**:44–9.

25 Chesnut RM, Marshall LF, Klauber MR, *et al.* The role of secondary brain injury in determining outcome from severe head injury. *J Trauma* 1993;**34**:216–22.
26 Pigula FA, Wald SL, Shackford SR, Vane DW. The effect of hypotension and hypoxia on children with severe head injuries. *J Pediatr Surg* 1993;**28**:315–6.
27 Gutling E, Gonser A, Imhof H-G, Landis T. EEG reactivity in the prognosis of severe head injury. *Neurology* 1995;**45**:915–8.
28 Jaffe KM, Polissar NL, Fay GC, Liao S. Recovery trends over three years following pediatric traumatic brain injury. *Arch Phys Med Rehab* 1995;**76**:17–26.
29 Kriel RL, Krach LE, Luxenberg MG, Jones-Saete C, Sanchez J. Outcome of severe anoxic/ischaemic brain injury in children. *Pediatr Neurol* 1994;**10**:207–12.
30 Heindl UT, Laub MC. Outcome of persistent vegetative state following hypoxic or traumatic brain injury in children and adolescents. *Neuropediatrics* 1996;**27**:94–100.
31 Ross BL, Temkin NR, Newell D, Dikmen SS. Neuropsychological outcome in relation to head injury severity. *Am J Phys Med Rehab* 1994;**73**:341–7.
32 Massagli TL, Michaud LJ, Rivara FP. Association between injury indices and outcome after severe traumatic brain injury in children. *Arch Phys Med Rehab* 1996;**77**:125–32.
33 Kriel RL, Krach LE, Jones-Saete C. Outcome of children with prolonged unconsciousness and vegetative states. *Pediatr Neurol* 1993;**9**:362–8.
34 Koskiniemi M, Kyykka T, Nybo T, Jarho L. Long-term outcome after severe brain injury in pre-schoolers is worse than expected. *Arch Pediatr Adolesc Med* 1995;**149**:249–54.

7: Perioperative management of infants with congenital heart disease

DUNCAN MACRAE, STEPHEN SCUPLAK

Congenital heart disease (CHD) is estimated to occur in between 0.55% and 0.86% of liveborn infants. Over half of these lesions are diagnosed in the first week of life and without treatment, mortality approaches 50% in the first year.

Presentation of congenital heart disease

Congenital heart disease, if not diagnosed by antenatal foetal ultrasound scanning, is usually diagnosed in the newborn period. Despite the variety of conditions, congenital heart disease presents in relatively few ways (table 7.1) and is the most frequent cause of admission of term neonates to intensive care.

Cyanosis due to congenital heart disease is usually suspected clinically and confirmed by blood gas analysis or pulse oximetry. Cyanosis caused by intrapulmonary shunting of blood is diminished by oxygen administration, whereas obligatory intra- or extracardiac shunting due to CHD is not (the basis for the so-called hyperoxic test). Neonates with persistent pulmonary hypertension of the newborn, but normal cardiac anatomy, present with severe cyanosis. Right to left shunting of blood is caused by failure of the pulmonary vascular resistance to fall at birth. In such infants, congenital heart disease can only be excluded reliably by echocardiography.

Neonates with CHD may present in the newborn period with congestive heart failure or severe circulatory shock. Presentation may be at birth or, more usually, delayed, often related to closure of the ductus arteriosus, e.g. aortic coarctation, or the postnatal fall in pulmonary vascular resistance,

TABLE 7.1—*Presentation of common congenital heart lesions*

	Causes
Central cyanosis	Transposition of the great vessels Fallot's tetralogy Critical pulmonary stenosis Pulmonary or tricuspid atresia Obstructed total anomalous pulmonary venous drainage (exclude persistent pulmonary hypertension of the newborn)
Congestive heart failure *Signs* Tachypnoea Tachycardia Hepatomegaly Cardiomegaly Cardiovascular collapse Failure to thrive	Patent ductus arteriosus Hypoplastic left heart syndrome Coarctation of the aorta Ventriculoseptal defects Unobstructed TAPVD AV fistulae/connections Critical aortic stenosis Congenital brady/tachyarrhythmias
Abnormal heart rate	Congenital heart block Congenital brady/tachyarrhythmias
Murmurs	Non-critical aortic or pulmonary stenosis All types of septal defect Patent ductus arteriosus "Innocent" murmurs
Tracheobronchial compression	Double aortic arch Anomalous left subclavian artery Absent pulmonary valve syndrome Pulmonary artery sling

e.g. abnormal AV connections, large septal defects. After basic resuscitative measures, the cardiac origin of shock should be confirmed and other causes of neonatal cardiorespiratory collapse, such as sepsis and metabolic abnormalities, excluded.

Other congenital abnormalities may occur in association with cardiac defects.[1] Of particular relevance to the paediatric intensivist is trisomy 21 (Down's syndrome), in which problems of upper airway obstruction and cervical spine instability may accompany the cardiac lesion. Di George syndrome, characterised by thymic aplasia, T cell deficiency and hypocalcaemia, is commonly associated with interrupted aortic arch and truncus arteriosus. Babies presenting with these lesions should be assumed to have associated Di George until normal lymphocyte subsets have been demonstrated. Plasma calcium levels must be carefully maintained and transfusion of viable leucocytes avoided by irradiation of cellular blood products to prevent graft versus host disease.

Early management of CHD

Neonates with a provisional diagnosis of congenital heart disease often require transportation to a regional paediatric cardiac centre for definitive diagnosis or further management. Transportation should never be undertaken without full resuscitation of the infant or by personnel not appropriately trained or equipped. Ideally, specialised transport teams should be used. All neonates should be transported in an incubator to facilitate temperature regulation, oxygen supplementation, and mechanical ventilation. Reliable venous access should be established prior to transfer. Temperature, ECG, and oximetric saturation must be monitored during transport of any infant. Invasive blood pressure measurement is recommended in all but the most stable cardiac transfers.

If there is any possibility of a duct dependent circulation, the infant must receive prostaglandin E1 (alprostadil) or E2 (dinoprostone) 5–30 ng/kg/min by continuous IV infusion to prevent duct closure. At higher doses prostaglandins may induce apnoea. Respiration must be closely monitored and if transfer to a regional centre is required, elective mechanical ventilation considered.

The general principles of resuscitation, *Airway-Breathing-Circulation*, should be applied to any critically ill neonate or child. The goals and limitations of resuscitation may require modification as the nature of the cardiac lesion is revealed. Babies presenting to specialist units must be rapidly assessed and resuscitated as clinically indicated, *before* further intensive investigation by echocardiography or cardiac catheterisation. The neonatal heart is significantly less compliant than that of the older child, being composed of a greater proportion of inelastic membrane mass and less contractile tissue. The immature neonatal myocardium cannot compensate well for increased afterload. The functional relationship of the ventricles is extremely close in the neonate and failure of one ventricle rapidly induces septal shift and consequent failure of the other ventricle. The small, non-compliant ventricles are limited in their ability to increase stroke volume and cardiac output is therefore increasingly dependent on heart rate. The unique pathophysiological problems of CHD are likely to be poorly tolerated by the neonate.

General postoperative considerations

Postoperatively, the patient should be transferred to the intensive care unit with minimal interruption in the monitoring of vital signs. Both surgeon and anaesthetist must communicate details of the surgical procedure and

163

patient status to the ICU team. The importance of good communication in the effective delivery of intensive care should not be underestimated. The admitting intensivist must follow this handover with a rapid assessment of the patient, as outlined in fig 7.1.

In the early postoperative period, a urinary catheter facilitates accurate monitoring of both fluid balance and renal function. Temporary atrial and ventricular pacing wires should be positioned intraoperatively during complex open heart surgery. These facilitate cardiac pacing and may also assist in the accurate ECG diagnosis (atrial electrocardiogram) and treatment (by overdrive pacing) of some postoperative rhythm disturbances.

Analgesia is required in patients of all ages following cardiac surgery[2] and may be provided by a continuous morphine infusion (neonates 5–15 µg/kg/h, children 10–40 µg/kg/h). Additional sedation may be safely achieved with midazolam (1–5 µg/kg/min by continuous IV infusion). Profound analgesia may be required in patients with acute haemodynamic instability, especially those with reactive pulmonary hypertension, and a suitable agent is the opioid fentanyl (5–20 µg/kg slow bolus followed by an IV infusion of 2–10 µg/kg/h). Neuromuscular blockade may occasionally be indicated in critically unstable patients after cardiac surgery. Intravenous infusions of vecuronium or atracurium achieve this with minimal haemodynamic perturbation.

Children with heart failure and those following cardiopulmonary bypass (CPB) are relatively fluid overloaded. We routinely restrict postoperative fluid intake as detailed in fig 7.2. Large potassium fluxes occur perioperatively, predisposing to rhythm disturbances. Plasma potassium should be closely monitored and maintained between 3.8 and 4.5 mmol/l. Ionised calcium levels frequently fall after CPB, especially in neonates with limited reserves, and intravenous supplementation must be guided by frequent blood analysis.

Many infants presenting for surgery are nutritionally depleted as a result of failure to thrive, induced by cardiac disease. Attempts to correct malnutrition must be made preoperatively and it is of paramount importance that nutrition is established at the earliest opportunity postoperatively. Enteral feeding can usually be reintroduced within 24 hours of surgery and if not tolerated, is an indication for early parenteral supplementation.

There is clear evidence that perioperative antibiotic cover reduces the incidence of wound infection. Antibiotics should be commenced prior to surgical incision and continued for 24 hours. A combination of flucloxacillin and gentamicin provides adequate prophylaxis against the bacterial pathogens commonly associated with wound infections.[3,4] In those sensitive to penicillin, alternatives are vancomycin or teicoplanin with gentamicin. There is little evidence to support longer term prophylaxis and clinical vigilance coupled with appropriate laboratory investigations should direct

Handover from operating team – surgeon and anaesthetist

Circulation
- Perform clinical examination
- Assess monitoring data
- Note current cardiovascular drug regime

Ventilation
- Clinical assessment
- Note mechanical ventilator settings
- Arterial blood gas analysis

Chest *x* ray
- Lung fields
  focal pathology
  perfusion
- Pleura
  effusion or pneumothorax
- Check "devices"
  endotracheal tube
  nasogastric tube
  chest drains
  pacing wires
  central venous/PA/LA lines

Laboratory data
- Arterial blood gas analysis
- Plasma potassium, calcium
- Glucose
- Haemoglobin
- Blood count and coagulation (only in bleeding patients)

Drugs
- Analgesia
- Sedatives
- Neuromuscular blockade

Parents
- Inform parents of admission status

FIGURE 7.1—*Postsurgical ICU admission checklist*

Normal daily fluid requirement

Body weight (kg)	Daily requirements
<10	100 ml/kg
10–20	1000 ml + 50 ml for each kg above 10 kg
>20	1500 ml + 20 ml for each kg above 20 kg

A. FLUIDS AFTER OPEN HEART SURGERY
Type of fluid
Age: 0–30 days 10% glucose 3 mmol KCl in each 50 ml
Over 30 days 5% glucose + KCl

Day 1 (Day of surgery)
Total fluid intake is restricted to 50% of normal

Subsequent days
(a) If pulmonary and/or systemic oedema are not present, fluid intake is gradually increased to achieve full maintenance requirements over a 2–3 day period.
(b) If pulmonary and/or systemic oedema are present, fluid restriction is maintained. Further management may indicate diuretics or peritoneal dialysis if renal function is impaired.

B. FLUIDS AFTER CLOSED HEART SURGERY
Type of fluid
10% glucose is used in infants and 0.18% saline in 4% glucose in children + KCl.

Day 1
Total fluid intake is restricted to 60% of normal maintenance in:
(a) infants with recent history of heart failure
(b) infants after shunt and/or valvotomy procedures with signs of increased pulmonary blood flow.

In others, total fluid intake is restricted to 75% of normal maintenance.

Subsequent days
Fluid intake is liberalised as indicated clinically.

Neonates
Fluid requirements of premature infants are higher than term neonates. Calculate as 120 ml/kg/day initially. Increase fluid intake of infants receiving phototherapy by 30%.

FIGURE 7.2—*Postoperative fluid requirements*

further therapy. Parents must be informed if there is a need for future antibiotic prophylaxis in the prevention of endocarditis.

Perioperative management of specific lesions

The general principles of resuscitation and intensive care are as relevant to cardiac patients as they are to other areas of children's intensive care. The intensivist, as part of a multidisciplinary medical team including surgeon and cardiologist, must not only apply these general principles, but also optimise treatment of specific lesions through knowledge of their individual pathophysiology.[5]

Pulmonary recirculatory ("left to right") shunts

By far the commonest grouping of congenital cardiac lesions are those such as patent ductus arteriosus (PDA), ventricular septal defect (VSD), atrial septal defect (ASD), and atrioventricular septal defect (AVSD) in which blood normally destined for the systemic circulation is shunted through the defect, resulting in increased pulmonary blood flow. The recirculation of shunted blood leads to volume loading of the left ventricle, progressive cardiomegaly and left ventricular failure. The pulmonary vascular bed responds to increased flow with vasoconstriction, leading to pulmonary hypertension and increased pulmonary arteriolar muscularisation. Failure to reduce the excessive pulmonary blood flow, by closure of the relevant lesion, encourages this muscularisation to progress to irreversible fibrosis and late reversal of the shunt, the Eisenmenger syndrome.

Isolated persistent ductus arteriosus

Persistence of the arterial duct (PDA) is unusual in term infants. It is often clinically silent, the classic machinery murmur only developing as infancy progresses. Ductal patency is much more common in premature infants in whom conservative management, consisting of fluid restriction, diuretics, and attempted induction of ductal closure with indomethacin, may be unsuccessful. In the symptomatic premature infant, failed medical therapy is an indication for prompt surgical closure. Surgical access is gained via a left thoracotomy and the duct clipped or ligated. PDA in an older child can be occluded surgically or during cardiac catheter, using a specifically designed occlusion device. After closure of the duct, recovery

167

of ventilator dependent premature neonates can be dramatic once the adverse respiratory consequences of the large shunt and left ventricular failure abate. Asymptomatic older children undergoing surgical duct closure rarely need intensive care, but the provision of effective analgesia and observation in a high dependency area are recommended.

Atrial septal defect

Usually this produces no symptoms and is diagnosed by the discovery of a murmur during routine medical examinations. Volume overload of the right atrium and ventricle results in dilation and hypertrophy. Pulmonary vascular disease can develop and for this reason, closure of the defect is usually undertaken before school entry.

Elective surgical closure of the defect is performed on cardiopulmonary bypass either through a median sternotomy or (especially in girls) a right thoracotomy. Recovery is usually uncomplicated and ventilation for more than four hours is unusual. Right atrial dilation may compromise sinus node function and atrial conduction, predisposing to arrhythmias that increase in incidence with age at repair.

Ventriculoseptal defects

Large VSDs which are not "restrictive" and therefore do not limit the amount of shunted blood present in early infancy with cardiac failure and failure to thrive. These lesions require surgical repair or occasionally palliation, by pulmonary artery banding during the first year of life and delayed definitive repair. Smaller "restrictive" defects, especially those of the muscular septum, may close spontaneously as the child grows. Late repair or very large shunts predispose to the problem of reactive pulmonary hypertension in the early postoperative period.

Atrioventriculoseptal defects (AVSD) include a spectrum of cardiac malformations characterised by varying degrees of incomplete development of the interatrial and interventricular septae and the atrioventricular valves. AVSD is the most common cardiac anomaly in children with Down's syndrome. In the "partial form" the predominant lesion is essentially a "primum" atrioseptal defect, with a natural history, surgical and intensive care course similar to simple ("secundum") ASD.

So-called "complete" AVSDs present in early infancy in a manner similar to unrestrictive VSDs. They are usually managed by repair on cardiopulmonary bypass in the first year of life. Of particular note for the intensivist are the possible association of Down's syndrome and preoperative

168

nutritional impairment as a result of failure to thrive. Postoperatively, acute elevations of pulmonary artery pressure may occur, particularly after "late" repair. Residual left AV valve regurgitation may compromise recovery by reducing effective left ventricular stroke volume and increasing pulmonary venous pressure. Reoperation for repair or replacement of the mitral valve may then be indicated.

Truncus arteriosus

This condition arises as a result of failure in the division between the aorta and the pulmonary artery. Usually a single multicusped valve opens into the aorta and is often stenosed and regurgitant. The lesion is always associated with a VSD. Physiologically, as PVR falls, there is unrestricted pulmonary blood flow resulting in pulmonary vascular disease and left ventricular volume overload. Repair is needed in the first months of life and involves reconstruction of the great vessels with the aid of a homograft between the right ventricle and pulmonary artery and closure of the VSD. In addition to pulmonary hypertension, postoperative problems can include ventricular failure due to truncal valve regurgitation.

Total anomalous pulmonary venous drainage

This occurs when the pulmonary veins are directed to the right side of the heart instead of the left atrium. An ASD is always present, allowing flow into the left ventricle. Pulmonary hypertension can develop rapidly from the increased pulmonary blood flow and particularly if pulmonary venous flow is obstructed. Obstructed venous flow usually presents preoperatively and gives rise to severe pulmonary oedema, hypoxaemia and pulmonary hypertension. Urgent surgery must be undertaken to relieve obstructive lesions. Postoperatively, increased pulmonary vascular reactivity and hypertension are major concerns.

Acyanotic obstructive lesions

Coarctation of the aorta

This condition, a congenital narrowing of the aorta in the periductal region, presents in two ways. Neonates present acutely with severe congestive heart failure and absent or diminished femoral pulses. Presentation is brought about by closure of the arterial duct and the key

169

to resuscitation is the administration of prostaglandin E1 in an attempt to reopen the duct. Other resuscitative measures include mechanical ventilation, intravascular volume expansion, and inotropic support. Provided the infant responds adequately, repair can be delayed 12–24 hours. Failure to respond implies failure of the duct to reopen and is an indication for immediate repair. Intraarterial monitoring cannulae must be placed in the right upper limb, as the aorta is crossclamped during repair and pressures lost in the other limbs.

In older children, coarctation rarely produces symptoms and is detected during routine medical examination. Elective repair is indicated to prevent the gradual onset of left ventricular failure.

Systemic hypertension frequently follows coarctation repair. In the neonate, hypertension can usually be managed with a continuous infusion of the vasodilator sodium nitroprusside (0.5–5 mg/kg/min) and resolution is expected within 24–48 hours. Hypertension is more persistent in older children and may require longer term antihypertensive therapy with β blockers. Paraplegia, secondary to spinal cord ischaemia, is a rare but devastating complication of coarctation repair. After repair the intensivist should observe the return of lower limb function, as well as noting the presence of good volume femoral pulses. In severely affected neonates, perioperative systemic hypoperfusion may precipitate renal failure or abdominal complications, such as ileus or necrotising enterocolitis. Postoperative ventilation and cardiovascular support are usually required in neonates to promote cardiovascular recovery, but are not required in older children.

Aortic stenosis

The presentation and intensive care management of neonatal aortic stenosis is similar to coarctation of the aorta. Critical aortic stenosis presents in the early neonatal period with severe cardiovascular compromise. In such cases, systemic perfusion is dependent on patency of the arterial duct. Critical aortic stenosis usually produces severe left ventricular dysfunction in combination with a relatively hypoplastic left ventricle and is still associated with a significant mortality.[6] Treatment is by surgical valvotomy or balloon dilation. A high level of cardiovascular support is to be expected in the perioperative period. Reoperation or valve replacement is often required later in life.

Children or young adults with less severe aortic valve disease are often asymptomatic, although left ventricular failure or angina may eventually develop. Older patients may undergo valvotomy, valve repair or replacement, with either a prosthetic valve or a pulmonary autograft (Ross procedure). Postoperative recovery is uneventful unless left ventricular function is severely compromised. Anticoagulation is required after all prosthetic valve implants, with heparin commenced on the second postoperative day, until oral anticoagulation is established.

Pulmonary valve stenosis

This is relatively common, representing approximately 10% of all cardiac malformations. It has both cyanotic and non-cyanotic presentations, depending on severity and associated lesions. Severe stenosis presents with cyanosis in the first days of life, as the arterial duct closes. In the presence of normal pulmonary arterial connections, severe stenosis is managed by surgical valvotomy. Persistent cyanosis after effective valvotomy suggests that the right ventricle is hypoplastic or failing to relax adequately. Under these circumstances, prostaglandin should be continued postoperatively to maintain duct patency and pulmonary blood flow, until RV function improves. A systemic–pulmonary shunt may ultimately be required. Serial echocardiographic examinations will assist in quantifying ductal and pulmonary blood flow.

Mild or moderate degrees of pulmonary stenosis are usually asymptomatic, but must be relieved before severe RV hypertrophy or failure occurs. Balloon dilation of the pulmonary valve performed under general anaesthesia has a high success rate, particularly in infants over 1 year of age. Children undergoing this procedure rarely require intensive care although temporary RV dysfunction can occur.

Vascular abnormalities

Abnormal branches of the aortic arch may encircle the trachea and oesophagus, presenting in various ways during infancy. Commonly, a double aortic arch is present, the two limbs combining to form the descending aorta. Tracheal compression results in respiratory symptoms and predisposes to recurrent chest infections. Other abnormalities include an anomalous pulmonary artery or sling and absent pulmonary valve syndrome (the dilated right ventricular outflow tract frequently compresses the main airways). Surgical correction of the vascular abnormality may not abolish all respiratory symptoms, as airway compression predisposes to tracheobronchomalacia. Symptomatic airway collapse may be managed with tracheal or nasal CPAP (continuous positive airway pressure). Bronchoscopy and dynamic airway imaging are useful in confirming the diagnosis and monitoring response to treatment. Occasionally the degree of tracheal and particularly bronchial pathology may prove unmanageable. Dysphagia, due to oesophageal compression, may present initially but rarely persists postoperatively.

171

Cyanotic lesions

Transposition of the Great Arteries

Transposition of the great arteries (TGA) is the commonest cyanotic lesion presenting in the newborn period. In this condition, the aorta arises from the right ventricle and the pulmonary artery from the left. This parallel arrangement of systemic and pulmonary circulations can only sustain life if mixing of blood from the two circulations occurs through a shunt. Possible shunts include a patent foramen ovale, arterial duct or a VSD. Although cyanosis is present at birth in the absence of associated VSD, severe circulatory insufficiency and severe hypoxaemia only occur once the arterial duct closes. Neonates with TGA without VSD (simple TGA) can be palliated by maintenance of duct patency with prostaglandin. Atrial mixing can be improved by percutaneous balloon atrial septostomy.[7] A simple TGA is usually repaired by arterial switch operation within the first two weeks of life, as late repair runs the risk of significant involution of the left ventricle. There is less urgency in cases of TGA-VSD as the left ventricle continues to be exposed to systemic pressure. TGA-VSD is usually repaired by arterial switch and closure of the VSD, before the second month of life.

Following repair, diastolic ventricular function is often poor and as a result, volume overload is poorly tolerated and cardiac output is relatively rate dependent. Left atrial pressures must be maintained at the lowest level consistent with a clinically adequate cardiac output, typically 4–8 mmHg, monitored with the aid of a surgically placed left atrial line. Pulmonary hypertension may complicate the postoperative period, especially after relatively late repair of TGA-VSD.

Correction of a transposition can be achieved at atrial level with a Mustard[8] or Senning "atrial switch" operation. These procedures result in the morphological right ventricle remaining permanently as the systemic ventricle and systemic venous blood diverted by intraatrial baffles into the left "pulmonary" ventricle. Following atrial switch operations, hypovolaemia, bradycardias, and non-sinus rhythms are poorly tolerated and right atrial pressures of 10–12 mmHg are desirable. The arterial switch operation is believed to give the best long term results, but may not be possible if presentation is delayed (as left ventricular involution ensues) or if the coronary artery anatomy is unfavourable.

Tetralogy of Fallot

Tetralogy of Fallot is a common malformation which combines a VSD, pulmonary stenosis, right ventricular hypertrophy, and overriding

172

aorta. Cyanosis may be present in the neonatal period, but is more commonly of gradual onset during the first year of life. Its severity is determined by the degree of right ventricular outflow obstruction, as this dictates the amount of right to left shunting of blood through the VSD. Right ventricular outflow obstruction occurs at the level of the pulmonary valve and also from hypertrophy of the infundibular musculature. Spasm of the muscular infundibulum gives rise to acute RV outflow obstruction and is responsible for the hypercyanotic "spells" which may threaten life. Treatment of hypercyanotic spells is aimed at increasing pulmonary blood flow by raising systemic vascular resistance and reducing infundibular spasm. This is achieved by placing the child in the knee–chest position, administering oxygen, sedation, and fluid to maintain RV filling. Vasopressors such as metaraminol (0.1 mg/kg) or noradrenaline by infusion (0.05–0.4 µg/kg/min) reduce right to left shunting by raising systemic vascular resistance, thereby improving oxygenation. The β blocker propranolol (0.1 mg/kg IV) may be used to reduce infundibular spasm.

Fallot's tetralogy is usually repaired surgically in infancy, before the onset of severe cyanosis or frequent hypercyanotic episodes. Severe right ventricular dysfunction may follow repair, especially if a pulmonary transannular patch or large right ventriculotomy has been performed. The latter problems are obviated, where possible, by avoiding transannular patches and by employing a transatrial approach to VSD closure and infundibular resection.

In the presence of a profoundly hypoplastic right ventricle or poorly developed central pulmonary arteries, complete repair is deferred. Under these circumstances a shunt is created from the systemic to pulmonary circulation (modified Blalock–Taussig shunt) to increase pulmonary blood flow. This palliative procedure enables growth to occur and encourages development of the pulmonary arteries. Complete repair can be performed later, if the central pulmonary arteries increase sufficiently in size.

Pulmonary atresia

This usually presents with cyanosis soon after birth because pulmonary blood flow is dependent on a PDA. Management is similar to that of a severe tetralogy of Fallot, with the creation of a systemic–pulmonary shunt. When there is no associated VSD the right ventricular cavity is often atretic.

Surgical procedures

Cardiopulmonary bypass

Ninety five percent of children admitted to our cardiac ICU undergo cardiac surgery, of whom 75% undergo open heart surgery. Such surgery is made possible by employing cardiopulmonary bypass (CPB) systems, consisting of an extracorporeal circuit encompassing a blood circulatory pump and artificial lung. CPB aims to support the circulation to vital organs, whilst isolating the heart and lungs to facilitate surgery. CPB brings blood into contact with non-biological surfaces and imposes additional strategies including haemodilution, hypothermia, and hypothermic circulatory arrest.[9]

Mechanical complications may occur during CPB, including air or particulate embolisation, with the potential for causing myocardial or neurological injury. CPB is widely recognised as a global inflammatory insult, triggering an acute stress response, manifesting as hyperglycaemia, increased systemic vascular resistance, tachycardia, and fluid retention.

A fulminant manifestation of this inflammatory reaction is seen as the "capillary leak syndrome" which can occur, particularly in infants, after prolonged cardiopulmonary bypass. Infants with capillary leak lose fluid from the circulation as a result of increased capillary permeability. Treatment is symptomatic, with the support of intravascular volume by colloid infusion and systemic perfusion by inotropes. It is sometimes necessary to drain pleural effusions and ascites. The condition usually resolves in parallel with the overall clinical progress of the baby.

Other problems, particularly electrolyte disturbances, occur as a result of surgery and CPB. Activation of the renin–angiotensin system, elevation in plasma aldosterone level, and elevated blood glucose levels all contribute to perioperative hypokalaemia. Hypokalaemia facilitates the emergence of arrhythmias and levels need to be closely monitored.

Ionised hypocalcaemia causes peripheral vasodilation, depresses myocardial contractility, and induces hypocalcaemic tetany. Ionised hypocalcaemia is seen in the sick newborn, in babies with hypoparathyroidism associated with the Di George anomaly, and following rapid infusion of citrated blood products. Symptomatic ionised hypocalcaemia should be corrected by administering 0.2 mmol/kg of calcium slowly intravenously and reassessing levels frequently.

Pulmonary artery banding

This is a palliative procedure to reduce excessive pulmonary blood flow by placement of a band or ligature around the main pulmonary artery. The operation aims to protect the pulmonary vasculature from the damaging long term effects of excessive pulmonary blood flow in infants with pulmonary recirculatory shunts. It is indicated in situations where immediate corrective surgery of the underlying shunt is contraindicated.

After banding, pulmonary blood flow is restricted, promoting the flow of blood from right to left and away from the lungs. Typical systemic saturations in babies with effective PA bands range from 70% to 85%. Vasodilators are not well tolerated in the face of a fixed obstruction to pulmonary blood flow. They reduce systemic vascular resistance and induce systemic hypotension, increasing cyanosis by diverting blood away from the lungs. In the absence of focal lung pathology or problems with mechanical ventilation, postoperative saturations below 70% imply excessive restriction to pulmonary blood flow and require urgent reassessment. Severe hypoxaemia, especially if accompanied by a metabolic acidosis, is usually an indication for early reoperation to loosen the band. High saturations (>90%) after PA banding suggest that the band is not sufficiently restrictive. These patients may continue to need treatment with diuretics and possibly require reoperation.

Systemic-pulmonary arterial shunts

These shunts are inserted to increase pulmonary blood flow in infants with lesions such as pulmonary or tricuspid atresia or severe Fallot's tetralogy. The most common are modified Blalock–Taussig shunts, in which a 4–6 mm Gore-Tex tube is anastomosed from the subclavian artery to the pulmonary artery, on the side opposite the aortic arch.

Pulmonary perfusion depends on systemic blood pressures exceeding pulmonary pressures and postoperative systemic hypotension must be avoided. Systemic arterial saturations are typically 70–85%, indicating that pulmonary and systemic blood flow are well balanced. If saturations fall below 70% in the absence of hypotension or abnormal lung function, occlusion of the shunt must be excluded by careful auscultation or Doppler echo. A heparin infusion (10–20 units/kg/h) can be used to maintain shunt patency in high risk cases.

Large shunts may result in excessive pulmonary blood flow, left ventricular failure and pulmonary oedema, which may be unilateral. This situation is usually managed with antifailure measures including fluid restriction and diuretic therapy.

Cannulation of neck veins on the side of a proposed shunt should be avoided, as accidental arterial puncture and subsequent haematoma may obscure the surgical field. Cannulation of the arteries of the ipsilateral arm should be avoided, as these will provide unreliable pressures both during and after the operative procedure.

Fontan operation

In 1968 Fontan successfully performed this procedure for the treatment of tricuspid atresia.[10] It involves connecting the systemic venous return directly onto the pulmonary artery, without an interposed ventricle. Indications for the Fontan and physiologically similar operations (such as the total cavopulmonary connection operation) have been extended to include many conditions with a "single" ventricle and conditions where, despite the presence of two ventricles, complex internal derangements prevent septation of the heart into a biventricular format.

Without a subpulmonary ventricle, blood flow across the lungs is critically dependent on a low transpulmonary gradient (TPG = mean central venous pressure – mean systemic atrial pressure). Preoperative selection of patients for Fontan type operations is crucial. It is imperative that pulmonary arteriolar resistance is low, with good ventricular function to minimise downstream pressure (ejection fraction >0.6 and competent AV valve).

Postoperatively, cardiac output is optimised by maximising systemic venous return. This is achieved with careful volume loading (typical CVP 10–15 mmHg) and by measures to minimise airway pressure, through the careful application of positive pressure ventilation and encouraging the early return of spontaneous ventilation. It is good cardiac intensive care practice to undertake separation from mechanical ventilation as soon as cardiorespiratory stability is achieved. Undue surgical fears about the adverse effects of positive pressure ventilation should be assuaged by the obvious detrimental effects of hypoventilation, atelectasis, and hypoxaemia which will ensue if "early" extubation is unsuccessful. Inotropic agents, such as dobutamine, improve ventricular function and thereby lower left atrial pressure and the transpulmonary gradient. Drugs which increase pulmonary vascular resistance should be avoided. A transpulmonary gradient exceeding 10 mmHg is associated with a high incidence of complications including low cardiac output syndrome and the consequences of raised CVP, which include ascites, pleural effusions, and the vicious circle of lymphatic hypertension, pulmonary oedema, and increased pulmonary vascular resistance. Some surgeons choose to offload high systemic venous pressures by deliberately creating a small fenestration in the atrial baffle, permitting a decompressive overflow into the systemic atrium.[11] The size of the fenestration (usually 4–6 mm) is such that up to one third of the systemic venous return may be delivered directly across the fenestration into the systemic ventricular atrium. The systemic ventricular output will be augmented, whilst CVP is lowered at the cost (assuming a mixed venous oxygen saturation of 60%) of mild systemic desaturation to 85%. It is clearly essential for the intensivist to be informed of the presence of such a fenestration and its physiological significance. As PVR falls postoperatively, shunting should decrease and the fenestration usually occludes spontaneously.

Hypoplastic left heart syndrome and the Norwood operation

Hypoplastic left heart syndrome (HLHS) is the most common cardiac malformation causing death from congenital heart disease in the first month of life. HLHS is a spectrum of left sided cardiac malformations including aortic atresia or stenosis, hypoplasia of the ascending aortic arch, and hypoplasia or absence of the left ventricle. The long term outlook for babies with this condition was until recently very poor. Two treatment options now offer hope: heart transplantation and the reconstructive surgery pioneered by Norwood.[12,13]

Physiologically, the right ventricle must sustain both pulmonary and systemic circulations. Survival in the neonatal period is dependent firstly on patency of the ductus arteriosus through which the right ventricle ejects blood to perfuse the aorta and secondly on mixing of blood at atrial level. Oxygenated pulmonary venous blood returns to the right ventricle, passing from left to right atrium through an ASD or patent foramen ovale.

The balance between the pulmonary (PVR) and systemic vascular resistance (SVR) and hence the balance of pulmonary (Qp) to systemic blood flow (Qs) is of paramount importance. Presentation of infants with HLHS is often precipitated by closure of the arterial duct or by the normal postnatal fall in PVR. The reduction in PVR leads to increased pulmonary blood flow, reduced systemic blood flow, and death from inadequate systemic and coronary perfusion. Although some babies with well balanced circulations (Qp = Qs) do not initially require intensive care, many present to the intensivist in a state of collapse with profound metabolic acidosis. General resuscitative measures must not be delayed. Further management is best guided by the precise diagnosis and dictated by the degree of duct patency and the presence of left atrial outlet obstruction, which may impede pulmonary blood flow.

Neonatal cardiac transplantation is only available in a few centres worldwide. Its development is not limited by absence of facilities or skilled personnel, but by the limited availability of suitably small donor hearts. The Norwood sequence of operations is therefore the only realistic option for most babies with HLHS. The first stage of this sequence aims to reconstruct the aortic arch, incorporating the right ventricular outflow. Adequate mixing of systemic and pulmonary venous return is ensured by means of an atrial septectomy and pulmonary blood flow secured with a central or modified Blalock–Taussig shunt. The aim of the intensivist should be to achieve, prior to surgery, a Qp:Qs as close to 1.0 as possible.

Duct patency must be maintained preoperatively with prostaglandin E1 or E2. Although many babies maintain a relatively balanced circulation, others require interventions to promote the desired Qp:Qs ratio. Excessive pulmonary blood flow (Qp:Qs>1) is heralded by saturations exceeding 85% (PaO$_2$>6 kPa). Pulmonary blood flow may be reduced by nursing or ventilating the baby in an FiO$_2$ of 0.21, avoiding alkalosis or by promoting respiratory acidosis with ventilatory manoeuvres, such as increasing ventilatory dead space or the addition of CO$_2$ to inspired gases. If pulmonary blood flow is inadequate (Qp:Qs<1, saturation <75%, PaO$_2$<3.5 kPa) due to a restrictive or inadequate ASD, the only rational approach is urgent surgery. It is of paramount importance that babies with HLHS are transported to the operating theatre in manner which ensures maintenance of ventilatory parameters, including FiO$_2$, so that a balanced Qp:Qs continues.

After a stage 1 Norwood operation the baby continues to have both pulmonary and systemic circulations supplied by the single ventricle and balanced flow must still be maintained. Excessive pulmonary blood flow is controlled using the techniques and measures described above. Inadequate postoperative pulmonary blood flow can be improved by measures that lower PVR (alkalosis, alveolar hyperoxia) and support shunt perfusion (volume and inotropic support).

The ultimate aim of the stage 1 operation is to allow palliation to an age and size at which a modified Fontan procedure can be undertaken, typically at 12–18 months. In preparation for this, a bidirectional cavopulmonary shunt (superior vena cava to pulmonary artery) is undertaken at 4–9 months of age, reducing volume load to the ventricle.

Respiratory implications of congenital heart disease

Infants are prone to respiratory insufficiency due to the small size of their airways, low lung compliance and functional residual capacity (FRC), relatively high oxygen consumption, and carbon dioxide production. The low FRC may result in airway collapse during tidal breathing, promoting atelectasis, ventilation perfusion mismatch, and infection. The infant has therefore little respiratory reserve and cardiac disease can readily induce additional respiratory demands and precipitate respiratory failure. Congenital heart disease itself may exert major stresses on the respiratory system, through delivery of either extremely low or excessively high pulmonary blood flow.[14]

Pulmonary blood flow is significantly reduced in children with right sided obstructive lesions such as Fallot's tetralogy and pulmonary atresia. Shunting from right to left in these and other cyanotic lesions results in low systemic oxygen saturations. The intensivist must understand the physiology underlying the specific cyanotic cardiac lesion to manage ventilation and oxygenation properly. Unless lung parenchymal disease coexists, the oxygenation of such patients is little influenced by inspired oxygen concentration. Cyanosis alone is an indication for neither increased oxygen supplementation nor continued mechanical ventilation.

Lesions resulting in excessive pulmonary blood flow and pulmonary hypertension have been described above. Excessive pulmonary blood flow due to pulmonary recirculatory shunts, obstructive left heart lesions or left heart failure is associated with pulmonary venous hypertension. Pulmonary venous and capillary hypertension induces pulmonary oedema resulting in ventilation perfusion mismatching and reduced lung compliance. Dilated pulmonary vessels can compress small airways and in longstanding left heart failure, dilation of the left atrium commonly causes left lower lobe atelectasis by compression of the left lower lobe bronchus. As previously noted, CPB increases lung water and further reduces lung compliance.

Postoperative respiratory compromise arises from the residual effects of anaesthetic drugs and wound pain, requiring a period of postoperative ventilation and careful titration of analgesia. Accidental phrenic nerve injury is common during cardiac surgery and may result in temporary or permanent paralysis of the associated hemidiaphragm. Diaphragmatic paralysis may not be apparent until the stenting effect of positive pressure ventilation and CPAP is removed. During weaning of ventilation the paradoxical movement of chest wall and abdomen becomes more obvious. The diagnosis is first suspected clinically or after radiographic evidence of a raised hemidiaphragm and confirmed by fluoroscopy, ultrasound or nerve conduction studies. Infants over 1 year of age usually tolerate loss of one hemidiaphragm. Below this age, assisted ventilation is required until phrenic nerve function recovers or the mechanical integrity of the hemidiaphragm is restored by surgical plication.

The majority of children undergoing open cardiac surgery are ventilated over the first postoperative night. The exceptions include simple repairs such as ASDs and VSDs in older children. Small infants require postoperative ventilation even if undergoing closed cardiac surgery due to the severity of illness and limited respiratory reserves.

The aim of ventilation in children without significant intracardiac shunting is to achieve a PaO_2 of 10–15 kPa, with saturations of 93–100%. Continuous monitoring of arterial oxygen saturation and frequent assessment of arterial $PaCO_2$ and pH should be performed for the duration of mechanical ventilation. In children with right to left shunts, saturations of 70–80% are normal and such levels of hypoxaemia are well tolerated.

Positive end expiratory pressure (PEEP) increases FRC during mechanical ventilation and improves oxygenation. The normal level of

179

PEEP required is 3–5 cmH$_2$O, but higher levels are useful to maintain lung volume or airway patency where there is atelectasis, pulmonary oedema or tracheobronchomalacia. High levels of PEEP increase mean intrathoracic and intraalveolar pressure and so hinder cardiac filling, resist pulmonary capillary blood flow, and reduce cardiac output. Therefore PEEP must be used cautiously in the presence of hypovolaemia and in the Fontan circulation where high PEEP may critically reduce pulmonary blood flow.

Weaning from mechanical ventilation should only be commenced once cardiovascular stability is achieved. Excessive oxygen requirement (FiO$_2$>0.45), peak inspiratory pressures (>25 cmH$_2$O) or a requirement for excessive sedation are relative contraindications to weaning from mechanical ventilation, as are residual hypothermia and continuing blood loss in the early postoperative period.

After extubation, oxygen can be delivered effectively only to an FiO$_2$ of 0.5 by face mask or nasal catheter. If necessary, after extubation, CPAP can be continued in infants up to 6 months of age by placement of a nasal prong or in older children by means of a face mask.

Low cardiac output and its management

Low cardiac output has many causes in the perioperative period. All exert their influence through one or more of the principal determinants of cardiac performance.

Preload

There is a well known relationship between ventricular preload, end diastolic volume and indices of ventricular ejection, such as stroke volume (fig 7.3). The energy of cardiac muscle contraction is proportional to the initial length of the muscle fibre, according to the Frank–Starling law. Within limits, as ventricular end diastolic volume increases, the force of contraction increases. If ventricular distension proceeds beyond a certain volume, myocardial performance declines and signs of cardiac failure appear. Relative hypovolaemia is by far the commonest cause of reduced preload. Other causes include cardiac tamponade, tachyarrhythmias and arrhythmias in which atrioventricular synchrony is lost.

Heart rate

A variety of rhythm disturbances commonly compromise cardiac output in the perioperative period. Sinus tachycardia may give insufficient time

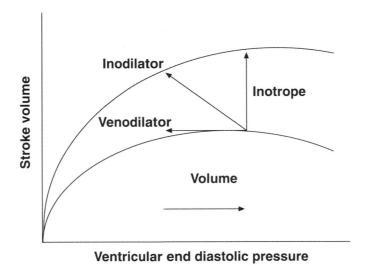

FIGURE 7.3—*Relationship between ventricular function and end diastolic volume*

for effective diastolic ventricular filling. In neonates, sinus bradycardia will reduce cardiac output, as the immature heart has only a limited ability to induce a compensatory increase in stroke volume.

Contractility

This may be reduced by the myocardial oedema and decreased ventricular compliance that follow damage to the heart during surgery. The myocardium may be further compromised by chronic volume or pressure overload, causing ventricular dilation, hypertrophy, and ischaemia. Coronary artery injury or compromise is an ever present risk in surgery for congenital heart disease, particularly in surgery involving coronary artery transfer, e.g. arterial switch operation. In addition, a variety of metabolic derangements may contribute to low cardiac output. These include hypoxaemia, acidosis, hypoglycaemia, and electrolyte disturbances, particularly of calcium, potassium or magnesium homoeostasis.

Afterload

Afterload is seen by the heart as impedance to ventricular ejection. High resistance to flow across either the pulmonary or systemic beds or ventricular outflow obstruction raises afterload. This may reduce stroke volume, raise ventricular end systolic volume, and detrimentally increase myocardial oxygen requirement, secondary to increased myocardial wall tension.

Diagnosis of low cardiac output syndrome

Despite the devilment of sophisticated cardiovascular monitoring devices, the intensivist will obtain much information helpful to the assessment of cardiac output from careful observation and examination of the child.

Clinical observation

In low cardiac output states, peripheral pulse volume is reduced, capillary refill slow (>2 s), and peripheral temperature reduced (>4°C below central temperature). Blood pressure may initially be normal, due to compensatory systemic vasoconstriction, although blood pressure will eventually fall if cardiac output continues to decline in the face of maximal vasoconstriction. Oliguria (urine output <1 ml/kg/h) is frequently seen as an early sign of low cardiac output, reflecting impaired renal perfusion. Restlessness may result from a reduction in cerebral perfusion and care should be taken not to misinterpret this as a sign of well being.

Metabolic indicators

In low cardiac output states there is a failure adequately to perfuse the tissues of the body. Anaerobic metabolism ensues and is reflected by the appearance of excessive hydrogen ion in arterial blood and a metabolic acidosis. Plasma lactate levels increase and in the absence of respiratory compensation, pH falls. Elevation in plasma lactate or the occurrence of a base deficit and fall in pH should stimulate the intensivist to search for other evidence of inadequate cardiac output.

In low cardiac output states, oxygen extraction from blood is increased and is reflected in falling mixed venous oxygen saturations. Serial measurement of mixed venous oxygen saturation gives a useful indication of trends towards improvement or deterioration in cardiac output and oxygen delivery.

Haemodynamic measurements

Blood pressure alone is not a reliable indicator of cardiac output. In physiological terms, the mean arterial blood pressure (MAP) can be expressed as the product of flow (cardiac output) and systemic vascular

182

resistance (MAP = CO × SVR). Systemic vascular resistance can vary widely under the influence of temperature, vasoactive mediators released during cardiac bypass, drugs, and metabolic status. Intense vasoconstriction can mask inadequate cardiac output in the normotensive or hypertensive child and conversely, hypotension may occur in a vasodilated child in the presence of an adequate cardiac output.

Central venous pressure (CVP) monitored by a catheter placed percutaneously, with the tip lying in the superior vena cava, estimates right ventricular filling pressure. Left atrial pressure (LAP) reflects left ventricular filling and is monitored postoperatively by a catheter placed in the atrium during the surgical procedure. CVP and LAP are the key to perioperative optimisation of preload.

Surgically placed or percutaneously introduced pulmonary artery catheters facilitate assessment of pulmonary artery pressure, sampling of mixed venous blood and, in the case of thermistor tipped catheters, cardiac output. Direct cardiac output measurement obtained by techniques such as thermodilution, dye dilution, and Doppler flow measurement are not continuous. Dilutional methods cannot be used in patients with uncorrected cardiac shunt lesions. However, in selected patients, cardiac output measurement is of great value in the diagnosis and further management of low cardiac output. Postoperatively, the pulmonary artery catheter may be useful in confirming residual left to right shunts.

Echocardiographic assessment

If a low cardiac output state is suspected, an urgent echocardiographic assessment should be obtained. As well as defining the structural integrity of the heart and surgical repair, the examination should reveal any evidence of impaired systolic ventricular function or pericardial tamponade and therefore guide further therapy.

Management of low cardiac output

As previously stated, cardiac output is influenced by a number of factors and in low output states these factors must be assessed and optimised. A practical approach to the management of low cardiac output is given in fig 7.4.

Preload

Cardiac output cannot be maximised unless optimal end diastolic ventricular filling is achieved. Low volume states are treated by careful

183

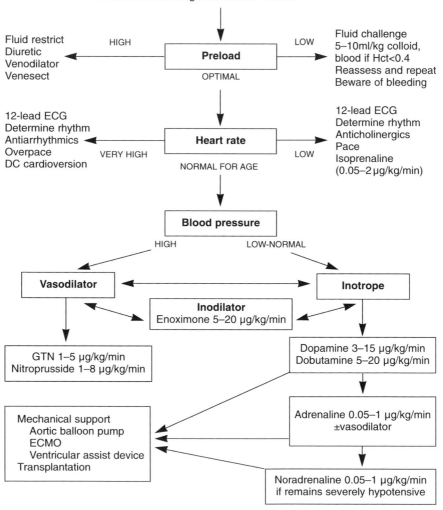

FIGURE 7.4—*Management of low cardiac output*

titration with boluses of colloid 5–10 ml/kg, the effects of which are monitored by measurement of CVP, LAP, and blood pressure, along with other clinical indices of perfusion. If no clinical improvement occurs, the process should be repeated. Fluid should not simply be administered to achieve arbitrary filling pressures, without regard to changes in perfusion or cardiac output. The loading conditions of the heart are probably adequate if filling pressures are seen to increase with no improvement in blood pressure or cardiac output. Fluid overload impairs ventricular performance and is managed by reducing end diastolic volume with fluid restriction, diuretic therapy or, more urgently, with vasodilators or venesection.

Heart rate

Excessive heart rates are detrimental to diastolic ventricular filling and must be controlled. Non-sinus tachyarrhythmias must be diagnosed and treated. Moderate degrees of sinus bradycardia are usually well tolerated but very slow rates, especially non-sinus rhythms, require treatment.

Contractility

Once preload and heart rate are optimised, further management of low cardiac output is undertaken through manipulation of contractility with inotropes and afterload reduction. In refractory cases, mechanical circulatory support or transplantation may be the final options.

The initial step in the augmentation of contractility is to establish a favourable metabolic environment. Hypoxia, hypercapnia, acidosis, hypoglycaemia, and electrolyte imbalance all adversely affect myocardial function and should be corrected.

Dopamine, an endogenous catecholamine, is a first line inotrope in the management of mild to moderate myocardial dysfunction. At low dosages (0.5–3 µg/kg/min) the drug stimulates dopaminergic D_1 receptors, resulting in dilation of renal, coronary, cerebral, and mesenteric vascular beds. At infusion rates between 2 and 10 µg/kg/min additional stimulation of adrenergic β_1 receptors occurs, with the predominant effect of augmenting myocardial contractility. At doses exceeding 10 µg/kg/min, stimulation of adrenergic α_1 receptors results in systemic and pulmonary vasoconstriction. These dose–response relationships are thought to vary with age, with higher doses necessary to achieve adequate inotropic support in infants.

Dopamine has been reported to result in an increased incidence of arrhythmias in children receiving doses in excess of 10 µg/kg/min. As with all potentially vasoconstricting agents, dopamine must be delivered into a large central vein to avoid local vasospasm and the risk of tissue damage.

185

One possible adverse effect of dopamine is the occurrence of pulmonary vasoconstriction at higher doses. Increased PVR may compromise right ventricular function and impair transpulmonary blood flow in the Fontan circulation.

Dobutamine activates β_1 and β_2 receptors, producing a dose related increase in stroke volume and heart rate and a reduction in systemic vascular resistance. It may be used as an alternative to dopamine in children with mild to moderate myocardial dysfunction. Dobutamine does not raise PVR at higher doses and may be the inotropic agent of choice in situations where a rise in PVR is not tolerated. As vasoconstriction does not occur, dobutamine may be administered via peripheral veins.

A perceived requirement for doses of dopamine or dobutamine in excess of 15–20 µg/kg/min suggests a need to consider more potent agents or strategies.

Adrenaline is a potent activator of α_1, β_1, and β_2 adrenoceptors. At doses less than 0.01 µg/kg/min, β_1 and β_2 activity predominates. At higher doses additional β_1 and β_2 effects are seen, combined with increasing α_1 mediated vasoconstriction. Adrenaline is indicated in the treatment of moderate to severe myocardial dysfunction, especially in the presence of hypotension. If used when systemic pressures are adequate, a vasodilator and renal dose dopamine should be added. This will reduce afterload and conserve blood flow to non-vital organs and the kidneys.

Noradrenaline is a potent endogenous catecholamine which predominantly exerts its effects through α_1 adrenoceptor activation. The major clinical effect of noradrenaline is powerful vasoconstriction, the drug having only limited α_1 mediated inotropic effects. Noradrenaline is used only in special situations that include the management of circulatory failure associated with very low systemic vascular resistance (e.g. sepsis) and as a pressor agent in the management of hypercyanotic episodes associated with tetralogy of Fallot.

Isoprenaline is a synthetic catecholamine with mixed β_1 and β_2 effects. Its use is reserved for situations where an increase in both heart rate and contractility is desirable and in which a degree of β_2 receptor mediated vasodilation can be tolerated. Isoprenaline is particularly useful in raising heart rate or facilitating AV conduction, when relative sinus bradycardia or first degree AV block occur postoperatively. Isoprenaline may lower elevated pulmonary vascular resistance. It should be noted, however, that by increasing heart rate and lowering diastolic pressure through vasodilation, isoprenaline can adversely affect myocardial oxygen balance, by both

186

increasing oxygen demand and reducing diastolic coronary perfusion pressure.

Administration of *calcium* has an inotropic effect when plasma ionised calcium is low. This situation occurs commonly in association with critical illness, especially in the neonate, and arises acutely with rapid transfusion of citrated blood products. Hypocalcaemia secondary to hypoparathyroidism is seen in Di George syndrome which is associated with various types of CHD, including truncus arteriosus and interrupted aortic arch. In low cardiac output states, ionised hypocalcaemia should be corrected, whilst hypercalcaemia should be avoided as it may induce unwanted peripheral vasoconstriction.

The selective *phosphodiesterase inhibitors* enoximone and amrinone act by direct competitive inhibition of phosphodiesterase type 3, resulting in increased levels of cAMP. These agents possess positive inotropic and to a lesser extent chronotropic actions, combined with potent vasodilating effects. Sometimes described as "inodilators", they are effective when given intravenously for the management of moderate to severe ventricular dysfunction and are frequently used in combination with β receptor agonists such as dobutamine or dopamine, with which synergy has been demonstrated. Inodilators appear to be particularly effective in patients with longstanding congestive heart failure, where β_1 receptor downregulation has occurred, as they produce a favourable combination of β receptor independent inotropy and vasodilation.

Reversible thrombocytopenia occurs in 2–4% of patients who receive amrinone. Elevation of liver enzymes has been reported with long term use of this drug. The half life of amrinone is known to be longer and clearance lower in neonates and infants than in older children and dosage must be altered accordingly. Enoximone (5–20 µg/kg/min) has been the inodilator of choice in our unit for a number of years, although there are few published data on its application in children.

Afterload

The compensatory increase in sympathetic activity that occurs in heart failure produces systemic vasoconstriction. If the failing heart cannot eject effectively against this higher resistance, stroke volume and cardiac output fall. In the absence of intraoperative vasodilator therapy, CPB also increases systemic vascular resistance. Judicious use of drugs to facilitate vasodilation, whilst maintaining adequate preload, will promote more complete ventricular ejection and lower myocardial oxygen demand by lowering myocardial wall stress.

Vasodilators have variable action on the arterial and venous vasculature. Reduction in afterload is achieved predominantly by reduction in arteriolar vessel tone and results in a fall in systemic vascular resistance.

The potential to reduce afterload is limited by the consequent fall in arterial blood pressure. Autoregulation of blood flow to vital organs ensures that small falls in perfusion pressure result in no change in flow, but if mean arterial pressure falls significantly, this mechanism is overwhelmed and cerebral, renal, and myocardial perfusion may be compromised. Venous dilation reduces preload and end diastolic volume, which is of benefit to an overdistended, failing ventricle.

The vasodilators most commonly used are sodium nitroprusside (SNP) and glyceryl trinitrate (GTN, nitroglycerine). SNP is a potent arteriolar vasodilator and can produce profound hypotension. It is administered intravenously and has a half life of minutes, which allows for accurate titration to response. Although safe when used appropriately, a break-down product is cyanide and the potential for toxicity exists. The maximum dose during prolonged use in intensive care should not exceed 5 µg/kg/min and its duration of use is limited to a few days. Signs of toxicity include unexplained metabolic acidosis, arrhythmias, and tachyphylaxis.

Intravenous GTN has a similar duration of action to SNP, but acts mainly on the venous capacitance vessels and produces significant arteriolar dilation only at high doses. Tolerance occurs quickly with continuous use. It has beneficial effects on the distribution of coronary blood flow and has more pronounced dilatory effect on pulmonary arterioles than other vasodilators.

Oral vasodilators can be used in the management of chronic heart failure. The angiotensin converting enzyme inhibitor captopril is particularly effective, with the absence of fluid retention, tolerance or compensatory tachycardias. The starting dose must be small to minimise any hypotensive effect and the daily requirement reduced, if there is coexistent renal impairment.

Diuretics are indicated in the treatment of fluid overload. Evidence of overload includes tachypnoea, cyanosis, tachycardia, gallop rhythm, cardiomegaly, and high atrial pressures with pulmonary oedema, hepatomegaly, and peripheral oedema. Frusemide 1 mg/kg IV is the usual first line therapy. Improvement should occur within 30 min, secondary to a diuresis and direct venous and arterial dilation, reducing both preload and afterload. Regular frusemide may be required, up to 4 mg/kg/day, and the addition of a potassium sparing diuretic (spironolactone or amiloride) helps prevent hypokalaemia. A frusemide infusion (0.1–0.2 mg/kg/h) has more potency and is titratable,[15] while the resultant controlled diuresis simplifies fluid balance. Ethacrynic acid or metalozone can be added if there is an inadequate response to frusemide alone.

Perioperative complications of congenital heart surgery

Pulmonary hypertension

Postoperative lability of the pulmonary vasculature is seen in children in whom preoperative conditioning of the pulmonary vasculature has occurred. This situation arises in lesions with either large pulmonary recirculatory (L–R) shunts or pulmonary venous obstruction. In spite of appropriate case selection and technically successful surgery, life threatening pulmonary hypertensive crises can occur. Postoperatively, vascular reactivity is increased as a result of CPB, through enhancement of the endothelial cell-smooth muscle interaction.

Pulmonary hypertensive episodes may be triggered by any of a number of factors known to promote pulmonary vasoconstriction (table 7.2), resulting in suprasystemic PA pressures. Pulmonary hypertension induces right ventricular failure and, through ventricular interdependence, LV failure and circulatory collapse. Pulmonary artery pressure monitoring is

TABLE 7.2—*Factors influencing pulmonary vascular resistance*

Factor	Pulmonary vascular resistance	
	increased	decreased
pH	Metabolic acidosis Respiratory acidosis	Metabolic alkalosis Respiratory alkalosis
Adrenergic drugs	α_1 adrenergic agonists (adrenaline, dopamine)	β_2 adrenergic agonists (isoprenaline)
Vasodilators		Prostacyclin (inhaled or IV) Nitroprusside Inhaled nitric oxide
Sympathetic tone	Pain and stress	Analgesia
Lung volume	Very low lung volume Very high lung volume Atelectasis	Normal lung volume
Perialveolar	Alveolar hypoxia Pulmonary oedema	Alveolar hyperoxia
Oxygenation	Low mixed venous saturation	High mixed venous saturation
Haematocrit	High	Low

extremely useful in the diagnosis and cardiovascular management of acute postoperative pulmonary hypertension. The aim is to limit PA pressures to <75% systemic levels. Care must be taken not to "overinterpret" PA pressure data, as PA pressures may transiently reach 50–75% of systemic levels during nursing procedures. Such pressures are usually well tolerated and in the absence of haemodynamic compromise, do not require treatment. Pulmonary vasoconstriction of a lesser degree can be of clinical significance if RV function is impaired or in the "Fontan" circulation in which a low PVR is essential.

Whether dealing with a child at risk of pulmonary hypertensive crises or the adverse effect of relative pulmonary hypertension on a dysfunctional right ventricle, the intensivist should aim to maintain a low PVR. This can be achieved by minimising the pulmonary constricting influences listed in table 7.2. Despite such measures, some infants will sustain acute reactive pulmonary hypertension. These episodes are managed by measures to reduce pulmonary vascular resistance: hyperoxia and alkalosis, induced with hyperventilation in 100% oxygen, provision of adequate analgesia and sedation, systemically administered non-selective vasodilators (nitrodilators, prostacyclin, phenoxybenzamine) and, more recently, the use of inhaled nitric oxide,[16,17] a selective pulmonary vasodilator. Additional measures are required to support the failing right ventricle, including optimising preload and contractility.

Postoperative bleeding

Bleeding in the postoperative period may be either the result of inadequate surgical haemostasis or an abnormality of the blood clotting mechanisms. Temporary blood clotting abnormalities after open heart surgery can be caused by incomplete heparin reversal, dilution or consumption of clotting factors, and alteration in platelet function. Consumptive coagulopathy is extremely rare in elective cardiac surgical practice, but may occur in the presence of sepsis.

An outline approach to the management of postoperative bleeding is detailed in table 7.3. Aprotinin, a proteolytic enzyme inhibitor acting on plasmin and kallikrein, is frequently used to reduce bleeding following extracorporeal circulation.[18] Surgical reexploration is mandatory if blood loss is substantial or persists in the face of near normal laboratory investigations. Failure to reexplore may result in cardiac tamponade or risk the hazards associated with "massive" transfusion. In our institution, a loss exceeding 10% total blood volume (TBV) in any hour or 20% TBV in a four hour period is an indication for reexploration.

TABLE 7.3—*Management of postoperative bleeding*

1. Replace blood losses. Use red cell preparations +/− plasma
2. Give protamine 1 mg/kg. Reverses residual heparin
3. Check clotting – PT, APTT, platelets, fibrinogen +/− FDPs
4. Infuse clotting factors if:
   platelets <50 (platelets 10 ml/kg)
   fibrinogen <1.0 (cryoprecipitate 3 ml/kg)
   PTT >1.5 control (fresh frozen plasma 10 ml/kg)
   APTT >1.5 (protamine 1 mg/kg if heparin effect)
5. Aprotinin. May reduce blood loss when infused intraoperatively
6. Observe carefully for cardiac tamponade. Monitor closely, especially if bleeding suddenly "stops". Echocardiology helpful in diagnosis
7. Surgical reexploration. Indicated for incessant bleeding: >10% total blood volume in 1 hour, >20% total blood volume in 4 hours

Patients with cyanotic heart disease, particularly those with a haematocrit greater than 0.6, frequently have deranged haemostasis. The cause of this defect is multifactorial and includes reduced plasma volume and altered platelet function. Aspirin should routinely be stopped two weeks prior to surgery so that the function of new platelets is unimpaired. Warfarin should be stopped and if continued anticoagulation is required, heparin can be commenced. Warfarin has a long half life and although vitamin K reverses its anticoagulant activity, it may take up to 12 hours to have effect. Urgent surgery will require the administration of fresh frozen plasma and therapy guided by the prothrombin time or INR.

Cardiac tamponade

Cardiac tamponade is an ever present threat in the postoperative cardiac surgery patient, but is also seen in association with penetrating chest wounds and inflammatory pericardial effusions such as the postcardiotomy syndrome. Cardiac function is severely compromised by increased pressure within the pericardial space, as this reduces venous return and effective ventricular preload. Classically, central venous pressure, left atrial pressure, and heart rate all rise, with a concomitant fall in systemic blood pressure and signs of shock.

Cardiac tamponade occurs most frequently in the early postoperative period. Its onset may be heralded by sudden cessation of chest drainage, leading to intrathoracic accumulation of blood. The removal of transthoracic pulmonary arterial or left atrial monitoring lines can occasionally result in bleeding of sufficient volume to produce tamponade, even if chest drains are *in situ*. For this reason crossmatched blood should be available prior to removal of these lines.

If clinical circumstances permit, the diagnosis of cardiac tamponade can be confirmed by 2D echo. Definitive management should not be delayed if haemodynamic instability is evident. The effusion must either be aspirated percutaneously or drained surgically. Prior to decompression of the tamponade, the circulation can be supported by augmentation of preload and the judicious use of inotropic drugs.

Perioperative arrhythmias

Disturbances of heart rate or rhythm are common in children with congenital heart disease, especially following cardiac surgery. All rhythm disturbances occurring in the intensive care unit should be documented by recording a surface multilead electrocardiogram. Additional information relating to atrial activity can be obtained from recordings via the temporary atrial pacing wire.

Arrhythmias may reflect global disturbances, such as hypoxia, pyrexia, hypovolaemia or electrolyte disturbances (particularly potassium, calcium, and magnesium). Correction of abnormal parameters may be all that is required to terminate many rhythm disturbances. Certain drugs, such as digoxin and catecholamines, are arrhythmogenic and may contribute to the abnormality.

Sinus tachycardia is the most common arrhythmia detected in the paediatric cardiac intensive care unit. Onset is gradual rather than paroxysmal, with a rate, even in neonates, of less than 230/min. The stress response to cardiopulmonary bypass may induce sinus tachycardia in the early postoperative period, particularly in neonates. Other precipitants include hypovolaemia, anxiety, pain, fever, and the use of chronotropic drugs. Postoperative sinus tachycardia, which is in a sense physiological, is not dangerous and typically settles over 4–8 hours, if precipitants are avoided.

Supraventricular tachycardias (SVT) are recognised by their sudden onset and regular rate, usually exceeding 240/min. If P waves are not seen, an atrial ECG lead trace will demonstrate atrial depolarisation and confirm a 1:1 atrioventricular relationship. The commonest cause is a concealed (normal P–R interval) accessory conduction pathway, leading to a reentry tachycardia. Occasionally this pathway is evident, as in Wolff–Parkinson–White syndrome, by shortening of the P–R interval. Automatic ectopic foci are an uncommon cause of SVT in the paediatric population.

192

SVT may revert with vagal stimulation (application of an ice pack to the face), overdrive atrial pacing, intravenous adenosine (0.25–2.5 mg/kg/dose) or synchronised direct current cardioversion (1 J/kg). If the SVT is recurrent, maintenance therapy with amiodarone or digoxin may be indicated.[19]

Atrial flutter and fibrillation compromise haemodynamics by reducing ventricular filling and producing variable AV block. DC cardioversion or overdrive pacing may terminate this rhythm and amiodarone can prevent recurrence. If the ventricular response rate is excessive, digoxin usefully slows AV conduction and enables improved ventricular filling.

His bundle tachycardia, also known as accelerated junction rhythm or junctional ectopic tachycardia, is characterised by atrioventricular dissociation with the ventricular rate (typically 170–250/min) exceeding the atrial rate. There is a beat to beat variability in blood pressure due to variable ventricular filling, resulting from atrial asynchrony. This rhythm is apt to occur in the immediate postoperative period, particularly after surgery near the His bundle conduction tissue, within the ventricular septum.

Stroke volume and cardiac output can be severely compromised. Treatment aims to reduce ventricular rate to 160–180/min, at which point AV synchrony may be imposed by temporary atrioventricular sequential pacing. Active cooling and antiarrhythmic drugs, such as amiodarone or propafenone, are used to control the heart rate. Plasma potassium should be raised to 4.5–5 mmol/l and catecholamine infusions reduced as tolerated. Hypovolaemia or excessive vasodilation should be avoided and combined with adequate sedation, reducing the detrimental release of endogenous catecholamines. Sinus rhythm normally returns within 3–7 days.

Sinus or nodal bradycardia can be physiological, due to either increased vagal tone or decreased sympathetic tone. Pathological causes include damage to the conduction system, hypoxaemia, and myocardial ischaemia. Bradycardia is managed by correcting hypoxaemia and inadequate myocardial perfusion. If unsuccessful, an isoprenaline infusion (0.05–2 µg/kg/m) can increase heart rate and promote AV conduction, while atropine or glycopyrrolate usefully abolish vagal influence. Ventricular or atrioventricular sequential pacing can be used if general and pharmacological measures are unsuccessful. Pacing provides the first line of therapy in the immediate postoperative period, when the wires are already *in situ*, and the aim is to achieve a heart rate appropriate for age.

Ventricular arrhythmias, such as ventricular tachycardia and ventricular fibrillation, are uncommon in children.

Complete heart block may be congenital or acquired during congenital heart surgery. Children separating from cardiopulmonary bypass in complete heart block are supported with AV sequential pacing using standard temporary epicardial pacing wires. Atrioventricular conduction usually returns within five days, as myocardial oedema resolves. Occasionally, when the surgical repair has resulted in irreversible disruption of the conducting pathway, a permanent pacemaker must be inserted.

Neurological complications

Critical illness associated with low cardiac output syndrome, cardiac surgery, and cardiopulmonary bypass contributes to postoperative brain injury in a small number of children. Some impairment can be detected in between 8% and 25% of children after cardiac surgery, but fewer than 1% of postsurgical children suffer from major irreversible and clinically important abnormalities.[20]

The risk of brain injury is greatest after aortic arch surgery, procedures incorporating deep hypothermic circulatory arrest, and following episodes of profound hypotension and hypoxia. Neurological injuries commonly manifest as seizures or motor disturbances such as choreoathetoid movements. More subtle damage may not be detected in the early postoperative period and the true incidence of neurodevelopmental problems resulting from congenital heart surgery is therefore underestimated.

Patients with suspected neurological complications must be investigated and treated urgently, preferably with the assistance of a paediatric neurologist. Brain imaging (CT or MRI) and an electroencephalogram are usually required. Seizure activity, fluid overload, hypoglycaemia, hypocalcaemia, and hypomagnesaemia require aggressive therapy.

Renal failure

Renal blood flow and function may be impaired perioperatively by hypotension, low cardiac output, hypoxia, sepsis or the inflammatory response to cardiopulmonary bypass. Factors specifically linked to postoperative renal impairment include coarctation of the aorta and similar duct dependent lesions, the use of nephrotoxic drugs and long periods of cardiopulmonary bypass or circulatory arrest. An additional nephrotoxic insult may be consequent to haemolysis during CPB, caused by excessively vigorous cardiotomy suction or overocclusion of roller pumps. If significant haemolysis is noted, renal function may be preserved by maintaining urine output with diuretics (mannitol, frusemide) and rendering the urine alkaline by the intravenous administration of sodium bicarbonate.

The commonest manifestation of incipient renal failure is with oliguria or anuria, often associated with hyperkalaemia and metabolic acidosis. Whilst oliguria or hyperkalaemia may respond to pharmacological interventions and optimisation of cardiac output and renal blood flow, established renal failure will necessitate renal replacement therapy with peritoneal dialysis or haemofiltration. If the overall condition of the child improves, renal function usually returns after 5–10 days. Long term renal support is rarely required.

1 Lenz W. Aetiology: incidence and genetics of congenital heart disease. In: Graham G, Rossi E, eds, *Heart disease of infants and children*. London: Edward Arnold, 1985:27–35.
2 Hatch D, Sumner E, Hellmann J, eds. Anaesthesia in patients with cardiac disease. In: *The surgical neonate: anaesthesia and intensive care*. London: Edward Arnold, 1995:183–96.
3 Pollock EMM, Ford-Jones EL, Rebeyka I, et al. Early nosocomial infections in paediatric cardiovascular surgery patients. *Crit Care Med* 1990;18:378–84.
4 Hall JC, Christiansen K, Carter MJ, et al. Antibiotic prophylaxis in cardiac operations. *Ann Thorac Surg* 1993;56:916–22.
5 Stark J, de Leval MR, eds. *Surgery for congenital heart defects*. Philadelphia: WB Saunders, 1993.
6 Turley K, Bove EL, Amato JJ, et al. Neonatal aortic stenosis. *J Thorac Cardiothorac Surg* 1990;99:679–83.
7 Javorski JJ, Hansen DD, Laussen PC, Fox ML, Lavoie J, Burrows FA. Paediatric cardiac catheterization: innovations. *Can J Anaesthesia* 1995;42:310–29.
8 Mustard WT. Successful two stage correction of transposition of the great vessels. *Surgery* 1964;55:469–72.
9 Hickey PR, Anderson NP. Deep hypothermic circulatory arrest: a review of pathophysiology and clinical experience as a basis for anaesthetic management. *J Cardiothorac Anaesthesia* 1987;1:137–55.
10 Fontan F, Baudet E. Surgical repair of tricuspid atresia. *Thorax* 1971;26:240–8.
11 Jacobs ML, Norwood WI. Fontan operation: influence of modifications on morbidity and mortality. *Ann Thorac Surg* 1994;58:945–51.
12 Piggott JD, Murphy JD, Barber G, Norwood WI. Palliative reconstructive surgery for hypoplastic left heart syndrome. *Ann Thorac Surg* 1988;45:122–8.
13 Gutgesell HP, Massaro TA. Management of hypoplastic left heart syndrome in a consortium of university hospitals. *Am J Cardiol* 1995;76:809–11.
14 Willson DF. Postoperative respiratory function and its management. In: Lake CL, ed, *Pediatric cardiac anaesthesia*. Connecticut: Appleton and Lange, 1993:445–64.
15 Martin SJ, Danziger LH. Continuous infusion of loop diuretics in the critically ill: a review of the literature. *Crit Care Med* 1994;22:1323–9.
16 Goldman AP, Delius RE, Deanfield JE, Macrae DJ. Nitric oxide is superior to prostacyclin for pulmonary hypertension after cardiac operations. *Ann Thorac Surg* 1995;60:300–5.
17 Miller OI, Celermajer DS, Deanfield JE, Macrae DJ. Very low dose inhaled nitric oxide: a selective pulmonary vasodilator after operations for congenital heart disease. *J Thorac Cardiovasc Surg* 1994;108:487–94.
18 Davis R, Whittington R. Aprotinin. A review of its pharmacology and therapeutic efficacy in reducing blood loss associated with cardiac surgery. *Drugs* 1995;49:954–83.
19 Deanfield J. Arrhythmias: paediatrics. *Curr Opin Cardiol* 1987;2:109–11.
20 Fallon P, Aparicio JM, Elliott MJ, Kirkham FJ. Incidence of neurological complications of surgery for congenital heart disease. *Arch Dis Child* 1995;72:418–22.

8: Clinical aspects of inhaled nitric oxide therapy

JAMES TIBBALLS

Introduction

The accidental discovery of an endothelial factor, essential for the vasodilatory action of acetylcholine,[1] has had many implications for intensive care medicine. This endothelium derived relaxing factor (EDRF) was subsequently identified[2,3] as a small highly reactive molecule, nitric oxide (NO). The additional observation that exogenous gaseous NO could not only mimic the vasodilatory action of endogenous NO but also selectively relax the pulmonary vascular bed provided clinicians with a new therapeutic substance.

While endogenous NO was discovered first in the cardiovascular system, it is present in many body systems. It plays a central role in numerous physiological and pathophysiological processes. Among these are vascular regulation, coagulation, neurotransmission and memory formation, host defence, and immune function, gastrointestinal function, genitourinary function, inflammation, and lung function. The diverse role of endogenous NO in the body may be examined in general reviews and editorials.[4-10] Its role in particular systems may also be examined in specialist reviews and editorials: circulation;[11-15] septic shock;[16-19] respiratory system;[20-23] platelet function;[5,24] neural function;[25-32] immune function and inflammation;[33-35] and gut function.[36] NO has a role in many disease states including septic shock, myocardial ischaemia, heart failure, hypertension, neuronal damage, and in many diseases of the lungs and of its pulmonary vasculature. The aim of inhaled NO therapy is to take advantage of its physiological actions and to avoid its pathophysiological effects.

This chapter summarises the current clinical applications and effects of inhaled NO therapy after a brief review of its action when administered in this manner. Other reviews of inhaled NO therapy have also been published.[37-45] At present, most applications are for pulmonary vascular and gaseous exchange disorders. Many of the effects of inhaled NO therapy on systems other than the pulmonary vasculature are unknown.

Physiology of endogenous nitric oxide

Endogenous NO is produced from the amino acid L-arginine by a group of enzymes, nitric oxide synthases (NOS). The reaction requires oxygen and also produces L-citrulline as a byproduct. It is known as the L-arginine–oxide pathway.[46] Different isoenzymes are found in different locations and serve different activities.[47] Their targets are guanylate cyclase, thiols, and iron containing proteins. Enzymes responsible for physiological functions are "constitutive" and produce NO briefly in picomolar amounts. This system contributes to control of vasodilator tone, central neurotransmission, platelet aggregation, cardiac contractility, and various respiratory, genitourinary, and gastrointestinal functions and is involved in host defence and immunological activities. Activators of the system include acetylcholine, glutamate, adenosine diphosphate, calcium ionophores, and shear stress. In contrast, "inducible" forms of NOS are responsible for continuous production of large amounts of NO, typically from macrophages in response to proinflammatory stimuli such as bacterial lipopolysaccharide or cytokines including tumour necrosis factor and interleukin 1. Glucocorticoids inhibit the inducible enzymes but both inducible and constitutive forms are inhibited by analogues of L-arginine. The pathways are illustrated in figs 8.1 and 8.2.

The mechanism of production of NO is the same in all tissues, but its actions are varied. Many actions are mediated by activation of guanylate cyclase which subsequently increases levels of cyclic guanosine monophosphate (cGMP) which in turn causes a decrease in intracellular calcium. Non-cGMP dependent actions of NO include cytotoxic effects by inhibition of mitochondrial enzymes, deamination, and disruption of nucleic acids, autoribosylation of glyceraldehyde-3-phosphate dehydrogenase, activation of ADP-ribosyltransferases and the formation of peroxynitrite with superoxide.

Clinical uses of nitric oxide

The aim of exogenous NO introduced via the lung is to mimic the action of endogenous NO on vascular smooth muscle cells, which is relaxation and consequent vasodilation. Because it is introduced to the pulmonary

197

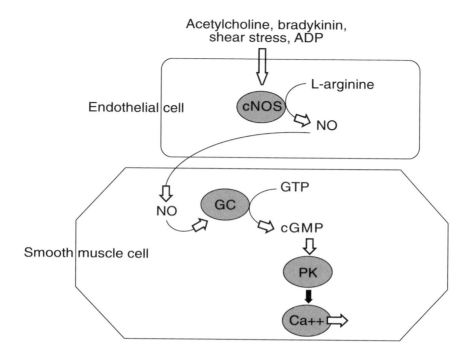

FIGURE 8.1—*Release and action of constitutive nitric oxide. ADP, adenosine diphosphate; cNOS, constitutive nitric oxide synthase; NO, nitric oxide; GC, guanylate cyclase; GTP, guanosine triphosphate; cGMP, cyclic guanosine monophosphate; PK, protein kinase; Ca + +, inoised calcium; unfilled arrows, facilitatory actions; filled arrows, inhibitory actions*

vascular smooth muscle cell from its abluminal surface, it has little opportunity to gain access to the systemic circulation and to cause systemic vasodilation. Nonetheless, some exogenous NO does enter the bloodstream where it is inactivated by formation of methaemoglobin.[48] All endogenous and exogenous inhaled NO eventually enters blood as NO or nitrite and is converted to nitrate via the formation of nitrosohaemoglobin or methaemoglobin. Nitrates are subsequently excreted in urine.[49] The plasma levels of nitrates increase during nitric oxide therapy[50] and may be used as markers of increased endogenous NO production such as occurs with sepsis.[51] The pharmacology of inhaled NO is illustrated in fig 8.3.

Treatment of pulmonary hypertension

NO has been used to treat various conditions associated with pulmonary hypertension, including idiopathic (primary) pulmonary hypertension,

198

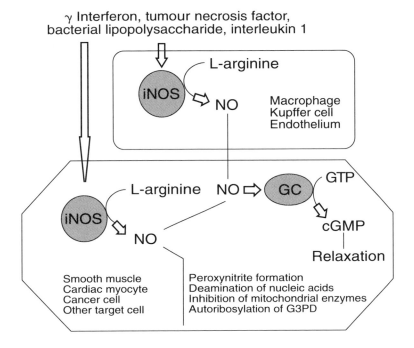

FIGURE 8.2—*Release and actions of inducible nitric oxide. iNOS, inducible nitric oxide synthase; NO, nitric oxide; GC, guanylate cyclase; GTP, guanosine triphosphate; cGMP, cyclic guanosine monophosphate*

pulmonary hypertension after cardiac surgery, persistent pulmonary hypertension of the newborn (PPHN), and pulmonary hypertension associated adult respiratory distress syndrome and heart-lung transplant candidates. Inhaled NO appears to dilate small resistance arteries and veins rather than larger capacitance arteries and veins.[52]

Primary pulmonary hypertension

The first clinical use of inhaled NO involved patients with idiopathic pulmonary hypertension.[53] In this study, eight patients spontaneously inspired 40 ppm NO for five-minute intervals from a Douglas bag. Pulmonary vascular resistance decreased in all patients by an average of more than 30% but there were no changes in systemic vascular resistance or pulmonary wedge pressure. In contrast, prostacyclin (PGI$_2$) caused reductions in both pulmonary and systemic vascular resistance. Not all patients with this condition, however, respond to inhaled NO. In another study,[54] a reduction of more than 30% in pulmonary resistance was observed

199

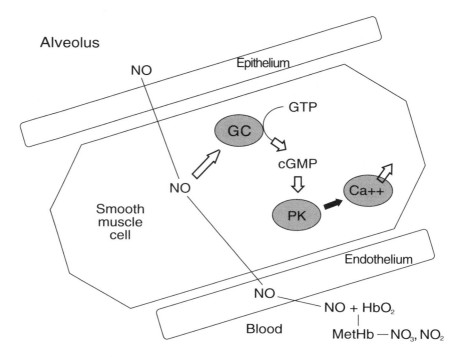

FIGURE 8.3—*Actions of inhaled nitric oxide. NO, nitric oxide; GC, guanylate cyclase; GTP, guanosine triphosphate; cGMP, cyclic guanosine monophosphate; PK, protein kinase; Ca + +, ionised calcium; HbO₂, oxyhaemoglobin; MetHb, methaemoglobin; NO₃, nitrate; NO₂, nitrite; unfilled arrows, facilitatory actions; filled arrows, inhibitory actions*

equally with the use of 10, 20 and 40 ppm NO and with PGI_2 in 13 patients (responders) but not in 22 (non-responders). Several case reports in children also report a selective pulmonary vasodilatory action in this condition. In one such report, NO at 3 ppm selectively reduced idiopathic pulmonary hypertension in a 2 year old infant[55] while in another report 6–40 ppm selectively reduced pulmonary hypertension in a 5 month old infant.[56] A fatal outcome in an adult with this condition during NO therapy at 5 ppm was attributed to a concomitant systemic hypotensive effect which reduced coronary perfusion pressure and caused myocardial ischaemia.[57] However, a direct effect on the heart could not be excluded.

Pulmonary hypertension after cardiac surgery

Children with congenital heart lesions with increased pulmonary blood flow (e.g. ventricular septal defect) or pulmonary venous obstruction develop pulmonary hypertension, which may persist after corrective surgery.

Several case reports[58-60] and several convenience studies with small or medium numbers of patients provide insights into the utility and therapeutic dose of NO.

Congenital cardiac defects NO was administered during spontaneous ventilation in several studies. Inhalation of NO for 30 min by 10 young children[61] with a variety of uncorrected congenital heart defects associated with high pulmonary flow caused a selective reduction in pulmonary vascular resistance (PVR) when inhaled in concentrations of 20, 40, and 80 ppm. No additional effect was observed with 90% oxygen while the maximum reduction in PVR was observed with 80 ppm. Pulmonary blood flow was also augmented by NO therapy. In a similar study of seven children with ventricular septal defects, seven-minute inhalations of 12 and 60 ppm NO selectively decreased PVR by 31% and 25% respectively.[62] In another study, the pulmonary vasodilatory effect of 40 ppm NO inhaled for 10 min was confined to children with increased vascular resistance who had a 34% reduction. Such effect was not observed at all in children with normal PVR.[63]

In the period immediately after surgery to correct congenital cardiac lesions, 20 ppm NO caused a mean reduction of 34% in pulmonary artery pressure in 17 children with a pulmonary hypertensive crisis, defined as acute pulmonary hypertension in excess of 75% of the systemic pressure and associated with a decrease in oxygenation. NO was effective after failure of conventional therapy which consisted of hyperventilation with 100% oxygen, deepening the level of anaesthesia and treatment of acidosis with sodium bicarbonate.[64] In another study, inhaled NO in an initial dose of 15 ppm was required for 4–16 days in a group of seven children with pulmonary pressure which was more than two thirds systemic pressure despite alkalotic hyperventilation after corrective cardiac surgery. Thereafter, complete weaning of NO was possible from approximately 4 ppm.[65]

Mitral valve disease Chronic mitral regurgitation or stenosis may cause pulmonary hypertension. The results of studies in several series of patients with this condition illustrate the value of inhaled NO. In a group of six adult patients after surgical repair, NO in a concentration of approximately 37–38 ppm inhaled for 10 min during mechanical ventilation decreased the mean pulmonary pressure by 10% but did not change the systemic arterial pressure or pulmonary wedge pressure.[66] In another group of 20 adult patients undergoing surgical repair, 20 ppm NO decreased the pulmonary artery pressure from a mean of 36 to 29 mmHg and from 32 to 27 mmHg before and after cardiopulmonary bypass respectively but did not alter central venous pressure, pulmonary artery occlusion pressure, cardiac output or systemic arterial pressure.[67] In another group of nine patients after repair of mitral valve regurgitation,[68] 40 ppm inhaled NO reduced the median systolic pulmonary artery pressure from 35 to 30 mmHg and the diastolic pressure from 17 to 12 mmHg after 20 min while the pulmonary capillary wedge pressure and systemic pressures remained unchanged and the cardiac index increased from 1.94 to 2.29 l/min/m². The major part of these changes were evident 10 min after commencement of therapy.

Cardiopulmonary bypass Cardiopulmonary bypass has long been suspected of exacerbating the problem of pulmonary hypertension, possibly by disrupting pulmonary endothelial cell function. Indeed, the pulmonary vasodilatory effect of intravenous acetylcholine was markedly attenuated by cardiopulmonary bypass after surgery for congenital heart lesions whereas inhalation of NO in a concentration of 80 ppm reduced the pulmonary vascular resistance by 33% and was accompanied by an increase in plasma cGMP levels.[69] In a canine model of myocardial ischaemia and reperfusion, intracoronary infusion of the nitric oxide donor compound SPM-5185 reduced myocardial necrosis. It also reduced adherence of neutrophils to the coronary endothelium, which may be the protective property of NO.[70] A subsequent study in isolated perfused rat hearts subjected to ischaemia and reperfusion[71] demonstrated that infusion of neutrophils alone caused a severe reduction in contractile function and that infusion of the NO donor CAS-754 or L-arginine largely restored contractile function. Moreover, NG-nitro-L-arginine methyl ester exacerbated contractile dysfunction while NO infusion alone without neutrophil infusion had no effect. In short, the post-ischaemic reperfusion myocardial dysfunction which was mediated by neutrophils was attenuated by NO.

Persistent pulmonary hypertension of the newborn (PPHN)

Persistent pulmonary hypertension of the newborn (PPHN) is a syndrome characterised by right to left shunting through the foramen ovale and ductus arteriosus secondary to abnormally persistent pulmonary hypertension in the newborn period. Severe hypoxaemia results. In addition, the elevated pulmonary vascular resistance causes right ventricular distention, tricuspid incompetence and impaired filling of the left ventricle with consequent limitation of cardiac output.

Studies in animals strongly suggest that NO is required for normal transition from foetal to adult circulation at birth and that persistence of foetal circulation is related to a failure of its activity. Inhibition of NO synthesis increases pulmonary blood flow and increased pulmonary vascular resistance in the perinatal period[72] and modulates the transition to adult circulation at birth.[73] Exogenous NO causes selective pulmonary vasodilation in the immature lamb[74] and can reverse pulmonary vasoconstriction caused by hypoxaemia and respiratory acidosis.[75] PPHN may be a consequence of reduced NO synthesis[76] since NO generating vasodilators and a cGMP analogue (8-bromo-cyclic GMP) inhibit mitogenesis and proliferation of vascular smooth muscle,[77] a feature of PPHN.

PPHN is associated with a variety of illnesses, but most notably meconium aspiration, congenital diaphragmatic hernia, hyaline membrane disease, and group B streptococcal sepsis. It may occur without obvious association (idiopathic) or be associated with uncommon conditions such alveolar capillary dysplasia or exomphalos. Since pulmonary artery catheterisation is not routinely used in this age group, blood gas evidence of right to left shunting or echocardiographic evidence of right ventricular distention with tricuspid incompetence is taken as a proxy for the presence of pulmonary hypertension. Conventional vasodilator therapy such as nitroprusside, nitroglycerine or tolazoline is prone to cause systemic hypotension as well as pulmonary vasodilation with no net benefit. Indeed, systemic hypotension exacerbates ductal right to left shunting and hypoxaemia. NO therapy may be the ideal therapy for this group of patients in whom selective pulmonary vasodilation reduces shunting without systemic hypotension. It may also improve pulmonary ventilation perfusion matching. The therapeutic dose among responders is, however, uncertain.

A concentration of 80 ppm NO for 10 min improved postductal SpO_2 in five of seven trials among six infants ventilated with 90% oxygen for PPHN. Lesser concentrations of NO were ineffective.[78] Nitric oxide in "low dose" (10–20 ppm) improved oxygenation in nine infant ECMO candidates with severe PPHN without reducing systemic blood pressure. The improvement was maintained by 6 ppm NO in six infants. These infants required therapy for 24 hours, avoided ECMO and recovered with no lung disease while the remaining three infants, whose outcome is unknown, required ECMO.[79] In another study, nine infant ECMO candidates with severe PPHN were treated initially with 20 ppm NO for four hours and subsequently with 6 ppm for 20 hours. All but one infant had sufficient improvement in oxygenation without systemic hypotension to avoid ECMO.[80]

Inhaled NO therapy reduces the requirement for ECMO in infants with PPHN. In such infants, improvement in oxygenation may be ascribed to a reduction in right to left cardiac or ductal shunting via reduction in pulmonary hypertension or to an improvement in ventilation perfusion matching or to both mechanisms. PPHN is, however, often associated with severe lung disease. Inhaled NO therapy appears to have a greater benefit if pulmonary hypertension is the predominant mechanism for severe hypoxaemia but less benefit if hypoxaemia is due to severe lung disease.

In a group of 23 infants referred for ECMO for a variety of conditions, 11 of 13 who had echocardiographic evidence of pulmonary hypertension responded to NO therapy while only three of 10 infants without pulmonary hypertension responded. Among the responders, there was no difference between a dose of 5 and 80 ppm. Of seven infants in the group with a congenital diaphragmatic hernia (CDH), five responded to NO and four required ECMO.[81] In another study of newborns with CDH, three of four responded to 5–10 ppm inhaled NO but developed tachyphylaxis and all required ECMO.[82] In a study of 10 infants with PPHN, five showed improvement in oxygenation but only two eventually avoided ECMO.[83]

Despite the apparent efficacy of NO therapy in the treatment of PPHN, many questions concerning its use remain.[43,44] PPHN is a consequence of a variety of diseases and the efficacy of NO among the different patient groups may be different. Moreover, the immaturity of the lung, particularly of the premature newborn, implies that NO therapy should be administered cautiously. Such patients usually require a high inspired oxygen and prolonged NO therapy, thus exposing them to risks of prolonged NO, NO_2, methaemoglobinaemia,[84] perioxynitrates, and possibly nitrates. On the other hand, the alternatives are prolonged mechanical ventilation with the risks of acute and chronic barotrauma, oxygen toxicity, and ECMO.

Acute respiratory distress syndrome

The acute respiratory distress syndrome (ARDS) is, in part, characterised by alveolar pulmonary infiltration by fluid and inflammatory cells, pulmonary hypertension, and a decrease in lung compliance. Hypoxic pulmonary vasoconstriction and microvascular occlusion contribute to intrapulmonary shunting. Reduction of PVR in this condition has several beneficial actions including improvement in right ventricular function. Reduction in capillary pressure may improve pulmonary oedema. Although intravenous vasodilators may reduce PVR, systemic vascular resistance is also reduced. This may cause systemic hypotension. Moreover, intravenous agents cause indiscriminate diffuse pulmonary vasodilation which may exacerbate intrapulmonary shunting. Inhaled NO therapy is an attractive alternative because its effects are confined to the pulmonary circulation and thus perfusion in ventilated non-perfused areas may be improved. Several convenience series of patients with ARDS have been published. These have added insight into the therapeutic dose and mode of action of inhaled NO.

Administration of 18 ppm NO to nine patients was associated with a reduction in pulmonary artery pressure from a mean of 37 ± 3 mmHg to 30 ± 2 mmHg, a decrease in intrapulmonary shunting from $36 \pm 5\%$ to

$31 \pm 5\%$ and an increase in the ratio of partial pressure of arterial oxygen to fraction of inspired oxygen (PaO_2/FiO_2) from 152 mmHg to 199 ± 23 mmHg. Mean systemic arterial pressure and cardiac output were unchanged. The duration of NO therapy was 3–53 days. An infusion of PGI_2 at 4 ng/kg/min also reduced the pulmonary artery pressure to the same degree as inhaled NO but in contrast, increased intrapulmonary shunting and decreased both the PaO_2/FiO_2 ratio and systemic arterial pressure.[85] In subsequent studies from the same clinic, the therapeutic dose and time course of action of inhaled NO were published for a total of 12

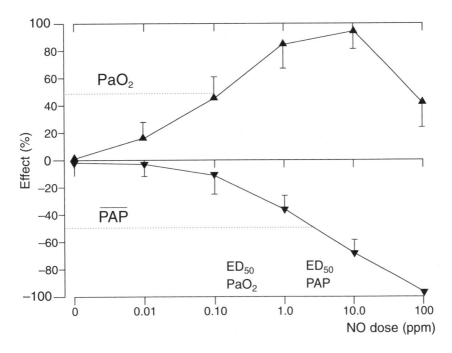

FIGURE 8.4—*Dose response for inhaled NO. Dose response for PaO_2 (upper panel) and PAP (lower panel) to inspiratory NO. (Reproduced with permission from Gerlach et al. Eur J Clin Invest 1993;23:499–502)*

patients (initially for three) with ARDS (fig 8.4). Enhanced oxygenation occurred within 1–2 min of the commencement of therapy and plateaued within 8–12 min. Upon cessation of therapy, baseline was attained within 5–8 min. The ED_{50} for improvement in oxygenation was approximately 100 parts per billion (ppb) (0.1 ppm) with a maximum effect at 10 ppm. Higher concentrations decreased oxygenation. The therapeutic dose of NO for improvement of oxygenation approximated the ambient atmospheric concentration – which stimulates speculation about the use of bottled gases.

The ED_{50} for reduction of mean pulmonary pressure was 2–3 ppm but progressive reduction was observed over the entire range from 0.01 to 100 ppm (10 to 100 000 ppb). Reductions in pulmonary artery pressure were observed after changes in oxygenation, leading to the conclusion that redistribution of blood flow, not the enhancement of pulmonary perfusion, caused better oxygenation.[86,87]

Another group of clinical investigators examined the oxygenation and pulmonary vasodilatory effects of inhaled NO in adults with acute respiratory failure with the aim of determining the therapeutic dose. Over the range 100–5000 ppb (0.1–5 ppm), the maximum decrease in pulmonary artery pressure (25%), increase in PaO_2, and reduction in intrapulmonary shunt all occurred in the range 100–2000 ppb (0.1–2.0 ppm).[88]

Yet another group has sought to determine the therapeutic dose of NO for ARDS. Seven patients inhaled 2–20 ppm for 2–27 days. This concentration decreased mean pulmonary artery pressure from 38 ± 7 to 31 ± 6 mmHg and increased PaO_2 from 79 ± 10 to 114 ± 27 mmHg.[89]

Inhaled NO also appears to be beneficial in children with ARDS. In a group of 10 children with ARDS, inhalation of 20 ppm decreased pulmonary pressure from a mean of 42 to 31 mmHg, decreased pulmonary shunt from 39% to 32% while cardiac index increased 14% and the systemic arterial pressure and pulmonary capillary wedge pressures were unchanged. The mean ratio of PaO_2/FiO_2 increased from approximately 75 to 90 with 10 ppm and further to 115 with 20 ppm.[90]

At variance with the previous studies, another conducted in 14 patients with acute respiratory failure found maximum improvements in oxygenation and pulmonary artery pressure with higher concentrations of NO: the mean increases in PaO_2 were 19, 38, and 22 mmHg while the decreases in pulmonary pressure were slight with means of 1.7, 3.2, and 3.3 mmHg with 8, 32, and 128 ppm respectively. It is difficult to interpret these findings in the light of the previous studies since smaller doses of NO were not tested and the accuracy of the concentrations is doubtful since they were calculated by flow ratios, not measured, in all but two of the patients.[91] Previously, the experimental group had established that the ED_{50} for inhaled NO in the treatment of induced pulmonary hypertension in sheep was 39 ppm during hypoxia and 48 ppm during *E. coli* endotoxaemia.[92]

Another study of the effects of inhaled NO on oxygenation and pulmonary hypertension in a convenience sample of 14 adults with ARDS[93] found that there was essentially no difference in the percentage increase in oxygenation caused by either 20 or 40 ppm (43% and 44% respectively) nor any difference in reduction of pulmonary artery pressure (17% and 18% respectively). No other significant haemodynamic or respiratory changes were observed. This study noted variable improvements in oxygenation (<20% to >50%) and pulmonary haemodynamics (<10% to >20%) among the group of patients.

Mechanisms of action

Improvement in oxygenation and intrapulmonary shunting during inhaled NO therapy may be attributed to various mechanisms. These include a reduction in pulmonary capillary pressure, a reversal of hypoxic induced vasoconstriction, an improvement in right ventricular function, and an improvement in ventilation perfusion matching.

Reduction in pulmonary capillary pressure   In acute lung injury, pulmonary vasoconstriction causes an increase in pulmonary capillary pressure which would be expected to increase the hydrostatic pressure difference across the capillary lumen and the interstitial thus increasing pulmonary oedema. As expected, inhaled NO (40 ppm) lowered PVR in a group of 18 patients with acute lung injury. It declined from 166 to 128 dyne/s/cm^5 and pulmonary artery pressure declined from 34 to 30 mmHg. When these changes were compartmentalised, pulmonary venous resistance decreased to a greater extent (from 76 to 50 dyne/s/cm^5) than did pulmonary arterial resistance (from 90 to 79 dyne/s/cm^5). Pulmonary capillary pressure declined from 25 to 22 mmHg but pulmonary capillary wedge pressure did not change. Thus NO appeared to have a predominant effect on the pulmonary venous vasculature, thereby lowering pulmonary capillary pressure.[94] The effect on pulmonary capillary pressure by inhaled NO was confirmed in a subsequent study of an additional nine patients with acute lung injury in which the pressure declined from 24 to 21 mmHg whereas pulmonary capillary wedge pressure did not change and moreover, the transvascular flux of technetium labelled albumin significantly decreased.[95] Although these studies demonstrated an effect on the pulmonary capillary pressure, the effect of inhaled NO on the PVR appears to be distributed throughout the entire pulmonary circulation. In a perfused animal lung model of pulmonary hypertension induced with the thromboxane A$_2$ mimetic U-46619 and the NO synthase inhibitor N^G-nitro-L-arginine methyl ester (L-NAME), NO reduced arterial resistance by 16%, middle or microvascular ("capillary") resistance by 14%, and venous resistance by 10%. There was no difference in the effects of 5, 20 or 80 ppm NO.[96]

Reversal of hypoxic pulmonary vasoconstriction   Inhaled NO (40 ppm) reversed acute pulmonary vasoconstriction caused by the thromboxane A$_2$ mimetic U-46619 and by inhalation of a hypoxic gas mixture in lambs.[97] Similar results were obtained by inhalation of 40–80 ppm NO after pulmonary hypertension was induced by infusion of protamine in heparin pretreated lambs.[98] Subsequently, inhaled NO was found to be efficacious in nine healthy human volunteers who breathed 12% oxygen in nitrogen. During inhalation of 12% oxygen in nitrogen, PaO_2 decreased to 47 mmHg, pulmonary artery pressure rose from 15 to 20 mmHg, cardiac output increased and systemic vascular resistance decreased. When NO was added to the hypoxic mixture, the pulmonary artery pressure returned to baseline values while the PaO_2, cardiac output, and systemic vascular resistance all remained unchanged.[99]

Improvement in right ventricular function The depression of right ventricular function in sepsis, a potent cause of ARDS, is probably related to elevated pulmonary artery pressure and increased right ventricular afterload.[100,101] In an animal model of endotoxaemic shock, 40 ppm of inhaled NO significantly decreased pulmonary hypertension and increased right ventricular ejection fraction and oxygen delivery without adverse effects.[102] Right ventricular failure and unacceptably high pulmonary vascular resistance after heart transplantation have been reported to improve with inhaled NO.[103,104]

Improvement of ventilation perfusion matching ARDS may be associated with smoke inhalation which is characterised by pulmonary inflammation, pulmonary hypertension, increased pulmonary capillary permeability, and oedema. In an animal model of this entity, inhaled NO in concentrations of 20 and 40 ppm significantly attenuated pulmonary hypertension and hypoxaemia.[105] The mechanism was subsequently determined to be improved ventilation perfusion matching by causing selective pulmonary vasodilation of ventilated areas without bronchodilation.[106]

Chronic obstructive lung disease

Pulmonary hypertension develops in animals and humans exposed to chronic hypoxaemia. This is due to an increase in pulmonary vasomotor tone and structural remodelling of the pulmonary vascular bed. In patients with chronic obstructive lung (airway) (pulmonary) disease [COL(A)(P)D], impairment of the L-arginine NO pathway may be responsible for pulmonary hypertension. *In vitro* endothelium dependent relaxation of pulmonary arteries is impaired in arteries from patients with end stage chronic hypoxic lung disease.[107] In a clinical study of 13 such patients, inhaled NO 40 ppm selectively decreased pulmonary artery pressure from a mean of 32 to 26 mmHg and increased PaO_2 from 57 to 69 mmHg. In two of these patients, acetylcholine infusion failed to cause the expected pulmonary vasodilation, leading to the suggestion that inadequate production of endogenous NO from the pulmonary endothelium is the cause of pulmonary hypertension in this condition.[108] This suggestion is supported by the observation that vasodilators which generate NO and the analogue of cGMP, 8-bromocyclic guanosine monophosphate, all inhibit the proliferation of cultured rat vascular smooth muscle cells.[77] Failure of endogenous NO might allow remodelling of the pulmonary vascular system so characteristic of COLD. It has been speculated that low dose inhaled NO therapy may become a domiciliary treatment.[109] This is ironic in the light of the aetiological associations between emphysema and cigarette smoking and between emphysema and NO. Cigarette smoke contains high concentrations of NO[110] and causes pulmonary vasodilation[111] even in the presence of hypoxic induced vasoconstriction.[112] Thus domiciliary NO therapy may exacerbate the destruction of alveolar septa but ameliorate the pulmonary hypertension in this condition.

The effects of inhaled NO among patients with COPD have not been entirely consistent. In another study of the effects of inhaled NO 40 ppm in 13 patients with advanced chronic obstructive pulmonary disease, although a reduction in pulmonary artery pressure from 26 to 22 mmHg was observed, the PaO_2 also decreased from 56 to 53 mmHg. The latter was due to a worsening of ventilation perfusion matching.[113] In yet another study, inhalation of 15 ppm NO by 14 hypoxic patients with COPD caused a mean 19% reduction of pulmonary vascular resistance but no change in the PaO_2 from 59 mmHg and no change in the ventilation/perfusion ratio.[114]

Although endogenous nitric oxide has an extensive role in lung function, inhaled NO does not appear to have a place in the treatment of bronchoconstriction. Inhaled nitric oxide has pronounced bronchodilator effects in animals but this has not been substantiated in humans. Inhaled NO in a concentration of 5–300 ppm and the NO releasing substance S-nitroso-N-acetylpenicillamine reversed metacholine induced broncho-constriction in rats.[115] Endogenous nitric oxide is exhaled in higher concentrations by asthmatic patients[116] and NO appears to be induced in patients with asthma.[117] However, inhaled NO 80 ppm did not affect specific airway conductance tone in healthy volunteers or patients with chronic obstructive pulmonary disease, although it modulated the response to metacholine provocation in subjects with hyperreactive airways and had only a weak bronchodilatory effect in subjects with asthma. In the latter group, inhalation of a β_2 agonist was considerably more efficacious.[118] Other investigators have also observed that a β sympathomimetic drug improves airway conductance better than inhaled NO.[119] In patients with ARDS, inhalation of 20 or 40 ppm NO did not significantly improve static or dynamic compliance.[93]

Systems used to administer nitric oxide

The supply of NO, instruments for its measurement, and the safety limits for exposure all have industrial origins. Specified concentrations of NO can be obtained. Medical grade quality, not industrial grade should be requested. Cylinders should be accompanied by a certificate stating the contamination with other higher oxides of nitrogen. Concentrations of 400–1000 ppm in nitrogen, an inert gas, are commonly used. These concentrations enable manageable administration of low volumes of 1–80 ppm without causing dilutional hypoxia. Tables and graphs are available which relate the source gas concentration and its flow rate to the inspired gas concentration and the minute ventilation.[120] Cylinders should be large enough to enable several days of continuous therapy.

NO can be administered to spontaneously breathing or mechanically ventilated patients. Some mechanical ventilators incorporate NO delivery and monitoring systems but numerous *ad hoc* techniques to administer NO have been devised by physicians intent upon using a potentially life saving therapy. All should be simple, reliable, and safe. They should incorporate a device for monitoring both NO and NO_2 and a means to prevent or warn of accidental overdose of NO. They should deliver a constant concentration of NO and minimise the formation of NO_2. A means to deliver NO should be available via a hand bagging circuit whenever the NO dependent patient is detached from the ventilator because pulmonary pressure may rise and oxygenation deteriorate rapidly.[121] Scavenging of exhaled gases and gases exhausted from the ventilator or its circuit is advisable but not universally practised because only insignificant amounts of NO and NO_2 are detectable in the vicinity of ventilated patients.[122]

Because NO reacts with O_2 rapidly to form NO_2, it must be added to air or oxygen enriched mixtures immediately before inspiration by the patient. NO cannot be premixed with oxygen since in static experiments, toxic amounts are formed rapidly at commonly used concentrations of NO and O_2. For example, 80 ppm NO mixed with 60% oxygen formed 5 ppm NO_2 in 1 min[123] or in 24 s.[124]

The performance of several systems has been evaluated using constancy of NO concentration and the generation of NO_2 as outcome measures.

Continuous flow of NO added to the inspiratory limb of a continuous (bias) flow ventilator[125]

A constant concentration of NO is obtained and the transit time in the circuit is short but in this systematic bench study, 5 ppm and 3 ppm NO_2

210

were generated when 80 ppm and 50 ppm respectively were added to 90% oxygen in the inspiratory limb of a continuous flow pressure limited infant ventilator (Drager Ltd, Babylog 8000). The addition of NO proximal to the humidifier lead to a small decrease in the NO delivery and a small rise in NO_2. A mixing chamber inserted into the inspiratory limb of the circuit allowed electrochemical monitoring of NO without interference by water.[126]

Continuous flow of NO and O_2 mixture to drive an intermittent flow ventilator via its low pressure inlet[127,128]

This system has the advantage of providing a constant concentration of inspired NO unaffected by changes in minute ventilation, but it may also impose the disadvantage of a longer reaction time and the possibility of higher NO_2 levels. In one study, 5 ppm NO_2 were generated when 100 ppm NO and 100% oxygen were employed to simulate infant respiratory settings while 3.2 ppm were generated with typical adult settings.[128] In that study, however, the influence of the ratio of fresh gas flow relative to the minute ventilation was not addressed. The ratio would be expected to influence the transit and reaction times of the gases. In a documentation of clinical experience, rather than a systematic study, this system[129] generated 3 ppm NO_2 when a low minute ventilation and the fresh gas flow into the ventilator were equivalent.

Continuous flow of NO and O_2 mixture to drive an intermittent flow ventilator via its high pressure inlet [130,131]

Inspired NO concentration would be constant but NO_2 generation may be problematic. The generation of NO_2 in the circuits of the Servo 900C and Puritan-Bennett 7200 ventilators has been studied with this technique. As expected, the amounts generated were related to the concentrations of NO and of O_2. In addition, greater amounts of NO_2 were generated at smaller minute ventilations. For example, with the Servo ventilator, at a minute ventilation of 5.0 l/min, 0.5–3.5 ppm NO_2 were generated when the FiO_2 exceeded 0.37 and when NO exceeded 50 ppm; when the minute ventilation was 10 l/min, 0.5–1.5 ppm NO_2 were generated when the FiO_2 exceeded 0.62 and when NO exceeded 60 ppm.[130]

Continuous NO added to the inspiratory limb of an intermittent flow ventilator

This is the simplest technique but creates peaks and troughs of inspired NO concentration because NO accumulates in the circuit during the expiratory phase.[127,132] Moreover, variation in inspired NO is expected if minute ventilation changes, as when pressure supported ventilation is used.

Intermittent flow of NO added to the inspiratory limb of an intermittent flow ventilator

In one system, a pneumotachograph in the inspiratory limb feeds back to a mass flow controller in the NO supply line to restrict NO flow to the inspiratory phase of the respiratory cycle.[133] In other systems, NO is injected via a magnetic valve into the inspiratory limb during inspiration[134] or administered by a nebuliser module during inspiration.[85,90]

Monitoring nitric oxide concentration

NO may be measured by spectroscopic and electrochemical methods.[135,136] The former include chemiluminescence detection, ultraviolet visible spectroscopy and electron spin spectroscopy. Mass spectrometry and gas chromatography are impractical for routine clinical use. Chemiluminescence and electrochemical methods have been adopted.

Chemiluminescence detection

The chemiluminescence method is based on the measurement of intensity of the fluorescent radiation emitted after chemical oxidation of NO with ozone. The product of this reaction is an excited molecule of nitrogen dioxide (NO_2^*) which emits a photon. Detectors incorporate a fluorometer, a reaction chamber, and a photomultiplier. The total number of photons emitted is proportional to the NO concentration. The detection limit is 10 nmol/l (0.25 ppm) and a signal response plot shows two linear regions with different slopes for concentrations between 2×10^{-8} to 2×10^{-7} mol/l and 3×10^{-7} to 3×10^{-6} mol/l. Breath by breath analysis of NO is not possible. The response time is less than 30 s at 25°C. The concentration of NO_2 may be derived from chemiluminescence detection of NO. Higher oxides of nitrogen (NO_2, N_2O_3, N_2O_5) are reduced in the reaction chamber to NO. NO_2 is derived as the difference between NO and total higher oxides of nitrogen.

Chemiluminescence detectors are intended for industrial use and are not ideal for clinical situations. They are bulky, noisy, and expensive. They aspirate a sample of gas which may be a significant part of the minute ventilation.

Electrochemical sensors

Electrochemical sensors are smaller and less expensive than chemiluminescence detectors and are silent. They may be placed in line but are subject to interference by condensed water and pressure changes. Like chemiluminescence detectors, they were adopted from industrial use. They also have long response times and cannot give breath by breath analysis. A NO electrochemical sensor is based on a modified oxygen electrode (Clark electrode). The anode is a platinum wire, the cathode is a silver wire. The electrodes are mounted in a capillary tube filled with a sodium chloride–hydrochloric acid solution. A constant potential of 0.9 V is applied and a direct current is measured secondary to the electrochemical oxidation of NO on the platinum anode. NO must diffuse through a gas permeable membrane and an analytic solution. The response time is thus relatively long (20–30 s). The detection limit of the electrode is 5×10^{-7} mol/l with a narrow linear response range. NO_2 is similarly analysed by a probe with electrodes. A constant voltage is maintained to oxidise NO_2 at the anode ($NO_2 + 2H^+ + 2e = NO + H_2O$). The magnitude of the electric current is directly proportional to the NO_2 content.

Although chemiluminescence detectors represent the gold standard for clinical use, electrochemical sensors are more practical. Several studies have compared the performances of such machines with the intention of replacing the chemiluminescence devices, but with mixed conclusions.[137–139] The differences between measurements made by the chemiluminescence and electrochemical devices are too large and too variable to permit reliable substitution. Electrochemical devices suffice as warning devices against overdosage of NO and toxic amounts of NO_2 but are not sufficiently sensitive to measure low concentrations of NO (1–3 ppm), which may ultimately be regarded as the therapeutic range.

Calculation of NO concentration

The concentration of inspired NO (NO_i) or flow of the source concentration (NO_s) may be calculated approximately by the following formula:

$$NO_i = NO_s \times [NO \text{ flow}/(NO \text{ flow} + \text{ventilator flow})]$$

Alternatively, the concentration of inspired NO may be calculated by dilution of the concentration of source oxygen to an inspired concentration:[127]

$$NO_i = NO_s \times [1\text{-inspired } O_2/\text{source } O_2]$$

Toxic effects of inhaled nitric oxide therapy

It is tempting to assume that because NO is an endogenous substance, administration of exogenous inhaled NO is not harmful. However, this practice has some recognised problems and some others which are far from clear.

Exposure to nitrogen dioxide

Nitrogen dioxide (NO_2) is well known as an environmental toxic gas and is formed rapidly when NO reacts with oxygen. Its effects are related to the concentration and duration of inhalation. Organisations for the maintenance of occupational health and safety have recommended that workers are not exposed to more than 5 ppm NO_2 during an eight hour period or to more than an average of 3 ppm over a five day working week.[140,141] However, these standards may not be applicable to clinical situations where patients have severe lung disease and in whom NO therapy may be required for many days.

Inhaled NO_2 causes lipoperoxidation of lung lipids.[142] Chronic exposure to NO_2 causes emphysema. In rats, exposure to 0.8 ppm caused tachypnoea alone, exposure to 2 ppm caused loss of cilia and of exfoliative activity, exposure to 4 ppm caused hyperplasia of bronchial epithelium while exposure to 10–25 ppm caused a two thirds reduction in alveoli and death by respiratory failure.[143] Brief exposure to high concentration causes destruction of bronchiolar epithelium.[144]

In adult humans, the effects of short term exposure are variable and a consequence of lipid peroxidation. Inhalation of 5 ppm NO_2 for 15 min caused a reduction in the diffusion capacity for carbon monoxide while 1.6–2.0 ppm caused an increase in airway resistance.[145] In another study, however, short term exposure to 4 ppm for 75 min produced no immediate effects.[146] The effects of low level NO_2 exposure are characteristically delayed. Exposure to 2.3 ppm caused reduction in glutathione peroxidase

214

(antioxidant) activity after 24 hours and a decrease in alveolar permeability after 11 hours.[147]

Preexisting respiratory illness increases susceptibilty to NO_2. The threshold to increase airway resistance is approximately 2.5 ppm in healthy subjects but 1.5 ppm in subjects with chronic bronchitis while in asthmatics, less than 1 ppm enhances airway responsiveness to various bronchconstrictor stimuli.[148] Exposure to 4 ppm adversely affects immune defence in the healthy lung.[149]

The margin of safety against NO_2 toxicity during inhaled NO therapy is relatively small. Indeed, several analyses of the performance of current delivery systems have revealed that the amount of NO_2 generated may exceed an environmentally safe amount (3 or 5 ppm) when 80–100 ppm NO is combined with oxygen in a concentration of 60% or more.[125,128]

Since evidence about long term exposure to NO_2 during severe lung disease and other potentially harmful therapies is lacking, it appears prudent to minimise amounts of inhaled NO_2. It cannot be eliminated by the use of soda lime. Although one study revealed that soda lime absorbs approximately 80% of NO_2 from the inspiratory line of a ventilator circuit in contrast to 15% of NO,[128] a systematic study of the efficacies of several preparations of soda lime found equivalent absorption of both NO_2 and NO.[150] Soda lime is therefore not a useful absorbent for NO_2 during NO therapy.

Nitric oxide toxicity

Little is known of the possible effects of inhaled nitric oxide beyond the respiratory and cardiovascular systems. In some observations, the effects are difficult to distinguish from those of NO_2. Nonetheless, the attribution of deleterious effects to NO_2 or NO is irrelevant in a clinical situation where NO is converted to NO_2 – both remain a consequence of NO therapy. An early account of NO toxicity cannot be attributed entirely to NO; exposure to very high concentrations of NO (20 000 ppm) in dogs caused acute pulmonary oedema and methaemoglobinaemia.[151,152] However, such concentration formed a brown gas within several seconds when mixed with oxygen, thus suggesting the formation of NO_2.

Short term inhalation of clinically relevant concentrations appears to have either nil or minor effects. Inhalation of 80 ppm for three hours in lambs did not increase extravascular lung water or modify lung histology.[97] Exposure to 43 ppm for six days in rabbits did not cause any lung histological changes[153] and indeed, nor did exposure to much greater concentrations of 1500 ppm for 15 min or to 1000 ppm for 30 min in rats.[154] Spontaneous inhalation of 20–30 ppm NO by healthy adults caused a reduction in PaO_2

215

of 8 mmHg, an increase in airway resistance but no change in diffusion capacity for CO. No changes in gas exchange or resistance were observed with less than 15 ppm.[155] A minor decrease in airway conductance was noted in healthy adults inhaling 1 ppm NO for two hours.[156]

Little is known of the effects of long term exposure of humans to NO. However, prolonged exposure of rats for nine weeks to 0.5 ppm with twice-daily one hour spikes to 1.5 ppm caused degeneration of interstitial cells, the interstitial matrix, and connective tissue fibres of alveolar septa. These changes resemble those observed in emphysema.[157]

In inflammation, ischaemia reperfusion and hyperoxic lung injury, the formation of oxidants exacerbates injury. Endogenous NO has a significant role in this process via the formation of peroxynitrite but it is not yet clear whether the role of NO is injurious or protective.[35] No information is available about the possible contribution of exogenous NO to the formation of peroxynitrite. The lung has antioxidant defences including superoxide dismutase (SOD) which converts superoxide (O_2^-) to hydrogen peroxide (H_2O_2), which in turn is converted to water and oxygen by catalase, thereby limiting the formation of more potent hydroxyl radicals (OH^-) formed when ferrous ions react with hydrogen peroxide. Hydroxyl radicals disrupt DNA strands and promote lipid peroxidation. Endogenous NO is an alternative target for superoxide to form peroxynitrite ($ONOO^-$) which can undergo any of three oxidative reactions, dependent on pH. These are reactions with protein and non-protein sulphydryl residues, the nitration of phenolic rings (e.g. of tyrosine) and, by protonation, the formation of peroxynitrous acid with its hydroxyl radical-like oxidant effects. Approximately 25% of $ONOO^-$ forms hydroxyl radicals.[158,159] Thus the formation of peroxynitrite may on one hand prevent the formation of hydroxyl radicals by diverting superoxide away from a reaction with iron but on the other contribute to the formation of hydroxyl radicals but to a lesser extent by a different route. Peroxynitrite is known to induce a lipoperoxidative injury to pulmonary surfactant[160] and there is indirect evidence that peroxynitrite is produced in ARDS; nitrotyrosine residues were demonstrable in postmortem lung tissue.[161]

NO radicals can be scavenged *in vitro* by nitecapone, which offers promise for this or related agents for the treatment of diseases associated with production of NO[162] and perhaps for scavenging of reactive species generated by NO therapy – if this proves to be real.

Formation of methaemoglobin

The selective pulmonary vasodilator activity of inhaled NO owes its efficacy to affinity with metallic irons. When NO gains access to blood, it reacts with the haem moiety of haemoglobin to form methaemoglobin by converting the ferrous state to ferric. The majority of methaemoglobin is converted back to haemoglobin by NADH dependent methaemoglobin reductase. A small amount of methaemoglobin is converted to haemoglobin by NADPH dependent methaemoglobin reductase. Autooxidation of haemoglobin causes a normal level of methaemoglobin of less than 1%. However, excessive administration of inhaled NO may overwhelm the enzymatic reconversion and cause high levels of methaemoglobin, which cannot carry oxygen or carbon dioxide and which prevent dissociation of oxyhaemoglobin. A state of severe hypoxaemia and acidosis may occur. Methaemoglobinaemia levels under 30% are tolerated by healthy persons whereas levels betwen 30–50% depress the central nervous and cardiovascular systems, 50–70% causes acidosis, bradycardia, respiratory depression, convulsions, and dysrhythmias while levels above 70% are usually fatal.[163]

A pharmacokinetic study in healthy adults predicted that maximum levels of approximately 1.0%, 1.8%, 3.8%, and 6.9% methaemoglobin would be formed after 3–5 hours by the continuous inhalation of 32, 64, 128, and 512 ppm respectively.[164] However, such limits may not apply to any patient with lung disease or to any infants. Newborns have reduced NADH dependent methaemoglobin reductase activity[165] while umbilical cord (haemoglobin F) may undergo autooxidation more readily than haemoglobin A.[166] Indeed, in many single case reports substantial levels of methaemoglobinaemia have been reported during NO therapy, particularly above 40 ppm. Brief therapy (15–30 min) with up to 80 ppm does not cause significant methaemoglobinaemia.[78,81] However, prolonged administration of 80 ppm NO is associated with significant methaemoglobinaemia. In one series using 80 ppm, several patients had methaemoglobin levels of 9.6% and 14%[129] while in another, 70 ppm NO was associated with 11.4% methaemoglobin.[167] Inhalation of 80 ppm for several hours by a premature newborn was associated with a rise to 3.5%.[84] High levels of methaemoglobinaemia should be managed with reduction of NO dose and intravenous administration of methylene blue (1.0–2.0 mg/kg) or ascorbic acid (500 mg) intravenously. The latter is less effective. Methylene blue is a cofactor for NADPH dependent methaemoglobin reductase.

The methaemoglobin level should be checked regularly by cooximetry, particularly if the therapeutic NO concentration exceeds 40 ppm, or less in newborns. A falling pulse oximetry reading should lead to a suspicion of a rising methaemoglobin level. Methaemoglobinaemia cannot be inferred from routine arterial blood gas tension measurements unless severe hypoxaemia is present, since the haemoglobin oxygen saturation calculated from these measurements is false. A decision to treat a raised methaemoglobin level with the antidote and by reduction in dose depends upon the absolute level and other factors which determine oxygen transport. A level of 10% or more should be treated with methylene blue. A level of less than 10% may require methylene blue depending on the haemoglobin and oxygenation status while a level of less than 5% may be manageable with reduction in the dose of NO alone. Elimination of NO follows first order kinetics with a time constant of 39–91 min in adults.[164]

Theoretically, administration of methylene blue may be expected to block the pulmonary dilatory action of NO therapy since it also inhibits guanylate cyclase.[168] Although administration of methylene blue did not reverse the pulmonary vasodilatory action of inhaled NO in pulmonary vasoconstricted hypoxaemic sheep,[169] it did increase both systemic and pulmonary artery pressure in humans with septic shock.[170]

Cardiac effects

Inhaled nitric oxide should be administered with caution to patients with left ventricular failure since there are several lines of evidence which suggest that both endogenous and exogenous NO have a negative inotropic effect, despite the observation that coronary blood flow is regulated by endogenous endothelial release of NO.[171]

Negative inotropic effect

Numerous experimental studies suggest that NO has a negative inotropic effect. Exogenous NO solution and nitroprusside depress guinea pig myocyte contraction and this effect was abolished by the L-arginine analogue N^G-nitro-L-arginine methyl ester.[172] The analogue of cGMP, 8-bromo-cGMP, also has a negative inotropic effect on ferret cardiac muscle.[173] The release of NO from the ferret endocardial endothelium raises myocardial cGMP and is associated with earlier myocardial relaxation and a decrease in peak force of contraction.[174] Endogenous NO from within rat myocytes causes a negative inotropic effect which is mimicked by 8-bromo-cGMP. Moreover, the L-arginine analogue NOS inhibitor (N^W-nitro-L-arginine) prevents this effect and increases the inotropic effect of the β adrenergic agonist isoproterenol.[175] In the isolated ejecting guinea pig heart, the NO donor nitroprusside and endogenous NO selectively modulate left ventricular relaxation.[176,177] Intracoronary infusion of an NOS inhibitor alone in patients with left ventricular dysfunction had no effect on left ventricular function but potentiated the inotropic action of dobutamine, thus suggesting that NO attenuates the inotropic response to β adrenergic stimulation.[178]

In heart failure there appears to be a decrease in the release of endogenous NO from the coronary vasculature. For example, in a canine model of heart failure induced by pacing, coronary arteries and microvessels produce less nitrite (the metabolite of nitric oxide) and are less responsive to acetylcholine dependent production of nitrite.[179] This is like endothelial dysfunction of peripheral arteries, well known in heart failure, and leads to greater peripheral vascular resistance.[180,181] Furthermore, infusion of the NOS inhibitor NG-monomethyl-L-arginine (L-NMMA) increased pulmonary and systemic resistance in patients with heart failure, suggesting that endothelial cells are incapable of producing NO or alternatively that NO production is at a maximum and that the increased vascular tone in heart failure represents a failure of a counterregulatory vasodilator system.[182] Endogenous NO appears to reduce contractility in the acutely ischaemic heart because infusion of L-NAME into the left anterior descending artery increased fractional shortening under ischaemic conditions but not under non-ischaemic conditions and the effects of L-NAME were prevented by infusion of L-arginine.[183] Thus endogenous NO production is depressed in heart failure but the mechanism by which this occurs is unknown.

Despite a decrease in activity of the constitutive NOS in cardiac endothelial tissue,[184] the plasma level of nitrates is raised in patients with heart failure,[185] thus suggesting that some other tissue has increased NOS activity. Perhaps this is due to an increased basal level of activity elsewhere to compensate for decreased vascular smooth muscle responsiveness to cGMP mediated vasodilation and neurohumoral vasoconstriction in heart failure.[181,186] Alternatively, high levels of plasma nitrate in heart failure may be due to the actions of cytokines such as tumour necrosis factor which is known to be elevated in heart failure[187] and which may activate inducible NOS in myocardial cells or the vasculature.

An obvious source of endogenous NO are the coronary vessel and endocardial endothelia. However, NO is probably also produced by cardiac myocytes since activated macrophages induce NOS within rat cardiac myocytes to depress the contractile response to β adrenergic agonist.[188] Of interest is the observation that endogenous NO is produced within skeletal muscle and that it also promotes relaxation via the cGMP pathway.[189]

Exogenous NO may also cause the same negative inotropic effect. Administration of an oral NO donor downregulated NOS gene expression in canine aortic endothelium[190] while NO and NO donors similarly inhibited NOS in bovine aortic endothelial cells[191] and in murine macrophages.[192] These observations of negative feedback may explain the difficulty sometimes observed in weaning patients from exogenous NO therapy.[85,86,89,103] This phenomenon has been labelled "rebound pulmonary hypertension".[193] Indeed, NO gas can inhibit the action of inducible NOS in aortic tissue.[194]

Inhaled NO does not appear to cause any problem in patients without cardiac failure. For example, in patients with lung injury but with mean cardiac output of 9.1 l/min, 40 ppm NO caused significant decreases in mean pulmonary pressure (34.1 to 29.6 mmHg) and mean PVR (166 to 128 dyne/s/cm^5) but insignificant changes in mean pulmonary artery wedge pressure (17.0 to 16.3 mmHg) and mean cardiac output.[94] Insignificant changes in cardiac output have also been observed in other studies of patients subjected to inhaled NO.[85,88,89,93,169]

NO therapy is sometimes used in the combined circumstances of pulmonary hypertension and heart failure. An overall benefit should not be assumed. It is established that NO lowers PVR in patients with primary or secondary pulmonary hypertension. However, in patients with left ventricular dysfunction, the reduction in PVR may be a result of a greater increase in left ventricular filling pressure rather than a lesser change (decrease or increase) in pulmonary artery pressure. These effects may not be obvious in the routine clinical setting since such changes may be accompanied by minor changes in systemic artery pressure and cardiac output. Several studies of inhaled NO in patients with heart failure illustrate these effects.

In a study of 19 patients with left ventricular dysfunction (mean cardiac output 2.3 l/min/m^2), inhaled 80 ppm NO caused a reduction in mean pulmonary vascular resistance from 226 to 119 dyne/s/cm^5 but an increase in mean pulmonary artery wedge pressure from 25 to 31 mmHg while the mean (systemic) and pulmonary artery pressures and cardiac index changed insignificantly.[195] In another study[196] of 12 heart transplantation candidates, inhalation of 20 ppm NO did not change systemic or pulmonary arterial pressure, cardiac output or systemic vascular resistance. However, PVR and transpulmonary gradient decreased 36% and 34% respectively. These decreases were explained by an increase in the mean pulmonary capillary wedge pressure from 28 to 33 mmHg. Sodium nitroprusside (SNP) 2 μg/kg/min also decreased the PVR, but in contrast to inhaled NO, the reduction in PVR was a result of decreases in the pulmonary artery pressure and pulmonary capillary wedge pressure and an increase in cardiac output. While SNP caused a significant decrease in systemic blood pressure, NO did not. The authors suggested that the NO induced increase in PCWP was due to pulmonary vasodilation rather than a negative inotropic effect. However, the latter seems a more plausible explanation. In yet another study of three patients, inhalation of 40 or 80 ppm was associated with reduction in PVR and an increase in cardiac output but clinical and radiological pulmonary oedema developed and in two patients the pulmonary capillary wedge pressure increased.[197]

Mechanism of negative inotropism

The question arises as to how NO modulates cardiac function. An interaction between cAMP and cGMP appears responsible (fig 8.5). The

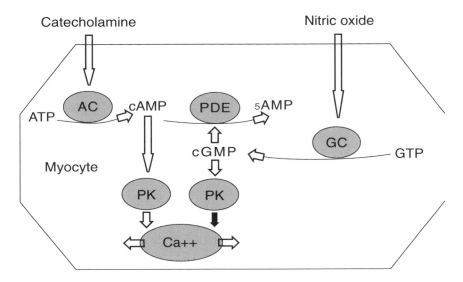

FIGURE 8.5—*Modulation of inotropic response by nitric oxide. ATP, adenosine triphosphate; AC, adenylate cyclase; cAMP, cyclic adenosine monophosphate; PDE, phosphodiesterase; 5AMP, 5 adenosine monophosphate; cGMP, cyclic guanosine monophosphate; PK, protein kinase; GC, guanylate cyclase; GTP, guanose triphosphate; Ca + +, ionised calcium; unfilled arrows, facilitatory actions; filled arrows, inhibitory actions*

positive inotropic effects of β adrenergic receptor stimulation are attributed to cAMP dependent phosphorylation of the Ca^{++} channel (Ica) via a protein kinase after adenyl cyclase converts ATP to cAMP. Cyclic AMP is degraded by cAMP phosphodiesterase. NO activates gaunylate cyclase to convert guanosine triphosphate (GTP) to cyclic (c)GMP which has a dual inhibitory action. It inhibits Ica by activation of cAMP phosphodiesterase and by activation of a cGMP protein kinase – an observation made in frog cardiac myocytes.[198] However, more recent work by the same group revealed that NO donors have both activatory and inhibitory effects on Ica which are mediated by cGMP sensitive cAMP phosphodiesterase. However, these opposing effects are dependent on the dose of NO donor and the state of the Ica. Basal Ica is not influenced by an NO donor alone but nanomolar amounts augment the effects of adrenergic stimulation whereas a millimolar amount reduced the adrenergic stimulated Ica.[199] In human cardiac myocytes, picomolar amounts of an NO donor exerted a profound

221

stimulatory effect on the basal calcium current, an effect which was similar to milrinone, a selective inhibitor of cGMP inhibited cAMP phosphodiesterase.[200]

Although NO appears to have a negative inotropic effect, other effects, including inhibition of leucocyte adhesion, may have important benefits. It is well known that coronary reperfusion after ischaemia contributes to myocardial cell injury. The reperfusion injury is probably due to neutrophils activated as a consequence of the inability of damaged coronary endothelium to release NO. Classic NO donors (nitrates) and novel NO donors (synonimines, molsidomine, cysteine containing agents, nonoates) may represent a new way of inducing vasodilation and inhibiting leucocyte adhesion in vascular tissues devoid of endogenous NO.[201] Such substances may eventually be employed in lieu of inhaled NO.

Antiplatelet effects

Endogenous NO and NO releasing vasodilators, such as nitroprusside, inhibit the aggregation of platelets and their adhesion to vascular endothelial cells.[202-205] Inhalation of NO 30 ppm for 15 min was associated with a 33% increase in the bleeding time ratio of six volunteers. In three of these, the bleeding time ratio was 14% above baseline 30 min after cessation of therapy and in the other three the ratio was 4% above baseline 60 min after cessation.[206] Agents that bind NO, such as purified crosslinked haemoglobin, increase platelet deposition at sites of subintimal injury.[207] These observations taken together suggest that the haematological effects of inhaled NO therapy are not confined to the formation of methaemoglobin and that coagulation should be monitored in patients receiving inhaled NO therapy. Thus far, serious problems with bleeding have not been reported in patients receiving inhaled NO therapy. This aspect of NO therapy requires more research.

Mutagenic and cytotoxic activities

Several mechanisms exist whereby elevated intracellular NO may potentially cause inheritable genomic alteration. These mechanisms are the formation of carcinogenic N-nitroso compounds, oxidation of DNA after formation of peroxynitrite and hydroxy radicals and the direct deamination of DNA bases.[208] The recognition of nitrosative deamination is not new but has been reactivated by studies which include NO among other nitrates, nitrites, and NO releasing compounds. NO in tobacco smoke may be another carcinogenic agent. It is present in a concentration of

700–1000 ppm.[110] The addition of aqueous NO to cultured human cells caused a 44-fold increase over spontaneous deamination mutation at a specified gene.[209] In another study, the addition of NO to human lymphoblastoid cells increased mutations 15–18-fold while addition to nucleic acids, DNA and RNA induced strand breakage and deamination of guanine and adenine.[210] In living *Salmonella typhimurium*, several NO releasing compounds, including nitroglycerine induced deamination of cytosine.[211] However, in direct contrast, NO did not cause deamination of cytosine in doublestranded DNA in *Escherichia coli*.[212] Although these studies indicate that NO is an important mediator of mutagenesis, there is no evidence related to inhaled NO therapy.

The oxidative actions of endogenously produced NO are important in defence against bacteria and tumour cells. It acts in conjunction with other free radicals including hydroxyl (OH^-), peroxide (H_2O_2), and superoxide (O_2^-). The free radical peroxynitrite ($ONOO^-$) forms from a reaction of NO with superoxide (O_2^-). This more active species is more bactericidal than both NO and O_2^-[213] and a more potent suppressant of mitochondrial respiration than NO in the cytotoxicity associated with immune stimulation.[214] The toxicity of inhaled NO towards native cells is unknown. However, NO donating agents enhance the damage to endothelial cells caused by H_2O_2 *in vitro*.[215]

Safety issues

Cylinders should be of aluminium alloy. Ancillary equipment such as regulators and flow meters should be constructed from stainless steel and other non-reactive substances. NO reacts with water to form corrosive acids but this has not appeared to be a practical problem when exposed to water in a humidifier.[127]

Cylinders of NO should be stored in a dedicated storage area, preferably open to the atmosphere. The availability of self-contained breathing apparatus is recommended in the case of accidental leakage.

Particular care should be taken when setting up a system to administer NO. There are no special measures, such as a pin index system, to prevent the accidental connection of other special gas mixtures, instead of a NO containing cylinder, to a ventilator circuit. Moreover, all cylinders of toxic non-flammable special gas mixtures appear identical with a yellow shoulder. For example, cylinders of nitric oxide, carbon monoxide and nitrogen dioxide are similar.

Although it is possible to administer NO and to calculate its concentration by use of accurate flow ratios or by dilution of another carrier gas,[127] the use of a monitoring device is highly recommended. Although the therapeutic dose of NO is probably less than 5 ppm for most purposes, concentrations of up to 80 ppm have been used, which may cause toxic levels of NO and of NO_2. The concentration of the latter cannot be calculated.

Ventilator circuits should incorporate an oxygen failure alarm, particularly those in which an $NO-O_2$ gas mixture drives the ventilator.

Alternatives to inhaled nitric oxide

An ideal pulmonary vasodilator must be selective to the pulmonary circulation and to the areas of lung which are ventilated.[216] Many systemically administered agents have been used to achieve pulmonary vasodilation. Among these are sodium nitroprusside, glyceryl trinitrate, isoprenaline, tolazoline, phenoxybenzamine, prostaglandin E1, and prostacyclin (PGI_2). All suffer from the disadvantage of causing both pulmonary and systemic vasodilation. Some of these agents with short half lives have been delivered into the pulmonary circulation in the forlorn hope that their effects will be contained in the pulmonary circulation. Moreover, they have increased blood flow to non-ventilated alveoli, thus increasing intrapulmonary shunting and decreasing oxygenation.

Inhaled aerosolised PGI_2 appears to be a pulmonary selective agent and an alternative to inhaled NO. Moreover, it appears free of serious toxic effects. Although its administration is simple, its delivery may be variable. It is a naturally occurring agent released from endothelial and other cells. It has a short half life of a few minutes and achieves vasodilation by activation of adenyl cyclase, which forms cAMP leading to a decrease in intracellular calcium via the effect of a protein kinase. Since it also causes release of NO from coronary artery endothelium,[217] a part of its effect may be via cGMP. Clinical experience is limited.

Inhalation of PGI_2 0.9 and 1.8 ng/kg/min ameliorated hypoxic induced pulmonary vasoconstriction in dogs to the extent similar to 50 ppm inhaled NO.[218] Inhalation of 50 µg/min by five healthy adult volunteers caused a decrease in (systemic) vascular resistance and inhibition of ADP induced platelet aggregation.[219] However, more recent reports of lower doses in patients have highlighted beneficial effects. In three adult patients with ARDS, doses of 17–50 ng/kg/min decreased mean pulmonary artery pressure from 40 to 32 mmHg while systemic pressure decreased from 77 to 75 mmHg and concomitantly, the PaO_2/FiO_2 ratio increased from 120 to 173 due to redistribution of blood flow from shunted areas.[220] In three children with ARDS, administration of inhaled NO in doses of 0.1, 1.0, and 10.0 ppm was compared to inhalation of PGI_2 in doses of 2, 10, and 20 ng/kg/min.[221] Although this was not a systematic study, NO reduced pulmonary artery pressure in all three patients at all doses except at 0.1 ppm in one patient and consistently raised the PaO_2/FiO_2 ratio in all patients at all doses. In contrast, PGI_2 had variable effects on pulmonary artery pressure and the PaO_2/FiO_2 ratio in all patients. The authors postulated that the delivery of PGI_2 may have been variable and called for a more extensive study. Administration of inhaled PGI_2 in doses of 20–50 ng/kg/min achieved a substantial improvement in oxygenation in one patient with amniotic fluid embolism while doses of 30–50 ng/kg/min achieved substantial reductions in pulmonary hypertension and a lesser improvement in alveolar-arterial oxygen difference which reverted when the drug was withdrawn.[222]

The effects of inhaled PGI_2 were compared among 12 patients mechanically ventilated for pneumonia with and without interstitial fibrosis.[223] In six of those with fibrosis, a dose of 33.6 ± 12 ng/kg/min reduced mean pulmonary artery pressure from 38 to 31 mmHg but decreased systemic arterial pressure from 80 to 71 mmHg, decreased the PaO_2/FiO_2 ratio from 74 to 66, and increased intrapulmonary shunt from 45% to 49%: In six without interstitial fibrosis, inhalation of 6.6 ± 3.0 ng/kg/min had comparable beneficial effects by decreasing mean pulmonary artery pressure from 35 to 31 mmHg and in addition, improved the PaO_2/FiO_2 ratio from 100 to 134 and decreased intrapulmonary shunt from 37% to 28% without adversely affecting systemic arterial pressure or cardiac output. In a single case report in a patient with pneumonia, inhalation of 5 ng/kg/min improved oxygenation and decreased pulmonary artery pressure.[224]

Administration of an unspecified dose of inhaled PGI_2 achieved a reduction in systolic pulmonary artery pressure from 60 to 50 mmHg and improvement in oxygenation in a newborn infant with right ventricular dyskinesia undergoing surgical repair of total anomalous venous drainage. Cessation of PGI_2 after 13 hours was associated with an increase in pulmonary artery pressure and a deterioration in oxygenation, which were both remedied with inhaled NO at 40 ppm.[225]

The relative economic costs of the two agents may ultimately determine which is preferable. The variable daily cost of PGI_2 at 20 ng/kg/min is approximately 50 times that of inhaled NO at 20 ppm.[226]

Inhaled aerolised PGI_2, like inhaled NO, is not approved for routine use and is regarded by regulatory and licensing bodies as an experimental substance. Its use therefore requires informed consent in a setting of a serious or life threatening condition.

Summary

Inhaled NO therapy has been widely adopted as a selective pulmonary vasodilator to reduce pulmonary hypertension and to improve ventilation perfusion matching and hence oxygenation, particularly during mechanical ventilation. However, no randomised controlled trials of its efficacy have yet been published. It remains an experimental substance and has not yet been licensed as a regular therapeutic substance. Nonetheless, it holds an enormous attraction for physicians who view it as an important advance in clinical therapeutics, supported by its existence as a naturally occurring potent substance.

1 Furchgott RF, Zawadzki JV. The obligatory role of endothelial cells in the relaxation of arterial smooth muscle by acetylcholine. *Nature* 1980;**288**:373–6.

2 Palmer RMJ, Ferrige AG, Moncada S. Nitric oxide release accounts for the biological activity of endothelium-derived relaxing factor. *Nature* 1987;**327**:524–6.

3 Ignarro LJ, Buga GM, Wood KS, Byrns RE, Chaudhuri G. Endothelium-derived relaxing factor produced and released from artery and vein is nitric oxide. *Proc Natl Acad Sci USA* 1987;**84**:9265–9.

4 Anggard E. Nitric oxide: mediator, murderer, and medicine. *Lancet* 1994;**343**:1199–206.

5 Moncada S, Palmer RM, Higgs EA. Nitric oxide: physiology, pathophysiology, and pharmacology. *Pharmacol Rev* 1991;**43**:109–42.

6 Bredt DS, Snyder SH. Nitric oxide: a physiologic messenger molecule. *Ann Rev Biochem* 1994;**63**:175–95.

7 Billiar TR. Nitric oxide. Novel biology with clinical relevance. *Ann Surg* 1995;**221**: 339–49.

8 Kuo PC, Schroeder RA. The multifaceted roles of nitric oxide. *Ann Surg* 1995;**221**: 220–35.

9 Snyder SH. Nitric oxide. More jobs for that molecule. *Nature* 1994;**372**:504–5.

10 Lowenstein CJ, Dinerman JL, Snyder SH. Nitric oxide: a physiologic messenger. *Ann Intern Med* 1994;**120**:227–37.

11 Tibballs J. The role of nitric oxide (formerly endothelium-derived relaxing factor – EDRF) in vasodilatation and vasodilator therapy. *Anaesth Intens Care* 1993;**21**:759–73.

12 Calver A, Collier J, Vallance P. Nitric oxide and the control of human vascular tone in health and disease. *Eur J Med* 1993;**2**:48–53.

13 Radomski MW, Moncada S. Regulation of vascular homeostasis by nitric oxide. *Thromb Haemost* 1993;**70**:36–41.

14 Ignarro LJ. Nitric oxide-mediated vasorelaxation. *Thromb Haemost* 1993;**70**:148–51.

15 Vane JR, Botting RM. Endothelium-derived vasoactive factors and the control of the circulation. *Semin Perinatol* 1991;**15**:4–10.

16 Brady AJ, Poole-Wilson PA. Circulatory failure in septic shock. Nitric oxide: too much of a good thing? *Br Heart J* 1993;**70**:103–5.

17 Weitzberg E. Circulatory responses to endothelin-1 and nitric oxide with special reference to endotoxic shock and nitric oxide inhalation. *Acta Physiol Scand Suppl* 1993;**611**:1–72.

18 Wolfe TA, Dasta JF. Use of nitric oxide synthase inhibitors as a novel treatment for septic shock. *Ann Pharmacother* 1995;**29**:36–46.

19 Booke M, Meyer J, Lingnau W, Hinder F, Traber LD, Traber DL. Use of nitric oxide synthase inhibitors in animal models of sepsis. *New Horizons* 1995;**3**:123–38.

20 Nijkamp FP, Folkerts G. Nitric oxide and bronchial reactivity. *Clin Exp Allergy* 1994;**24**: 905–14.

21 Barnes PJ. Nitric oxide and airways. *Eur Respir J* 1993;**6**:163–5.

22 Rossaint R, Pison U, Gerlach H, Falke KJ. Inhaled nitric oxide: its effects on pulmonary circulation and airway smooth muscle cells. *Eur Heart J* 1993;**14** (suppl 1):133–40.

23 Gaston B, Drazen JM, Loscalzo J, Stamler JS. The biology of nitrogen oxides in the airways. *Am J Respir Crit Care Med* 1994;**149**:538–51.

24 Luscher TF. Platelet-vessel wall interaction: role of nitric oxide, prostaglandins and endothelins. *Baillière's Clin Haematol* 1993;**6**:609–27.

25 Lipton SA, Singel DJ, Stamler JS. Neuroprotective and neurodestructive effects of nitric oxide and redox cogeners. *Ann NY Acad Sci* 1994;**738**:382–7.

26 Grozdanovic Z, Brunig G, Baumgarten HG. Nitric oxide – a novel autonomic neurotransmitter. *Acta Anat* 1994;**150**:16–24.

27 Bennett MR. Nitric oxide release and long term potentiation at synapses in autonomic ganglia. *Gen Pharmacol* 1994;**25**:1541–51.

28 Brosnan CF, Battistini L, Raine CS, Dickson DW, Casadevall A, Lee SC. Reactive nitrogen intermediates in human neuropathology: an overview. *Dev Neurosci* 1994;**16**: 152–61.

29 Dawson TM, Zhang J, Dawson VL, Snyder SH. Nitric oxide: cellular regulation and neuronal injury. *Prog Brain Res* 1994;**103**:365–9.

30 Lipton SA, Singel DJ, Stamler JS. Nitric oxide in the central nervous system. *Prog Brain Res* 1994;**103**:359–64.

31 Snyder SH. Nitric oxide: first in a new class of transmitters? *Science* 1992;**257**:494–6.

32 Dawson TM, Dawson VL. ADP-ribosylation as a mechanism for the action of nitric oxide in the nervous system. *New Horizons* 1995;**3**:86–92.

33 Albina JE, Reichner JS. Nitric oxide in inflammation and immunity. *New Horizons* 1995; **3**:46–64.

34 Pastor CM, Billiar TR. Regulation and function of nitric oxide in the liver in sepsis and inflammation. *New Horizons* 1995;**3**:65–72.

35 Royall JA, Kooy NW, Beckman JS. Nitric oxide-related oxidants in acute lung injury. *New Horizons* 1995;**3**:113–22.

36 Salzman AL. Nitric oxide in the gut. *New Horizons* 1995;**3**:33–45.

37 Zapol WM, Rimar S, Gillis N, Marletta M, Bosken CH. Nitric oxide and the lung. NHBI Workshop Summary. *Am J Respir Crit Care Med* 1994;**149**:1375–80.

38 Pearl PG. Inhaled nitric oxide. The past, the present, and the future. *Anesthesiology* 1993;**78**:413–16.

39 Edwards AD. The pharmacology of inhaled nitric oxide. *Arch Dis Child Fetal Neonatal Ed* 1995;**72**:F127–F130.

40 Cioffi WG, Ogura H. Inhaled nitric oxide in acute lung disease. *New Horizons* 1995;**3**: 73–85.

41 Adatia I, Wessel DL. Therapeutic use of inhaled nitric oxide. *Curr Opin Pediatr* 1994;**6**: 583–90.

42 Zapol WM. Minidose inhaled nitric oxide: less is better. *Intens Care Med* 1993;**19**:433–4.

43 Geggel RL. Inhalational nitric oxide: a selective pulmonary vasodilator for treatment of persistent pulmonary hypertension of the newborn. *J Pediatr* 1993;**123**:76–9.

44 Davidson D. No bandwagon yet. Inhaled nitric oxide (NO) for neonatal pulmonary hypertension. *Am Rev Respir Dis* 1993;**147**:1078–9.

45 Mupanemunda RH, Edwards AD. Treatment of newborn infants with inhaled nitric oxide. *Arch Dis Child Fetal Neonatal Ed* 1995;**72**:F131–F134.

46 Moncada S, Higgs A. The L-arginine–nitric oxide pathway. *N Engl J Med* 1993;**329**: 2002–12.

47 Szabo C. Alterations in nitric oxide production in various forms of circulatory shock. *New Horizons* 1995;**3**:2–32.

48 Rimar S, Gillis CN. Selective pulmonary vasodilation by inhaled nitric oxide is due to hemoglobin inactivation. *Circulation* 1993;**88**:2884–7.

49 Wennmalm A, Benthin G, Edlund A, *et al.* Metabolism and excretion of nitric oxide in humans. An experimental and clinical study. *Circ Res* 1993;**73**:1121–7.

50 Valvini EM, Young JD. Serum nitrogen oxides during nitric oxide inhalation. *Br J Anaesth* 1995;**74**:338–9.

51 Shi Y, Li H-Q, Shen C-K, *et al.* Plasma nitric oxide levels in newborn infants with sepsis. *J Pediatr* 1993;**1213**:435–8.

52 Roos CM, Rich GF, Uncles DR, Daugherty MO, Frank DU. Sites of vasodilation by inhaled nitric oxide vs. sodium nitroprusside in endothelin-constricted isolated rat lungs. *J Appl Physiol* 1994;**77**:51–7.

53 Pepke-Zaba J, Higenbottam TW, Dinh-Xuan AT, Stone D, Wallwork J. Inhaled nitric oxide as a cause of selective pulmonary vasodilation in pulmonary hypertension. *Lancet* 1991;**338**:1173–4.

54 Sitbon O, Brenot F, Denjean A, *et al*. Inhaled nitric oxide as a screening agent in primary pulmonary hypertension. *Am J Respir Crit Care Med* 1995;**151**:384–9.

55 Radermacher P, Rammos S. Low dose inhaled nitric oxide causing selective pulmonary vasodilatation in child with idiopathic pulmonary hypertension. *Eur J Pediatr* 1994;**153**: 691–3.

56 Kinsella JP, Toews WH, Henry D, Abman SH. Selective and sustained pulmonary vasodilation with inhalational nitric oxide therapy in a child with idiopathic pulmonary hypertension. *J Pediatr* 1993;**122**:803–6.

57 Partanen J, Nieminen MS. Death of a young woman suffering from primary pulmonary hypertension during inhaled nitric oxide therapy (letter). *Arch Intern Med* 1995;**155**: 875–6.

58 Schranz D, Huth R, Wippermann C-F, Ritzerfeld S, Schmitt FX, Oelert H. Nitric oxide and prostacyclin lower suprasystemic pulmonary hypertension after cardiopulmonary bypass. *Eur J Pediatr* 1993;**152**:793–6.

59 Haydar A, Mauriat P, Pouard P, *et al*. Inhaled nitric oxide for postoperative pulmonary hypertension in patients with congenital heart defects (letter). *Lancet* 1992;**340**:1545.

60 Girard C, Neidecker J, Laroux M-C, Champsaur G, Estanove S. Inhaled nitric oxide in pulmonary hypertension after total repair of total anomalous pulmonary venous return (letter). *J Thorac Cardiovasc Surg* 1993;**106**:369–82.

61 Roberts JD, Lang P, Bigatello LM, Vlahakes GJ, Zapol WM. Inhaled nitric oxide in congenital heart disease. *Circulation* 1993;**87**:447–53.

62 Day RW, Lynch JM, Shaddy RE, Orsmond GS. Pulmonary vasodilatory effects of 12 and 60 parts per million inhaled nitric oxide in children with ventricular septal defect. *Am J Cardiol* 1995;**75**:196–8.

63 Winberg P, Lundell BPW, Gustafsson LE. Effect of inhaled nitric oxide on raised pulmonary vascular resistance in children with congenital heart disease. *Br Heart J* 1994; **71**:282–6.

64 Journois D, Pouard P, Mauriat P, Malhere T, Vouhe P, Safran D. Inhaled nitric oxide as a therapy for pulmonary hypertension after operations for congenital heart defects. *J Thorac Cardiovasc Surg* 1994;**107**:1129–35.

65 Beghetti M, Habre W, Friedli B, Berner M. Continuous low dose inhaled nitric oxide for treatment of severe pulmonary hypertension after cardiac surgery in paediatric patients. *Br Heart J* 1995;**73**:65–8.

66 Girard C, Lehot J-J, Pannetier J-C, Filley S, Ffrench P, Estanove S. Inhaled nitric oxide after mitral valve replacement in patients with chronic pulmonary artery hypertension. *Anesthesiology* 1992;**77**:880–3.

67 Rich GF, Murphy GD, Roos CM, Johns RA. Inhaled nitric oxide. Selective pulmonary vasodilation in cardiac surgical patients. *Anesthesiology* 1993;**78**:1028–35.

68 Snow DJ, Gray SJ, Ghosh S, *et al*. Inhaled nitric oxide in patients with normal and increased pulmonary vascular resistance after cardiac surgery. *Br J Anaesth* 1994;**72**: 185–9.

69 Wessel DL, Adatia I, Giglia TM, Thompson JE, Kulik TJ. Use of inhaled nitric oxide and acetylcholine in the evaluation of pulmonary hypertension and endothelial function after cardiopulmonary bypass. *Circulation* 1993;**88**:2128–38.

70 Lefer DJ, Nakanishi K, Johnston WE, Vinten-Johansen J. Antineutrophil and myocardial protecting actions of a novel nitric oxide donor after acute myocardial ischemia and reperfusion in dogs. *Circulation* 1993;**88**:2337–50.

71 Pabla R, Buda AJ, Flynn DM, *et al*. Nitric oxide attenuates neutrophil-mediated myocardial contractile dysfunction after ischaemia and reperfusion. *Circ Res* 1996;**78**: 65–72.

72 Abman SH, Griebel JL, Parker DK, Schmidt JM, Swanton D, Kinsella JP. Acute effects of inhaled nitric oxide in children with severe hypoxemic respiratory failure. *J Pediatr* 1994;**124**:881–8.

73 Cornfield DN, Chatfield BA, McQueston JA, McMurtry IF, Abman SH. Effects of birth-related stimuli on L-arginine-dependent pulmonary vasodilation in ovine fetus. *Am J Physiol* 1992;**262**:H1474–H1481.

74 Kinsella JP, McQueston, Rosenberg AA, Abman SH. Hemodynamic effects of exogenous nitric oxide in ovine transitional pulmonary circulation. *Am J Physiol* 1992;**263**: H875–H880.

75 Roberts JD, Chen T-Y, Kawai N, *et al.* Inhaled nitric oxide reverses pulmonary vasoconstriction in the hypoxic and acidotic newborn lamb. *Circ Res* 1993;**72**:246–54.

76 Castillo L, de Rojas T, Chapman T, Burke JF, Tannenbaum S, Young VR. Nitric oxide synthesis is decreased in persistent pulmonary hypertension of the newborn. *Pediatr Res* 1993;**33**:20A.

77 Garg UC, Hassid A. Nitric oxide-generating vasodilators and 8-bromo-cyclic guanosine monophosphate inhibit mitogenesis and proliferation of cultured rat vascular smooth muscle cells. *J Clin Invest* 1989;**83**:1774–7.

78 Roberts JD, Polaner DM, Lang P, Zapol WM. Inhaled nitric oxide in persistent pulmonary hypertension of the newborn. *Lancet* 1992;**340**:818–19.

79 Kinsella JP, Neish SR, Shaffer E, Abman SH. Low-dose inhalational nitric oxide in persistent pulmonary hypertension of the newborn. *Lancet* 1992;**340**:819–20.

80 Kinsella JP, Neish SR, Ivy DD, Shaffer E, Abman SH. Clinical responses to prolonged treatment of persistent pulmonary hypertension of the newborn with low doses of inhaled nitric oxide. *J Pediatr* 1993;**123**:103–8.

81 Finer NN, Etches PC, Kamstra B, Tierney AJ, Peliowski A, Ryan C. Inhaled nitric oxide in infants referred for extracorporeal membrane oxygenation: dose response. *J Pediatr* 1994;**124**:302–8.

82 Shah N, Jacob T, Exler R, *et al.* Inhaled nitric oxide in congenital diaphragmatic hernia. *J Pediatr Surg* 1994;**29**:1010–15.

83 Muller W, Kachel W, Lasch P, Varnholt V, Konig SA. Inhaled nitric oxide for avoidance of extracorporeal membrane oxygenation in the treatment of severe persistent pulmonary hypertension of the newborn. *Intens Care Med* 1996;**22**:71–6.

84 Ahluwalia JS, Kelsall AWR, Raine J, *et al.* Safety of inhaled nitric oxide in premature neonates (letter). *Acta Paediatr* 1994;**83**:347–8.

85 Rossaint R, Falke KJ, Lopez F, Slama K, Pison U, Zapol WM. Inhaled nitric oxide for the adult respiratory distress syndrome. *N Engl J Med* 1993;**328**:399–405.

86 Gerlach H, Pappert D, Lewandowski K, Rossaint R, Falke KJ. Long-term inhalation with evaluated low doses of nitric oxide for selective improvement of oxygenation in patients with adult respiratory distress syndrome. *Intens Care Med* 1993;**19**:443–9.

87 Gerlach H, Rossaint R, Pappert D, Falke KJ. Time-course and dose-response of nitric oxide inhalation for systemic oxygenation and pulmonary hypertension in patients with adult respiratory distress syndrome. *Eur J Clin Invest* 1993;**23**:499–502.

88 Puybasset L, Rouby JJ, Mourgeon E, *et al.* Inhaled nitric oxide in acute respiratory failure: dose–response curves. *Intens Care Med* 1994;**20**:319–27.

89 Bigatello LM, Hurford WE, Kacmarek RM, Roberts JD, Zapol WM. Prolonged inhalation of low concentrations of nitric oxide in patients with severe adult respiratory distress syndrome. Effects on pulmonary hemodynamics and oxygenation. *Anesthesiology* 1994; **80**:761–70.

90 Abman SH, Chatfield BA, Hall SL, McMurtry IF. Role of endothelium-derived relaxing factor during transition of pulmonary circulation at birth. *Am J Physiol* 1990;**259**; H1921–H1927.

91 Young JD, Brampton WJ, Knighton JD, Finfer SR. Inhaled nitric oxide in acute respiratory failure in adults. *Br J Anaesth* 1994;**73**:499–502.

92 Dyar O, Young JD, Xiong L, Howell S, Johns E. Dose-response relationship for inhaled nitric oxide in experimental pulmonary hypertension in sheep. *Br J Anaesth* 1993;**71**: 702–8.

93 McIntyre RC, Moore FA, Moore EE, Piedalue F, Haenel JS, Fullerton DA. Inhaled nitric oxide variably improves oxygenation and pulmonary hypertension in patients with acute respiratory distress syndrome. *J Trauma* 1995;**39**:418–25.

94 Benzing A, Geiger K. Inhaled nitric oxide lowers pulmonary capillary pressure and changes longitudinal distribution of pulmonary vascular resistance in patients with acute lung injury. *Acta Anaesthesiol Scand* 1994;**38**:640–5.

95 Benzing A, Brautigam P, Geiger K, Loop T, Beyer U, Moser E. Inhaled nitric oxide reduces pulmonary transvascular albumin flux in patients with acute lung injury. *Anesthesiology* 1995;**83**:1153–61.

96 Lindeborg DM, Kavanagh BP, van Meurs K, Pearl RG. Inhaled nitric oxide does not alter the longitudinal distribution of pulmonary vascular resistance. *J Appl Physiol* 1995; **78**:341–8

97 Frostell C, Fratacci M-D, Wain JC, Jones R, Zapol WM. Inhaled nitric oxide: a selective pulmonary vasodilator reversing hypoxic pulmonary vasoconstriction. *Circulation* 1991; **83**:2038–47.

98 Fratacci M-D, Frostell CG, Chen T-Y, Wain JC, Robinson DR, Zapol WM. Inhaled nitric oxide. A selective pulmonary vasodilator of heparin-protamine vasoconstriction in sheep. *Anesthesiology* 1991;**75**; 990–9.

99 Frostell CG, Blomqvist H, Hedenstierna G, Lundberg J, Zapol WM. Inhaled nitric oxide selectively reverses human hypoxic pulmonary vasoconstriction without causing systemic vasodilation. *Anesthesiology* 1993;**78**:427–35.

100 Reuse C, Frank N, Contempre B, Vincent J-L. Right ventricular function in septic shock. *Intens Care Med* 1988;**14**:486–7.

101 Sibbald WJ, Driedger AA. Right ventricular function in acute disease states: pathophysiologic considerations. *Crit Care Med* 1983;**11**:339–45.

102 Offner PJ, Ogura H, Jordan BS, Pruitt BA, Cioffi WG. Effects of inhaled nitric oxide on right ventricular function in endotoxin shock. *J Trauma* 1995;**39**:179–86.

103 Girard C, Durand PG, Vedrinne C, et al. Inhaled nitric oxide for right ventricular failure after heart transplantation. *J Cardiothorac Vasc Anesth* 1993;**7**:481–5.

104 Foubert L, Latimer R, Oduro A, et al. Use of inhaled nitric oxide to reduce pulmonary hypertension after heart transplantation. *J Cardiothorac Vasc Anesth* 1993;**7**:506–7.

105 Ogura H, William G, Jordan BS, et al. The effect of inhaled nitric oxide on smoke inhalation injury in an ovine model. *J Trauma* 1994;**37**:294–302.

106 Ogura H, Saitoh D, Johnson AA, et al. The effect of inhaled nitric oxide on pulmonary ventilation-perfusion matching following smoke inhalation injury. *J Trauma* 1994;**37**: 893–8.

107 Dinh-Xuan AT, Higenbottam TW, Clelland CA, et al. Impairment of endothelium-dependent pulmonary artery relaxation in chronic obstructive lung disease. *N Engl J Med* 1991;**324**:1539–47.

108 Adnot S, Kouyoumdjian C, Defouilloy C, et al. Hemodynamic and gas exchange responses to infusion of acetylcholine and inhalation of nitric oxide in patients with chronic obstructive lung disease and pulmonary hypertension. *Am Rev Respir Dis* 1993; **148**:310–16.

109 Adatia I, Thompson J, Landzberg M, Wessel DL. Inhaled nitric oxide in chronic obstructive lung disease. *Lancet* 1993;**341**:307–8.

110 Norman V, Keith CH. Nitrogen oxides in tobacco smoke. *Nature* 1965;**205**:915–16.

111 Alving K, Fornhem C, Weitzberg E, Lundgren JM. Nitric oxide mediates cigarette smoke-induced vasodilatory responses in the lung. *Acta Physiol Scand* 1992;**146**:407–8.

112 Dupuy PM, Lancon J-P, Francoise M, Frostell CG. Inhaled cigarette smoke selectively reverses human hypoxic vasoconstriction. *Intens Care Med* 1995;**21**:941–4.

113 Barbera JA, Roger N, Roca J, Rovira I, Higenbottam TW, Rodriguez-Roisin R. Worsening of pulmonary gas exchange with nitric oxide inhalation in chronic obstructive pulmonary disease. *Lancet* 1996;**347**:436–40.

114 Moinard J, Manier G, Pillet O, Castaing Y. Effect of inhaled nitric oxide on hemodynamics and V/Q inequalities in patients with chronic obstructive pulmonary disease. *Am J Respir Crit Care Med* 1994;**149**:1482–7.

115 Dupuy PM, Shore SA, Drazen JM, Frostell C, Hill WA, Zapol WM. Bronchodilator action of inhaled nitric oxide in guinea pigs. *J Clin Invest* 1992;**90**:421–8.

116 Kharitonov SA, Yates D, Robbins RA, Logan-Sinclair R, Shinebourne EA, Barnes PJ. Increased nitric oxide in exhaled air of asthmatic patients. *Lancet* 1994;**343**:133–5.

117 Hamid Q, Springall DR, Riveros-Moreno V, et al. Induction of nitric oxide synthase in asthma. *Lancet* 1993;**342**:1510–13.

118 Hogman M, Frostell CG, Hedenstrom H, Hedenstierna G. Inhalation of nitric oxide modulates adult human bronchial tone. *Am Rev Respir Dis* 1993;**148**:1474–8.

119 Sanna A, Kurtansky A, Veriter C, Stanescu D. Bronchodilator effect of inhaled nitric oxide in healthy men. *Am J Respir Crit Care Med* 1994;**150**:1702–4.

120 Young JD, Dyar OJ. Delivery and monitoring of inhaled nitric oxide. *Intens Care Med* 1996;**22**:77–86.

121 Grover R, Murdoch I, Smithies M, Mitchell I, Bihari D. Nitric oxide during hand ventilation in patient with acute respiratory failure (letter). *Lancet* 1992;**340**:1038–9.

122 Goldman AP, Cook PD, Macrae DJ. Exposure of intensive-care staff to nitric oxide and nitrogen dioxide (letter). *Lancet* 1995;**345**:923–4.

123 Foubert L, Fleming B, Latimer R, *et al.* Safety guidelines for use of nitric oxide. *Lancet* 1992;**339**:1615–16.

124 Bouchet M, Renaudin M-H, Raveau C, Mercier J-C, Dehan M, Zupan V. Safety requirement for use of inhaled nitric oxide in neonates. *Lancet* 1993;**341**:968–9.

125 Miller OI, Celermajer DS, Deanfield JE, Macrae DJ. Guidelines for the safe administration of inhaled nitric oxide. *Arch Dis Child* 1994;**70**; F47–F49.

126 Tang SF, Symonds J, Miller OI. A simple method of nitric oxide delivery and analysis. *Anaesth Intens Care* 1996;**24**; 126–7.

127 Tibballs J, Hochmann M, Carter B, Osborne A. An appraisal of techniques for administration of gaseous nitric oxide. *Anaesth Intens Care* 1993;**21**:844–7.

128 Stenqvist O, Kjelltoft B, Lundin S. Evaluation of a new system for ventilatory administration of nitric oxide. *Acta Anaesthesiol Scand* 1993;**37**:687–91.

129 Wessel DL, Adatia I, Thompson JE, Hickey PR. Delivery and monitoring of inhaled nitric oxide in patients with pulmonary hypertension. *Crit Care Med* 1994;**22**:930–8.

130 Nishimura M, Hess D, Kacmarek RM, Ritz R, Hurford WE. Nitrogen dioxide production during mechanical ventilation with nitric oxide in adults. *Anesthesiology* 1995;**82**:1246–54.

131 Channick RN, Newhart JW, Johnson FW, Moser KM. Inhaled nitric oxide reverses hypoxic pulmonary vasoconstriction in dogs. A practical nitric oxide delivery and monitoring system. *Chest* 1994;**105**:1842–7.

132 Moors AH, Pickett JA, Mahmood N, Latimer RD, Oduro A. Nitric oxide administration (letter). *Anaesth Intens Care* 1994;**22**:310–12.

133 Young JD. A universal nitric oxide delivery system. *Br J Anaesth* 1994;**73**:700–2.

134 Benzing A, Beyer U, Kiefer P, Geiger K. Inhaliertes stickstoffmonoxid. Anwendung und kontinuierliche konzentrationmessung. *Anaesthesist* 1993;**42**:175–8.

135 Archer S. Measurement of nitric oxide in biological models. *FASEB J* 1993;**7**:349–60.

136 Kiechle FL, Malinski T. Nitric oxide biochemistry, pathophysiology and detection. *Am J Clin Pathol* 1993;**100**:567–75.

137 Petros AJ, Cox P, Bohn D. A simple method for monitoring the concentration of inhaled nitric oxide. *Anaesthesia* 1994;**49**:317–19.

138 Mercier J-C, Zupan V, Dehan M, Renaudin M-H, Bouchet M, Raveau C. Device to monitor concentration of inhaled nitric oxide (letter). *Lancet* 1993;**342**:431–2.

139 Moutafis M, Hatahet Z, Castelain MH, Renaudin MH, Monnot A, Fischler M. Validation of a simple method assessing nitric oxide and nitrogen dioxide concentrations. *Intens Care Med* 1995;**21**:537–41.

140 Commonwealth Government of Australia. *Worksafe Australia. Exposure standards for atmospheric contaminants in the occupational environment.* Canberra: Australian Government Publishing Service, 1991.

141 Centers for Disease Control. Recommendations for occupational safety and health standard. *MMWR Morb Mortal Wkly Rep* 1988;**37** (suppl 7):21.

142 Thomas HV, Mueller PK, Lyman RL. Lipoperoxidation of lung lipids in rats exposed to nitrogen dioxide. *Science* 1967;**159**:532–4.

143 Freeman G, Crane SC, Stephens RJ, Furiosi NJ. Environmental factors in emphysema and a model system with NO_2. *Yale J Biol Med* 1968;**40**:566–75.

144 Kawakami M, Yasui S, Yamawaki I, Katayama M, Nagai A, Takizawa T. Structural changes in airways of rats exposed to nitrogen dioxide intermittently for seven days. *Am Rev Respir Dis* 1989;**140**:1754–62.

145 Von Nieding G, Wagner HM. Vergleich der Wirkung von Stickstoffdioxid und Stickstoffmonoxid auf die Lungenfunktion des Menschen. *Staub-Reinhalt* 1975;**35**; 175–8.

146 Linn WS, Solomon JC, Trim SC, *et al.* Effects of exposure to 4 ppm nitrogen dioxide in healthy and asthmatic volunteers. *Arch Environ Health* 1985;**40**:234–9.

147 Rasmussen TR, Kjaergaard SK, Tarp U, Pedersen OF. Delayed effects of NO_2 exposure on alveolar permeability and glutathione peroxidase in healthy humans. *Am Rev Respir Dis* 1992;**146**:654–9.

148 Magnussen H. Experimental exposures to nitrogen dioxide. *Eur Respir J* 1992;**5**:1040–2.

149 Sandstrom T, Helleday R, Bjermer L, Stjernberg N. Effects of repeated exposure to 4 ppm nitrogen dioxide on bronchoalveolar lymphocyte subsets and macrophages in healthy men. *Eur Respir J* 1992;**5**:1092–6.

150 Pickett JA, Moors AH, Latimer RD, Mahmood N, Ghosh S, Oduro A. The role of soda lime during administration of inhaled nitric oxide. *Br J Anaesth* 1994;**72**:683–5.

151 Greenbaum R, Bay J, Hargreaves MD, *et al.* Effects of higher oxides of nitrogen on the anaesthetized dog. *Br J Anaesth* 1967;**39**:393–403.

152 Shiel F O'M. Morbid anatomical changes in the lungs of dogs after inhalation of higher oxides of nitrogen during anaesthesia. *Br J Anaesth* 1967;**39**:413–23.

153 Hugod C. Effect of exposure to 43 ppm nitric oxide and 3.6 ppm nitrogen dioxide on rabbit lung. *Int Arch Occup Environ Health* 1979;**42**:159–67.

154 Stavert DM, Lehnert BE. Nitric oxide and nitrogen dioxide as inducers of acute pulmonary injury when inhaled at relatively high concentrations for brief periods. *Inhalation Toxicol* 1990;**2**:53–67.

155 Von Nieding G, Wagner HM, Krekeler H. Investigation of the acute effects of nitrogen monoxide on lung function in man. Proceedings of the Third International Clean Air Congress, Dusseldorf, October 8–12. Verlag des Vereins Deutcher Ingenieure 1973; A14–A16.

156 Kagawa J. Respiratory effects of 2-hr exposure to 1.0 ppm nitric oxide in normal subjects. *Environ Res* 1982;**27**:485–90.

157 Mercer RR, Costa DL, Crapo JD. Effects of prolonged exposure to low doses of nitric oxide or nitrogen dioxide on the alveolar septa of adult rat lung. *Lab Invest* 1995;**73**: 20–8.

158 Gryglewski RJ, Palmer RMJ, Moncada S. Superoxide anion is involved in the breakdown of endothelium-derived vascular relaxing factor. *Nature* 1986;**320**:454–6.

159 Graham A, Hogg N, Kalyanaraman B, *et al.* Peroxynitrite modification of low-density lipoprotein leads to recognition by the macrophage scavenger receptor. *FEBS Lett* 1993; **330**:181–5.

160 Haddad IY, Ischiropoulos H, Holm BA, Beckman JS, Baker JR, Matalon S. Mechanisms of peroxynitrite-induced injury to pulmonary surfactants. *Am J Physiol* 1993;**265**: L555–L564.

161 Kooy NW, Royall JA, Ye YZ, Kelly DR, Beckman JS. Evidence for in vivo peroxynitrite production in human acute lung injury. *Am J Respir Crit Care Med* 1995;**151**:1250–4.

162 Marcocci L, Maguire JJ, Packer L. Nitecapone: a nitric oxide radical scavenger. *Biochem Mol Biol Int* 1994;**34**:531–41.

163 Ellenhorn MJ, Barceloux DG. *Medical toxicology. Diagnosis and treatment of human poisoning.* New York: Elsevier, 1988.

164 Young JD, Dyar O, Xiong L, Howell S. Methaemoglobin production in normal adults inhaling low concentrations of nitric oxide. *Intens Care Med* 1994;**20**:581–4.

165 Choury D, Reghis A, Pichard AL, Kaplan JC. Endogenous proteolysis of membrane-bound red cell cytochrome-b5 reductase in adults and newborns: its possible relevance to the generasation of the soluble "methemoglobin reductase". *Blood* 1983;**61**:894–8.

166 Pavri RS, Gupta AD, Baxi AJ, Advani SH. Further evidence for oxidative damage to hemoglobin and red cell membrane in leukemia. *Leuk Res* 1983;**7**:729–33.

167 Tibballs J. Clinical applications of nitric oxide. *Anaesth Intens Care* 1993;**21**:866–71.

168 Gruetter CA, Gruetter DY, Lyon JE, Kadowitz PJ, Ignarro LJ. Relationship between cyclic guanosine 3′:5′-monophosphate formation and relaxation of coronary arterial

smooth muscle by glyceryl trinitrate, nitroprusside, nitrite and nitric oxide: effects of methylene blue and methemoglobin. *J Pharmacol Exp Ther* 1981;**219**:181–6.

169 Young JD, Dyar OJ, Xiong L, Zhang J, Gavaghan D. Effects of methylene blue on the vasodilator action of inhaled nitric oxide in hypoxic sheep. *Br J Anaesth* 1994;**73**:511–16.

170 Gachot B, Bedos JP, Veber B, Wolff M, Regnier B. Short-term effects of methylene blue on hemodynamics and gas exchange in humans with septic shock. *Intens Care Med* 1995; **21**:1027–31.

171 Losano G, Pagliaro P, Gattullo D, Marsh NA. Control of coronary blood flow by endothelial release of nitric oxide. *Clin Exp Pharmacol Physiol* 1994;**21**:783–9.

172 Brady AJ, Warren JB, Poole-Wilson PA, Williams TJ, Harding SE. Nitric oxide attenuates cardiac myocyte contraction. *Am J Physiol* 1993;**265**:H176–H182.

173 Shah AM, Lewis MJ, Henderson AH. Effects of 8-bromo-cyclic GMP on contraction and on inotropic response of ferret cardiac muscle. *J Mol Cell Cardiol* 1991;**23**:55–64.

174 Smith JA, Shah AM, Lewis MJ. Factors released from the endocardium of the ferret and pig modulate myocardial contraction. *J Physiol (Lond)* 1991;**439**:1–14.

175 Balligand J-L, Kelly RA, Marsden PA, Smith TW, Michel T. Control of cardiac cell function by an endogenous nitric oxide signaling system. *Proc Natl Acad Sci USA* 1993; **90**:347–51.

176 Grocott-Mason RM, Fort S, Lewis MJ, Shah AM. Myocardial relaxant effect of exogenous nitric oxide in the isolated ejecting heart. *Am J Physiol* 1994;**266**:H1699–H1705.

177 Grocott-Mason R, Anning P, Evans H, Lewis MJ, Shah AM. Modulation of left ventricular relaxation in isolated ejecting heart by endogenous nitric oxide. *Am J Physiol* 1994;**267**:H1804–H1813.

178 Hare JM, Loh E, Creager MA, Colucci WS. Nitric oxide inhibits the positive inotropic response to β-adrenergic stimulation in humans with left ventricular dysfunction. *Circulation* 1995;**92**:2198–203.

179 Wang J, Seyedi N, Xu X-B, Wolin MS, Hintze TH. Defective endothelium-mediated control of coronary circulation in conscious dogs after heart failure. *Am J Physiol* 1994; **266**:H670–H680.

180 Drexler H, Hayoz D, Munzel T, Just H, Zelis R, Brunner HR. Endothelial dysfunction in chronic heart failure. Experimental and clinical studies (review). *Arzneimittelforschung* 1994;**44**(3A):455–8.

181 Katz SD, Schwarz M, Yuen J, LeJemtel TH. Impaired acetylcholine-mediated vasodilation in patients with congestive heart failure. *Circulation* 1993;**88**:55–61.

182 Habib F, Dutka D, Crossman D, Oakley CM, Cleland JGF. Enhanced basal nitric oxide production in heart failure: another failed counter-regulatory vasodilator mechanism? *Lancet* 1994;**344**:371–3.

183 Node K, Kitakaze M, Kosaka H, *et al.* Increased release of NO during ischaemia reduces myocardial contractility and improves metabolic dysfunction. *Circulation* 1996; **93**:356–64.

184 de Belder AJ, Radomski MW, Why HJF, *et al.* Nitric oxide synthase activities in human myocardium. *Lancet* 1993;**341**:84–5.

185 Winlaw DS, Smythe GA, Keogh AM, Schyvens CG, Spratt PM, Macdonald PS. Increased nitric oxide in heart failure. *Lancet* 1994;**344**:373–4.

186 Drexler H, Hayoz D, Munzel T, *et al.* Endothelial function in chronic congestive heart failure. *Am J Cardiol* 1992;**69**:1596–601.

187 Levine B, Kalman J, Mayer L, Fillit HM, Packer M. Elevated circulating levels of tumour necrosis factor in severe chronic heart failure. *N Engl J Med* 1990;**323**:236–41.

188 Balligand J-L, Ungureanu D, Kelly RA, *et al.* Abnormal contractile function due to induction of nitric oxide synthesis in rat cardiac myocytes follows exposure to activated macrophage-conditioned medium. *J Clin Invest* 1993;**91**:2314–19.

189 Kobzik L, Reid MB, Bredt DS, Stamler JS. Nitric oxide in skeletal muscle. *Nature* 1994; **372**:546–8.

190 Smith CJ, Sun D, Hoegler C, *et al.* Reduced gene expression of vascular endothelial NO synthase and cyclooxygenase-1 in heart failure. *Circ Res* 1996;**78**:58–64.

191 Buga GM, Griscavage JM, Rogers NE, Ignarro LJ. Negative feedback regulation of endothelial cell function by nitric oxide. *Circ Res* 1993;**73**:808–12.

192 Assreuy J, Cunha FQ, Liew FY, Moncada S. Feedback inhibition of nitric oxide synthase activity by nitric oxide. *Br J Pharmacol* 1993;**108**:833–7.

193 Miller OI, Tang SF, Keech A, Celermajer DS. Rebound pulmonary hypertension on withdrawal from inhaled nitric oxide (letter). *Lancet* 1995;**346**:51–2.

194 Kiff RJ, Moss DW, Moncada S. Effect of nitric oxide gas on the generation of nitric oxide by isolated blood vessels: implications for inhalation therapy. *Br J Pharmacol* 1994; **113**:496–8.

195 Loh E, Stamler JS, Hare JM, Loscalzo J, Colucci WS. Cardiovascular effects of inhaled nitric oxide in patients with left ventricular dysfunction. *Circulation* 1994;**90**:2780–5.

196 Kieler-Jensen N, Ricksten S-E, Stenqvist O, *et al*. Inhaled nitric oxide in the evaluation of heart transplant candidates with elevated pulmonary vascular resistance. *J Heart Lung Transplant* 1994;**13**:366–75.

197 Bocchi EA, Bacal F, Costa JO, *et al*. Inhaled nitric oxide leading to pulmonary oedema in stable severe heart failure. *Am J Cardiol* 1994;**74**:70–2.

198 Mery P-F, Lohmann SM, Walter U, Fischmeister R. Ca^{++} current is regulated by cyclic GMP-dependent protein kinase in mammalian cardiac myocytes. *Proc Natl Acad Sci USA* 1991;**88**:1197–201.

199 Mery P-F, Pavoine C, Belhassen L, Pecker F, Fischmeister R. Nitric oxide regulates cardiac Ca^{++} current. *J Biol Chem* 1993;**268**:26286–95.

200 Kirstein M, Rivet-Bastide M, Hatem S, Beenardeau A, Mercadier J-J, Fischmeister R. Nitric oxide regulates the calcium current in isolated human atrial myocytes. *J Clin Invest* 1995;**95**:794–802.

201 Lefer DJ. Myocardial protective actions of nitric oxide donors after myocardial ischemia and reperfusion. *New Horizons* 1996;**3**:105–12.

202 Ignarro LJ. Biological actions and properties of endothelium-derived nitric oxide formed and released from artery and vein. *Circ Res* 1989;**65**:1–21.

203 Radomski MW, Palmer RMJ, Moncada S. Endogenous nitric oxide inhibits human platelet adhesion to vascular endothelium. *Lancet* 1987;**2**:1057–8.

204 Bassenge E. Antiplatelet effects of endothelium-derived relaxing factor and nitric oxide donors. *Eur Heart J* 1991;**12** (suppl E):12–15.

205 Golino P, Cappelli-Bigazzi M, Ambrosio G, *et al*. Endothelium-derived relaxing factor modulates platelet aggregation in an in vivo model of recurrent platelet activation. *Circ Res* 1992;**71**:1447–56.

206 Hogman M, Frostell C, Arnberg H, Hedenstierna G. Bleeding time prolongation and NO inhalation. *Lancet* 1993;**341**:1664–5.

207 Olsen SB, Tang DB, Jackson MR, Gomez ER, Ayala B, Alving BM. Enhancement of platelet deposition by cross-linked hemoglobin in a rat carotid endarterectomy model. *Circulation* 1996;**93**:327–32.

208 Liu RH, Hotchkiss JH. Potential genotoxicity of chronically elevated nitric oxide: a review. *Mutat Res* 1995;**339**:73–89.

209 Routledge MN, Wink DA, Keefer LK, Dipple A. Mutations induced by saturated aqueous nitric oxide in the pSP189 supF gene in human Ad293 and E. coli MBM7070 cells. *Carcinogenesis* 1993;**14**:1251–4.

210 Nguyen T, Brunsen D, Crespi CL, Penman BW, Wishnok JS, Tannenbaum SR. DNA damage and mutation in human cells exposed to nitric oxide *in vitro*. *Proc Natl Acad Sci USA* 1992;**89**:3030–4.

211 Wink DA, Kasprzak KS, Maragos CM, *et al*. DNA deaminating ability and genotoxicity of nitric oxide and its progenitors. *Science* 1991;**254**:1001–3.

212 Schmutte C, Rideout WM III, Shen JC, Jones PA. Mutagenicity of nitric oxide is not caused by deamination of cytosine or 5-methylcytosine in double-stranded DNA. *Carcinogenesis* 1994;**15**:2899–903.

213 Brunelli L, Crow JP, Beckman JS. The comparative toxicity of nitric oxide and peroxynitrite to *Escherichia coli*. *Arch Biochem Biophys* 1995;**316**:327–34.

214 Szabo C, Salzman AL. Endogenous peroxynitrite is involved in the inhibition of mitochondrial respiration in immuno-stimulated J774.2 macrophages. *Biochem Biophys Res Commun* 1995;**209**:739–43.

215 Volk T, Ioannidis I, Hensel M, deGroot H, Kox WJ. Endothelial damage induced by nitric oxide: synergism with reactive oxygen species. *Biochem Biophys Res Commun* 1995; **213**:196–203.

216 Wetzel RC. Aerosolized prostacyclin. In search of the ideal pulmonary vasodilator. *Anesthesiology* 1995;**82**:1315–17.

217 Shimokawa H, Flavahan NA, Lorenz RR, Vanhoutte PM. Prostacyclin releases endothelium-derived relaxing factor and potentiates its action in coronary arteries of the pig. *Br J Pharmacol* 1988;**95**:1197–203.

218 Welte M, Zwissler B, Habazettl H, Messmer K. PGI2 aerosol versus nitric oxide for selective pulmonary vasodilation in hypoxic pulmonary vasoconstriction. *Eur Surg Res* 1993;**25**:329–40.

219 Burghuber OC, Silberbauer K, Haber P, Sinzinger H, Elliot M, Leithner C. Pulmonary and antiaggregatory effects of prostacyclin after inhalation and intravenous infusion. *Respiration* 1984;**45**:450–4.

220 Walmrath D, Schneider T, Pilch J, Grimminger F, Seeger W. Aerosolised prostacyclin in adult respiratory distress syndrome. *Lancet* 1993;**342**:961–2.

221 Pappert D, Busch T, Gerlach H, Lewandowski K, Radermacher P, Rossaint R. Aerosolized prostacyclin versus inhaled nitric oxide in children with severe acute respiratory distress syndrome. *Anesthesiology* 1995;**82**:1507–11.

222 Van Heerden PV, Webb SAR, Hee G, Corkeron M, Thompson WR. Inhaled aerosolized prostacyclin as a selective pulmonary vasodilator for the treatment of severe hypoxaemia. *Anaesth Intens Care* 1996;**24**:87–90.

223 Walmrath D, Schneider T, Pilch J, Schermuly R, Grimminger F, Seeger W. Effects of aerosolized prostacyclin in severe pneumonia. Impact of fibrosis. *Am J Respir Crit Care Med* 1995;**151**:724–30.

224 Bein T, Pfeifer M, Riegger GA, Taeger K. Continuous intraarterial measurement of oxygenation during aerosolized prostacyclin administration in severe respiratory failure (letter). *N Engl J Med* 1994;**331**:335–6.

225 Zwissler B, Rank N, Jaenicke U, *et al.* Selective pulmonary vasodilation by inhaled prostacyclin in a newborn with congenital heart disease and cardiopulmonary bypass. *Anesthesiology* 1995;**82**:1512–16.

226 Tibballs J. Inhaled prostacyclin (PGI$_2$) versus nitric oxide (NO). *Anaesth Intens Care* 1996;**24**:515–16.

9: Management of septic shock in children

WARWICK BUTT

Introduction

Infection remains a common problem in modern medicine. Improved resuscitation and emergency transport, improved survival of children with immunodeficiency, leukaemia, cancer, and the prolonged use of intravascular devices have contributed to the increasing problem of infection in hospital and its sequelae. Ten to fifteen percent of children in hospital are admitted because of infection or will develop an infection at some point during their hospital stay. The sepsis syndrome occurs in less than 25% of children with documented bacteraemia and blood cultures are negative in 40% of children with sepsis.[1] The mortality rate for children with septic shock varies but approximates 40%.

Definitions

The term "systemic inflammatory response syndrome" (SIRS) was proposed by the American College of Chest Physicians and Society of Critical Care Medicine to describe the non-specific inflammatory process occurring in adults after trauma, infection, burns, pancreatitis, and other diseases. The criteria developed for use in adults[2] have been modified for

236

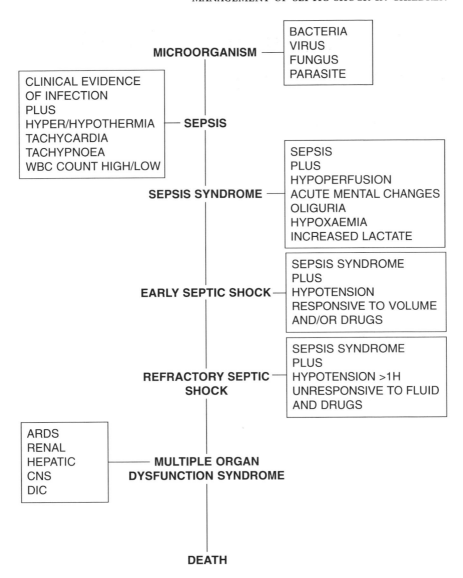

FIGURE 9.1—*Systemic inflammatory response syndrome*

use in children[3] (fig 9.1). SIRS encompasses several stages of infection from sepsis to sepsis syndrome, early septic shock, and refractory shock, which can lead to multiple organ dysfunction and death.[4]

237

Sepsis occurs when there is a systemic response to an infection. Evidence of bacteraemia or an infective focus is not required. When sepsis is accompanied by altered organ perfusion, as manifested by hypoxaemia, elevated plasma levels of lactate, oliguria or acute changes in mental status, *sepsis syndrome* is diagnosed. *Septic shock* ensues when systolic blood pressure drops below the fifth percentile for age. If shock responds promptly to parenteral fluid administration and pharmacologic treatment, it is defined as *early septic shock*. Shock that lasts for more than one hour despite vigorous therapeutic measures and necessitates vasopressor support is regarded as *refractory septic shock*. Finally, the presence of impaired organ perfusion accompanied by any combination of derangements such as disseminated intravascular coagulation, adult respiratory distress syndrome, and acute renal, hepatic or neurologic dysfunction is called *multiple organ dysfunction syndrome*.

Epidemiology

The natural history of SIRS in adults has been evaluated in a multicentre prospective study of 3708 patients admitted to an ICU with infection: 69% developed SIRS (7% of these patients died); 20% developed sepsis (16% of these patients died); 18% developed severe sepsis (20% of these patients died); and 4% developed septic shock (46% of these patients died). A similar prospective study[5] in 1058 children admitted to a PICU showed that 82% developed SIRS, 23% developed sepsis, 4% severe sepsis, 2% septic shock, and the overall mortality was 6%.

Septic shock arises in a variety of clinical settings that are either host or treatment related (table 9.1). Septic shock occurs in children with impaired immunity such as neonates and those children with congenital immunodeficiencies, leukaemia, cancer or after chemotherapy. Children with congenital urinary tract abnormalities, congenital heart disease, extensive burns, multiple trauma or critically ill children with prolonged

TABLE 9.1—*Risk factors for septic shock*

Host related	Treatment related
Prematurity	Surgical invasive procedure
Malnutrition	Invasive devices
Immunodeficiency, cancer	Antibiotics
Chronic health problems (hepatic dysfunction, cardiac and renal disease, diabetes mellitus)	Immunosuppression (cytotoxic drugs, steroids, irradiation)
	Hypothermia
Traumatic/thermal wounds	Hospital environment (virulent organisms)

stay in ICU are also at increased risk. In adults and adolescents translocation of bacteria from the gastrointestinal tract can complicate virtually any critical illness and lead to septic shock; this is uncommon in infants. Septic shock also occurs *de novo* in otherwise healthy children and can be rapidly fatal. Infection with polysaccharide escapulated organisms such as meningococcus, pneumococcus, and *H. influenzae* are frequently complicated by septic shock. These organisms have a particular predilection for children less than 2 years of age who cannot make T cell independent antibody which is necessary to kill polysaccharide escapulated organisms. The pathogens responsible for initiating septic shock in children vary with age (table 9.2).

TABLE 9.2—*Pathogens responsible for septic shock*

Neonates
Group B β-haemolytic streptococci
Enterobactericeae
Listeria monocytogenes
Staph. aureus
N. meningitidis

Infants
H. influenzae
S. pneumoniae
Staph. aureus
N. meningitidis

Children
S. pneumoniae
N. meningitidis
Staph. aureus
Enterobacteriaceae

Immunocompromised
Enterobacteriaceae
Staph. aureus
Pseudomonadaceae
Candida albicans

Pathophysiology

A microorganism in the blood (bacteria, virus, fungus or parasite) initiates an inflammatory response; the process is similar irrespective of the organism.[6,7] There are a heterogeneous group of molecules (lipopolysaccharide) in the outer membrane of all Gram-negative bacteria known as endotoxin. Lipopolysaccharide consists of a lipid A and polysaccharide core linked to an "O-polysaccharide" side chain that comprises repeating units of sugars, which vary for each specific Gram-

239

negative organism. Lipid A appears to be the key piece of the endotoxin molecule involved in this interaction. A model is emerging about the details of this interaction.

1. Lipopolysaccharide binds to receptors found on mononuclear leucocytes (monocytes and macrophages).
2. This interaction results in the release of cytokines from these mononuclear cells. It appears that the primary adverse cytokines involved are interleukin (IL) 1 and tumour necrosis factor (TNF).
3. IL-I and TNF influence the physiology of the septic state by their effects on temperature control (fever induction, hypothermia), vascular resistance and permeability, cardiovascular function, bone marrow (increased WBC, etc.), and many enzyme systems such as lactate dehydrogenase and lipoprotein lipase, which adversely affect energy utilisation. At some point, a specific cardiodepressant factor appears to be elaborated, although the identify of this molecule is unclear. This process can also proceed in the absence of endotoxin, as occurs in Gram-positive septic shock.
4. Many effects of cytokines are mediated at the end organs by nitric oxide, arachidonic acid metabolites (prostaglandins, eicosanoids, platelet activating factor), and/or lipoxygenase derivatives.
5. IL-I and/or TNF stimulate a complex cytokine cascade with amplification and modulation. Of special importance may be the local production of IL-8 by the cells of various organs, which has the function of recruiting and activating polymorphonuclear leucocytes, which then cause tissue damage and organ dysfunction. *In vitro* data have documented significant IL-8 production in response to extremely small concentrations of IL-I (amplification).
6. The complement, coagulation, and kinin cascades are also activated and play important roles in the septic state.
7. The last aspect of this model is that specific anticytokine substances are concomitantly produced, including IL-I receptor antagonist and soluble cytokine receptors. Also, some liberated cytokines (IL-4, IL-10) appear to have predominantly antiinflammatory effects, such as decreased synthesis of IL-I and TNF in response to lipopolysaccharide. Although antibiotics are crucial in treating infection they may also exacerbate SIRS by causing rapid death and lysis of microorganisms with massive release of endotoxin.

Clinical signs of septic shock

Sepsis may present dramatically (as in fulminant meningococcaemia) or insidiously, such as candidaemia in an immunosuppressed patient. Clinical manifestations of septic shock are the result of activation of endogenous physiologic processes (described in detail above) in response to endotoxin which lead to hypotension and multiorgan failure. It is the host's response to multiplying microorganisms and their active metabolites that causes most of the tissue injury. As cellular injury continues, sepsis progresses to the recognisable entity of septic shock.

The initial mediators of inflammation (cytokines, kinins) lead to a marked reduction in systemic vascular resistance; in response to the decrease in systemic vascular resistance, cardiac output increases. Heart rate increases early, particularly in younger children where cardiac output is more dependent on increases in heart rate than stroke volume. At this stage the patient is warm, dry and well perfused and pulses are usually bounding. This hyperdynamic circulatory state is also referred to as "warm shock". Mean arterial blood pressure may be normal, but the pulse pressure is characteristically widened as vasodilation decreases diastolic pressure and increased cardiac output heightens the systolic pressure. Patients are tachypnoeic with deep, non-laboured respiratory efforts (table 9.3).

TABLE 9.3—*Warm septic shock*

Early clinical signs	Early physiologic/biochemical markers
Hyper or hypothermia	Decreased peripheral vascular resistance
Flushed, warm, dry skin	Increased cardiac output
Widened pulse pressure	Decreased oxygen consumption
Tachycardia	Normal oxyhaemoglobin saturation

Decreased cerebral perfusion and decreased CNS pH are potent stimuli to the chemoreceptors located in the medulla. Chemoreceptor stimulation increases minute ventilation by increasing both tidal volume and respiratory rate. Hyperventilation with respiratory alkalosis is frequently seen in early shock. However, arterial PO_2 usually falls as a result of pulmonary ventilation perfusion mismatch, due to pulmonary arteriovenous shunting of blood.

Subtle changes in mental status occur early in septic shock. Adults and adolescents may demonstrate changes in mental status before any change in haemodynamic variables. Irritability, restlessness or feeding difficulty may be the only manifestations in infants.

Despite the increased cardiac output, tissue injury continues secondary to impaired cellular metabolism and compromised tissue perfusion. A progression from warm shock to cold shock occurs as hypovolaemia and ventricular dysfunction occur. In adults the progression from warm shock to cold shock can take 2–12 hours, but in small children and newborn infants this progression can be very rapid because of their limited ability to maintain the increased cardiac output. Heightened autonomic responses to stress result in increased catecholamine levels and, in the face of hypovolaemia, vasoconstriction. Systemic vascular resistance becomes progressively elevated in an attempt to maintain blood pressure as increased vascular permeability results in fluid flux out of the vascular space. Increasing vasoconstriction and decreased cardiac output compromise oxygen delivery and lead to increased production of lactic acid. Local acidosis causes compensatory changes in the capillary beds, the arterioles dilate and the venules constrict, causing pooling and stasis of blood. Hypotension develops as intravascular volume is further depleted from ongoing capillary leak and capillary pooling and progressive myocardial depression occurs.

In cold shock the patient has an elevated heart rate, low blood pressure, and a narrowed pulse pressure. Extremities are cold and clammy. Pulses are thready and peripheral cyanosis develops. Respiratory rate remains elevated with shallow, laboured efforts as acidosis increases and muscle fatigue develops (table 9.4).

TABLE 9.4—*Cold septic shock*

Late clinical signs	Late physiologic/biochemical markers
Hypotension	Increased peripheral vascular resistance
Tachycardia with thready pulses	Decreased cardiac output
Narrow pulse pressure	Low CVP, low PCWP
Cold clammy skin	Hypoxia
Cyanosis	Metabolic acidosis
Rapid, shallow breaths	Increased lactate
Oliguria	Thrombocytopenia, DIC

Depleted intravascular volume, poor tissue perfusion, impaired oxygen utilisation, exhausted metabolic energy supplies, and myocardial dysfunction lead to ongoing severe acidosis. If this cycle is not broken, the patient will progress to vascular collapse, irreversible multiple system organ failure, and death (see box 9.1).

Decreased tissue perfusion can be identified by changes in body surface temperature, capillary refill, and impaired function of several organ systems. Body surface temperature is a simple and effective method of assessing the adequacy of tissue perfusion. Cold extremities or an increased peripheral–core temperature gradient (greater than 2°C) indicate intact homoeostatic mechanisms that have decreased non-essential cutaneous perfusion in the face of contracted intravascular volume. Decreased capillary refill is a sensitive indicator of tissue perfusion. The rate of refill after firm compression of soft tissues and nail beds for five seconds is related to the site of determination, the temperature, and the amount of circulation through microvasculature; in general, refill over the face is faster than that over the chest which is faster than that over the hands and feet. Normally a blanched area disappears in less than three seconds. Capillary refill that

Box 9.1—*Pathophysiological events of SIRS*

MICROORGANISM
Immune stimulation
Release of catecholamines and other vasoactive substances
Impaired cellular metabolism
Transient peripheral vasodilation

WARM SHOCK
Continued cell injury
Decreased intravascular volume
Vasoconstriction
Decreased tissue perfusion

COLD SHOCK
Hypoxia
Hypovolaemia
Systemic metabolic acidosis
Tissue ischaemia
Endstage damage
   vasomotor collapse
   lysosomal rupture
   cellular autolysis

MULTISYSTEM ORGAN DYSFUNCTION
CHF
Renal failure
ARDS
DIC
Coma
Irreversible ischaemic injury

DEATH

---

takes longer than five seconds is abnormal. In addition, stasis due to peripheral vasoconstriction may lead to peripheral cyanosis. Although peripheral hypoperfusion is the physiologic response to intravascular volume contraction, it does not in itself indicate shock; however, it clearly precedes

243

it. Vital organ hypoperfusion can be assumed to occur if there is oliguria from renal hypoperfusion or if there is altered mentation, from CNS hypoperfusion.

It is important to remember that changes in blood pressure are a late manifestation of hypovolaemia and blood pressure only falls when haemodynamic compromise is severe. Initially, pulse pressure is decreased, often because of a minor decrease in systolic pressure and an increase in diastolic pressure. As stroke volume falls because of decreased preload, systolic pressure slowly falls, but the increased tone of the arterial circulation initially maintains diastolic pressure. Eventually, systolic and diastolic pressures fall. Pulsus paradoxus occurs with decreased lung compliance but may also indicate impaired myocardial contractility or myocardial tamponade.

Prediction of outcome/severity of illness

Scoring systems may be used objectively to assess the severity of illness of critically ill children and to predict outcome, e.g. Paediatric Risk of Mortality (PRISM),[8] Paediatric Index of Mortality (PIM).[9] Although not sufficiently accurate for individual patient outcome prediction, such scoring systems may be useful to guide the level of intervention, to assess the outcome of a group of patients or to justify the use of other salvage therapies. Specific scoring systems or prognostic factors for meningococcaemia have been developed by a number of groups.[10–12] The Stiehm and Damrosh scoring system[10] included the following criteria.

- Onset of petechiae within 12 hours prior to admission
- Normal or low leucocyte count
- Normal or low erythrocyte sedimentation rate
- Absence of meningitis
- Shock

At the time of publication, the presence of three or more of these features indicated a greater than 85% chance of dying whereas children with two or less had a less than 10% chance of dying.

A review of several scoring systems by Gedde Dahl et al.[11] concluded that:

- blood pH <7.35 was the best single factor predicting fatal outcome followed by:
    thrombocytopenia
    low WBC count ($<10 \times 10^9$/l)

hypotension
clinically observed cyanosis and ecchymoses;
- fatality rate amongst those aged 5–19 years was less than half of that in younger and older patients with meningococcal disease;
- onset of skin haemorrhage within 12 hours before admission to hospital appeared to be no better indicator than the presence of skin haemorrhage on admission.

The Glasgow Meningococcal Septicaemia Prognostic Score (GMSPS) includes the following criteria.

BP <75 mmHg systolic, age <4 yr <85 mmHg systolic, age <4 yr	3
Skin/rectal temperature difference >3°C	3
Modified coma scale score <8 or deterioration of <3 points in 1 hr	3
Deterioration in perceived clinical condition in the hour before scoring	2
Absence of meningism	2
Extending purpuric rash or widespread ecchymoses	1
Base deficit (capillary or arterial >8.0)	1
Maximum score	15

In the original study by Sinclair et al.,[13] a GMSPS of greater than seven had a specificity of 100% and positive predictive value of 100% for mortality; in a subsequent evaluation, however, a score of nine or more had a specificity of 95% and a positive predictive value for death of 74%.

McManus,[13] in a retrospective review of meningococcaemia and infectious purpura, found that severe coagulopathy (partial thromboplastin time greater than 50 s, serum fibrinogen concentration less than 150 mg/dl) was a good predictor of poor outcome (death or serious morbidity).

It is important to realise that any scoring system should be evaluated by any hospital considering using it; differences will occur over time, in different units, and perhaps with different organism virulence or host factors.

Monitoring

In children with septic shock it is important to monitor the adequacy of cardiac output and oxygenation and the ability of oxygen delivery to meet the metabolic demands of vital organs. The goals of haemodynamic monitoring are to aid in diagnosis, guide therapy, provide warning of physiological deterioration, and predict outcome. Bedside monitoring includes heart rate, indices of perfusion, respiratory rate, conscious state,

245

urine output, invasive haemodynamics (blood pressure, central venous pressure and pulmonary artery pressure), cardiac output, echocardiography, and gastric tonometry.

Heart rate

Continuous monitoring of heart rate and ECG is essential. Bradycardia is an ominous sign and a predictor of imminent cardiac arrest. Tachycardia may have a number of causes; accurate diagnosis is essential for appropriate treatment.

Causes of sinus tachycardia

- Inadequate cardiac output
- Hypoventilation/hypoxia
- Seizures
- Fever
- Pain/awareness
- Drugs (pancuronium, catecholamines)

Respiratory rate

It is useful to monitor respiratory rate; low respiratory rate indicates fatigue, profound shock, and poor CNS perfusion and is a warning sign of imminent respiratory arrest. Tachypnoea is related to fever, metabolic acidosis, and CNS hypoperfusion.

Perfusion

As shock progresses, blood flow is diverted from the less vital tissues to the heart, brain, and lungs. Monitoring the perfusion of less vital tissues may provide an early indication of significant tissue hypoperfusion.

A widened gradient between the surface temperature of the great toe and ambient temperature has been reported to be a more sensitive marker of severe systemic hypoperfusion than conventional haemodynamic parameters and even arterial lactate concentration. With the onset of shock and peripheral hypoperfusion, toe temperature decreases and approaches ambient levels. Patients recovering from shock demonstrated widening of the toe–ambient gradient to more than 4°C whereas the gradient remained less than 1–2°C in patients who ultimately died from shock.[14] Although core–peripheral temperature gradients do not predict cardiac output or systemic vascular resistance,[15] failure to increase temperature of the toe after open heart surgery has been associated with increased mortality.[16]

Hypoperfusion of the gastrointestinal system occurs early in septic shock. Monitoring of gastric intramucosal pH (pHi) is advocated as a way of evaluating splanchnic perfusion. Several studies[17,18] suggest that clinical measurement of gastric intramucosal pH is an index of systemic hypoperfusion and has implications with regard to outcome and the development of organ failure. Titration of therapy to maintain normal gastric intramucosal pH also may be associated with improved survival.[18] pHi is now being evaluated in paediatric intensive care. In 19 septic children studied in our unit (eight of whom died), pHi measured at 24 hours barely distinguished those who died from those who survived; the area under the ROC curve for pHi as a predictor of survival was 0.71. There are problems with pHi measurement including the reliability and reproducibility of saline filled tonometer CO_2 measurements and the equilibration time required (60–90 min). Nonetheless, PHi may in time provide useful information about the adequacy of regional perfusion and therefore a guide to global perfusion.

Urine output

Urine output is a useful measure of adequacy of cardiac output and insertion of a urinary catheter is essential in children with septic shock. Normal urine output is 2–3 ml/kg/h; less than 1 ml/kg/h implies hypoperfusion.

Invasive haemodynamic monitoring

Blood pressure

It is essential to use intra-arterial pressure monitoring rather than a sphygmomanometer in children with septic shock to ensure accurate measurement of blood pressure. Normal blood pressure is important for adequate organ perfusion, although blood pressure should not be the only focus of attention. Blood pressure is an unreliable measure of cardiac output and systemic oxygen delivery;[19] only at extremely low blood pressure does blood flow become pressure dependent.

247

Central venous pressure (CVP) and pulmonary capillary wedge pressure (PCWP)

Insertion of a Swan Ganz catheter may provide a reasonably accurate assessment of cardiac performance (as determined by cardiac output) and also both right and left heart filling pressures and alterations in pulmonary vascular resistance. Total circulating blood volume is one contributing factor to both right and left atrial filling pressures: other determinants of atrial pressure are ventricular function and compliance. With a constant intravascular volume, changes in right ventricular contractility, afterload (pulmonary vascular resistance), and compliance will markedly affect central venous pressure. A similar argument applies to left atrial and pulmonary capillary wedge pressures. A low CVP indicates hypovolaemia; a normal or high CVP, however, does not exclude hypovolaemia.

Insertion of a Swan Ganz catheter in young infants may be difficult, has a significant risk of complications, and often fails to yield information that alters management. We rarely use them in children less than 5 years and only occasionally in older children.

Cardiac output

Cardiac output is difficult to measure accurately in children and the main issue is not what the cardiac output is but whether it is adequate. The focus is therefore usually directed towards perfusion assessment and not the absolute value of cardiac output.

There are a number of methods for measurement of cardiac output (table 9.5). Non-invasive measurement of cardiac output with thoracic bioimpedance and Doppler ultrasound provides simple, safe and repeatable measures of cardiac output; unfortunately there are wide limits of agreement (35–65%). Invasive methods of measurement of cardiac output are reliable and accurate to within 15% but have other problems. Fick is difficult to perform because a cuffed ETT is essential, as is a pulmonary artery catheter and a ventilator circuit with no leaks. Dye dilution is probably the easiest method to do but can be inaccurate at low cardiac output because of coronary recirculation; thermodilution systematically overreads the cardiac output by up to 600 ml/min and also requires a pulmonary artery catheter.

Echocardiography

Echocardiography is useful in children with sepsis. It is non-invasive, easy to perform, and repeatable. It gives a general guide to the contractile state of the heart including diastolic function, whether the heart is adequately

TABLE 9.5—*Techniques of cardiac output determination*

Method	Advantage	Problem
Bioimpedance	Non-invasive Repeatable Continuous	Inaccurate
Doppler	Non-invasive Easy Repeatable	Operator dependent Limits of agreement (38%)
Fick	Reliable	Circuit leaks Needs cuffed ETT Complex Needs PA catheter
Thermodilution	Reliable Repeatable	Overestimates Needs PA catheter Inaccurate with intracardiac shunt
Dye dilution	Reliable Repeatable	Inaccurate at low CO because of recirculation and intracardiac shunt

filled or dilated and finally whether a pericardial effusion is present. All of these findings have major implications for therapy. In our unit rapid, reliable echocardiography is available and we rarely use the Swan Ganz catheter.

Laboratory diagnosis and markers of sepsis

Haematology

Neutrophilia (>15 000) and neutropenia (<1000) are suggestive of infection; an increase in the immature to total neutrophil ratio (ITR) is strongly suggestive of sepsis. Daily monitoring is useful in children with sepsis.

Thrombocytopenia may suggest the diagnosis of sepsis or be associated with disseminated intravascular coagulation (DIC). DIC with low fibrinogen and elevated fibrin degradation products is common in septic shock.

Blood chemistry

The most frequently performed and most valuable laboratory investigation is the arterial blood gas and acid–base analysis. Arterial oxygen and carbon dioxide tensions aid in evaluation of the adequacy of oxygenation and ventilation and pH and base deficit provide information regarding the

249

adequacy of tissue perfusion. Serum lactate is very useful to monitor efficacy of treatment – failure of lactate to decrease with therapy is predictive of a fatal outcome. Ionised hypocalcaemia and hypomagnesaemia are common. Hyperkalaemia is not infrequent, especially if renal failure is present. Urea, creatinine, and liver function tests are measured on a daily basis.

Measurement of inflammatory response

Erythrocyte sedimentation rate (ESR) and C-reactive protein (CRP)[20] are increased in the early phase of sepsis and are useful in the differentiation of the cause of fever; a CRP greater than twice normal or rising suggests infection.

Cultures

It is essential to obtain adequate cultures before antibiotics, in an attempt to identify the infecting microorganism and its antibiotic sensitivities.

In children with community acquired infections, nasopharyngeal aspirates, blood, urine, and CSF are mandatory. If the patient is intubated and pneumonia is suspected tracheal aspiration, bronchoscopic or non-bronchoscopic alveolar lavage and possibly lung biopsy are indicated. Punch biopsy of a skin lesion with microscopy and culture may rapidly identify an organism.

In children with nosocomial infections the usual cultures include those mentioned above as well as blood cultures taken via the central venous catheter and possibly arterial blood culture if endocarditis is suspected.

Bacterial antigens

These are useful for diagnosis of *H. influenzae* infections but are less reliable for *S. pneumoniae* and *N. meningiditis* (60% specificity).

Treatment

The standard treatment of a child with sepsis involves initial resuscitation, accurate diagnosis of the infecting microorganism, appropriate choice and dose of antimicrobial (bacterial, fungal, viral) chemotherapy, adequate monitoring, and rapid correction of physiological derangements.

Resuscitation

Initial resuscitation should be rapid and adequate to restore blood pressure. All children with sepsis are hypovolaemic (relative or absolute) and require intravenous plasma expanders.[21] Initially the type of fluid is not critical: colloid or crystalloid fluids may be used. Inadequate volume resuscitation is a common problem in children. A total volume of 60–100 ml/kg may be needed over the first 12 hours to restore circulating volume adequately. This should be given in 5–10 ml/kg aliquots with repeated assessment of response. Volume expansion also decreases haemoglobin, clotting factors, and serum protein concentrations. Catecholamines have a vital role in treating impaired myocardial contractility but only after blood volume has begun to be reestablished. Children usually have no chronic myocardial impairment and normal coronary vasculature so that early use of catecholamines is safe and appropriate. Oxygen should be given to all children with sepsis by either face mask or intranasal cannula.

Antibiotic therapy

Several studies have demonstrated that choosing an antibiotic regimen with *in vitro* killing capability against the infecting organism is important. If one chooses antibiotics that kill the isolated microorganism, the prognosis of a septic shock patient is significantly better than if one chooses antibiotics that do not kill the microorganism.[22] Four to six hours after antibiotics have been given systemic vasodilation and hypotension may occur. This is thought to be caused by the release of large amounts of endotoxin (bacterial cell wall) due to the antibiotics killing large numbers of bacteria. Some authors advocate a small dose of steroids (25–50 mg of hydrocortisone or 1 mg/kg of prednisolone) before or within one hour of initial antibiotic therapy. The evidence is equivocal but I favour giving a single small dose of steroids with or before the first dose of antibiotics.

Acidosis

In infants and young children, acute acidosis with a pH less than 7.25 is associated with decreased force of ventricular ejection and catecholamine unresponsiveness and it is therefore important to treat acidosis. In children with sepsis, metabolic acidosis is initially related to hypovolaemia. If the base deficit is less than 10, volume therapy alone should suffice; for larger base deficits intravenous bicarbonate should be used. Bicarbonate supplementation can be given by repeated slow boluses

251

of sodium bicarbonate of 1–2 mmol/kg. The formula required to half correct acidosis [0.3 × (body weight in kg) × (base deficit)/2 = mmol of NaHCO$_3$] may serve as an approximate guide.[23] If bolus therapy is not effective or the metabolic acidosis persists or becomes more severe, a continuous intravenous sodium bicarbonate infusion may be required. The major limitation in bicarbonate replacement therapy is sodium overload and hyperosmolarity. Close monitoring of serum sodium is required if massive bicarbonate replacement (more than 10 mmol/kg) is undertaken. If sodium bicarbonate supplementation is ineffective, dialysis or haemofiltration may be necessary to remove excess acid, lactate, phosphate, and hydrogen ion, as well as to correct hypernatraemia and to allow further bicarbonate administration.

When correcting acidosis with bicarbonate replacement, it is important to remember that other electrolyte abnormalities may occur. As pH returns toward normal, serum potassium levels also fall as potassium reenters the cells. The principal cause of metabolic acidosis is poor tissue perfusion and only improvement of tissue blood flow will lead to a sustained improvement of pH. If the patient is being artificially ventilated, then lowering PaCO$_2$ by increasing minute ventilation is a very useful short term option to correct acidosis (respiratory component). If severe lung disease is present this option may not be appropriate; lung injury and impairment of cardiac function by high intrathoracic pressure may limit this strategy.

Hypocalcaemia

Ionised hypocalcaemia is common in children with sepsis because of parathyroid ischaemia. Hypocalcaemia can lead to hypotension, tachycardia, myocardial depression, seizures and tetany. Thus if low, extra calcium should be given by a combination of bolus calcium gluconate (0.22 mmol/kg over 30 min) and infusion (2 mmol/kg/24 h). There is now some evidence that independent of calcium level, ventricular contraction improves if serum calcium is increased. It may therefore be used as an additional inotropic agent in children with sepsis and has the advantage of being the only one not to increase myocardial oxygen demands. Calcium is a vasoconstrictor which can be useful in children with sepsis. However, it should also be remembered that calcium is the final common pathway to cell death and is important in reperfusion injury. Calcium should only be used as an inotrope if large doses of dopamine (greater than 10 µg/kg/min) or adrenaline (greater than 0.5 µg/kg/min) are being used or where severe ionised hypocalcaemia is present.

Circulatory support

Rate and rhythm

Ensuring adequate cardiac rate and rhythm is essential to life support. Treatment of arrhythmias includes correction of hypoxia, acidosis, hypocalcaemia, hypomagnesaemia and hypokalaemia or hyperkalaemia.

Preload

Ongoing capillary leak and vasodilatory mediators lead to hypovolaemia. Red blood cells remain in the circulation longer than albumin when capillary permeability is increased and therefore packed red blood cells are the blood volume expander of choice in this situation. However, the amount of packed red blood cells that can be given is limited by the haemoglobin level and its effect on viscosity. Combinations of albumin and saline solutions (5% or 20% albumin in saline) are used. Hypovolaemia is often present (despite massive tissue oedema and high filling pressures due to poor ventricular function and compliance). The only limitation to the administration of extra volume is the demonstrated lack of response to volume, that is, a persistent elevation in ventricular filling pressures without an increase in cardiac output. At that stage, further preload augmentation does not improve peripheral perfusion and may, by increasing venous pressure and tissue oedema, decrease perfusion pressure to the myocardium or other critical vascular beds. Increased venous pressures will increase vascular leak, leading to increased tissue oedema, especially pulmonary oedema, pleural effusion, and ascites. In patients with ARDS, the target central filling pressure should be the lowest compatible with adequate cardiac output (usually CVP 8–10 mm Hg) to minimise or reduce interstitial pulmonary and tissue oedema.

Myocardial contractility

Poor myocardial contractility is common in sepsis and inotropic drugs are required to improve ventricular function.[24]

Dopamine is the most commonly used therapeutic agent in shock states in children. Dopamine has dose related a, β, and dopaminergic sympathetic affects. In low doses (0.5–4 µg/kg/min) it may act by causing renal and splanchnic vasodilation and as a natriuretic drug, thus causing diuresis, and may promote renal perfusion. In medium doses (4–10 µg/kg/min) increasing inotropy is seen with increased stroke volume and cardiac output. In larger doses (more than 10 µg/kg/min) increasing vasoconstrictor activity is seen, with decreased peripheral and renal perfusion and increased left

253

ventricular afterload. The exact degree to which these effects occur in an individual varies.

Dobutamine was synthesised as a drug to provide an inotropic effect without the untoward effects of isoproterenol. Peripheral vasodilation, pulmonary vasodilation, attenuated pulmonary vascular hypoxic vasoconstriction and, occasionally, unwanted tachycardia can occur. Dobutamine (5–10 µg/kg/min) has been shown to enhance myocardial performance but if falling blood pressure and increased myocardial oxygen consumption occur concurrently, myocardial ischaemia is still a serious threat. Dobutamine is the intravenous drug that is at present closest to being a pure inotropic agent but it still causes vasodilation and hence is not the ideal agent to restore blood pressure.

Adrenaline stimulates both α and $\beta_{1,2}$ receptors. The response to adrenaline mimics that of generalised autonomic stimulation. In general, increased cardiac output, blood pressure, and heart rate, a hypermetabolic state, CNS stimulation, and increased myocardial oxygen consumption occur. Both pulmonary and systemic vascular resistances are elevated and renal ischaemia is a potential complication. Adrenaline can certainly be expected to enhance myocardial contractility and is usually used in the sickest patients. Many believe that adrenaline is the inotrope of choice in septic shock.

Noradrenaline is predominantly an α agonist and has potent peripheral vasoconstrictor effects and positive inotropic effects. Severe systemic, pulmonary, peripheral, renal, and splanchnic vasoconstriction occur with its use. The combination of enhanced contractility and a return to normal systemic vascular resistance rapidly restores blood pressure and perfusion to multiple beds. This drug is increasingly being used in septic patients with encouraging results. Both adrenaline and noradrenaline can be started at 0.1 µg/kg/min and increased as required.

In early sepsis dopamine is the standard drug. If hypotension continues despite adequate volume expansion and dopamine 10–15 µg/kg/min then note the systolic and diastolic blood pressure. If the diastolic pressure is low commence noradrenaline 0.1 µg/kg/min and increase by 0.1 µg/kg/min every few minutes until a satisfactory blood pressure is achieved. If the systolic pressure is also low, then commence adrenaline 0.1 µg/kg/min and increase by 0.1 µg/kg/min until a satisfactory blood pressure is achieved. Often a combination of adrenaline and noradrenaline is useful. Echocardiography at this stage will usually reveal a dilated, poorly contracting heart; if the heart is poorly filled and contracting well then colloid/blood infusion and/or noradrenaline should be used for treatment of hypotension. It is also important to remember that the myocardium may be insensitive/unresponsive to catecholamines in the presence of severe metabolic acidosis (pH less than 7.25).

Afterload reduction

Afterload reduction may play a role in improving myocardial performance in children in the vasoconstrictive (late) stage of septic shock, with high systemic vascular resistance, poor peripheral perfusion, and decreased cardiac output. However, vasodilators may cause profound hypotension, particularly if hypovolaemia has not been fully corrected. The combination of afterload reduction with inotropic support may provide benefit for a profoundly impaired myocardium. Both nitroprusside and nitroglycerine lower systemic vascular resistance in children; these agents act via generation of nitric oxide (NO), endothelium derived relaxing factor (EDRF). Nitroglycerine is a more potent venodilator and pulmonary vasodilator than nitroprusside, whereas nitroprusside has more potent peripheral arteriolar vasodilating effects. Both drugs should be used very cautiously as hypotension is likely, especially if hypovolaemia is present. Nitroglycerine (1–5 µg/kg/min) is the safer agent. Mild hypotension will respond rapidly to plasma volume expansion; profound hypotension will necessitate cessation of the vasodilator (which is the reason that only short acting drugs should be used, if at all).

Pulmonary hypertension

In sepsis syndrome with ARDS, pulmonary hypertension may become a major problem. A selective pulmonary vasodilator, such as inhaled nitric oxide, can be safely used to deal with this problem or to improve ventilation perfusion matching and correct hypoxaemia.

Respiratory therapy for the child with septic shock

In children with septic shock, work of breathing (WOB) may represent 15–30% of oxygen consumption and therefore contributes to the development of lactic acidosis. The early use of mechanical ventilation aided by sedation and paralysis provides a number of advantages. It removes the WOB and allows redistribution of limited cardiac output to vital organs. Improved conditions are provided for the safe establishment of invasive haemodynamic monitoring; this is particularly useful in the irritable young child. Mechanical ventilation allows manipulation of the respiratory component of acid-base balance (i.e. respiratory alkalosis is used to counteract metabolic acidosis and restore pH). Mechanical ventilation with PEEP may also improve oxygenation, lower PVR and reduce LV afterload. However, care is required in the presence of persisting hypovolaemia.

255

A rapid sequence induction with cricoid pressure should be employed to establish mechanical ventilation. Choice of induction agents and dose should aim to minimize cardiovascular depression and achieve rapid paralysis. Great care should be exercised with thiopentone. Ketamine (1 mg/kg) and suxamethonium (1 mg/kg) is a useful approach, as is a narcotic, benzodiazepine and muscle relaxant combination. *Caution with dosage and speed of administration is more important than the choice of any particular drug.*

Adjunctive therapies in septic shock

Children with severe sepsis may develop septic shock, refractory to conventional medical management. In such circumstances, adjunctive therapies such as ECMO, plasma exchange, immunotherapy, corticosteroids, and granulocyte transfusion, although unproven, may offer additional benefit either alone or in combination.

Intravenous immunoglobulin (IVIG) therapy in newborns

IVIG appears to be a safe agent which can be administered to term and premature newborns in doses of 500–750 mg/kg over 4–6 hours without serious side effects in most instances. This results in a rise in serum IgG concentrations to near those found in adults and results in a significant increase in the concentration of specific antibodies. Not all of the IVIG preparations contain the same amount of specific antibodies against the main pathogens in neonatal sepsis. Several studies have confirmed improved outcome in septic neonates treated with IVIG.

Exchange transfusion

In infants less than 5 kg, two blood volume exchange transfusions have been used for many years as a therapy for septic shock (table 9.6). Theoretically, exchange transfusions can remove or dilute circulating bacteria and endotoxin and provide control of circulatory shock by improving both pulmonary and peripheral perfusion. An exchange transfusion may also improve the humoral and cellular immune status of the newborn infant by increasing opsonic activity and by delivering functional and mature granulocytes. An exchange transfusion can also improve acidosis, coagulopathy, and electrolyte abnormalities.

TABLE 9.6—*Outcome of newborn infants receiving exchange transfusion*

	Survivors/total	
Author	Transfused	Not transfused
Prodholm[25] (1974)	7/8	0/8
Xanthou[26] (1975)	8/20	8/40
Tollner[27] (1977)	10/10	5/10
Pearse[28] (1978)	13/19	7/17
Belchiradsky[29] (1978)	37/74	60/132
Courtney[30] (1979)	23/34	4/14
Lemos[31] (1981)	8/8	0/19
Bossi[32] (1981)	12/22	7/13
Naranyan[33] (1982)	25/44	18/62
Mathur[34] (1993)	13/20	3/10
	156/259 (60%)	116/325 (36%)

There are a number of potential problems with exchange transfuion:

- imbalance between volumes of blood removed and given;
- the need for relatively fresh blood with near normal K^+ concentration;
- citrate toxicity: anticoagulant citrate binds calcium and 0.5 ml 10% calcium gluconate should be given with each 25 ml of blood exchanged.

A continuous exchange transfusion with blood removed via a peripheral arterial catheter and blood infused via a venous catheter is relatively easily performed and generally well tolerated; it is important to increase inotropic drug therapy and inspired oxygen concentration during the exchange.

Granulocyte transfusions

Neutropenia is common in life threatening infections and septic neonates who are neutropenic are less likely to survive. The neutrophils from stressed term and preterm infants exhibit decreased chemotaxis, opsonisation, phagocytosis, and intracellular bactericidal activity. These findings suggest that the transfusion of functional neutrophils from adult donors could improve the survival of septic, neutropenic neonates. The neutrophil storage pool (NSP) of the adult is 14 times larger than the size of the circulating granulocyte pool whereas the NSP in neonates is only twice as large as the circulating pool. In addition, neonatal stem cells may be unable to increase proliferation in the presence of infection.

Complication rates in newborns receiving granulocyte transfusions are low and benefit is suggested in a number of small trials or anecdotal reports (table 9.7). There are, however, several potentially life threatening complications of granulocyte transfusions in neonates. These include the transmission of hepatitis virus, CMV, and HIV; sensitisation to human lymphocyte antigen (HLA) and leucocyte, erythrocyte, and platelet antigens; pulmonary leucoagglutination reactions; and graft versus host disease, particularly with non-irradiated products. In neonates, the reported complication rate has thus far been minimal, including a transient decrease in PaO_2, polycythaemia, and thrombocytosis. A follow up study of 33 infants treated with granulocyte transfusions did not demonstrate the development of alloantibodies or abnormal immunoglobulin levels or clinical evidence of graft versus host disease.

TABLE 9.7—*Outcome of infants receiving granulocyte transfusion*

Author	Survival/total	
	Transfused	Not transfused
Laurenti[35,36]	18/20	11/18
Christensen[37]	7/7	1/9
Cairo[38]	13/13	6/10
Wheeler[39]	4/4	2/5
Baley[40,41]	8/12	10/13
	50/56 (89%)	30/55 (55%)

In older children with cancer the debate about granulocyte transfusion has diminished because of the advent of recombinant human granulocyte colony stimulating factor (GCSF). The number of hospital days due to treatment of febrile neutropenia, the number of days on broad spectrum antibiotics, and the duration of neutropenia are significantly reduced with the use of GCSF. In the treatment of documented fungal superinfection, it may be beneficial if GCSF and an antifungal drug are used as combination therapy. GCSF is non-toxic and well tolerated in children.

Antibody/mediator antagonists

As SIRS is initiated by endotoxin and potentiated by inflammatory mediators, antibodies that neutralise or block receptors to some of these substances have been developed and trialled in adults and children. None of these different antimediator/antibody regimes have been shown to improve survival.[42] Different types of antibody (polyclonal core directed, monoclonal E5, human monoclonal HA-IA) have been tried and although retrospective analysis in shock states due to infection shows some benefit, prospective evaluation of groups of patients shows no sustained benefit and perhaps increases the risk of death in those patients who prove not to have Gram-negative bacteraemia. Anti-TNF and anti-IL therapies are effective in animal models but have not yet proven effective in clinical trials. Although based on sound scientific rationales these therapies have not proven useful.[43,44,45]

Corticosteroids

Evidence from animal models of sepsis suggests that when corticosteroids are given early and in adequate dosage for brief periods, they are associated with a significant decrease of the inflammatory response, improvement in survival rates, and a decrease in morbidity. These drugs inhibit the production of TNF and IL-1 and decrease complement and polymorphonuclear activation.

Two multicentre, prospective, randomised trials of methylprednisolone in adults with sepsis syndrome and septic shock failed to show decreased mortality rates.[46,47] In infants and children with bacterial meningitis, most of whom had bacteraemia when first seen, two prospective, double blind, randomised trials have demonstrated beneficial effects of dexamethasone in improving outcome.[48,49] Dexamethasone exerts its effects by modulating similar pathophysiologic mechanisms that may be operative in patients with sepsis. In a retrospective review of children with pneumococcal meningitis, dexamethasone therapy was associated with a significant reduction in haemodynamic instability in the six hours after initiation of antibiotic therapy, which presumably resulted from release of bacterial cell wall products, compared with patients receiving placebo. Currently, in children it is reasonable to give two doses of IV or IM dexamethasone (0.1–0.6 mg/ kg) before the first and 12 hours after the first dose of antibiotic.

Toxin/mediator removal

Death from septic shock is primarily due to uncontrolled inflammation which is initiated by toxin and amplified and propagated by endogenous mediators. It is attractive to hypothesise that removal of these toxins/ mediators might influence the outcome. Various extracorporeal techniques including haemofiltration, plasmapheresis, and absorption (charcoal, polymyxin) remove these toxins/mediators. A number of animal/human reports are summarised in table 9.8.

Anecdotal reports of survival after haemofiltration/plasmapheresis[63] and apparent improvement in the survival of children with sepsis compared to historical controls after receiving plasmapheresis do not prove that toxin/ mediator removal should be a standard therapy. However, in our unit, plasmafiltration is used as adjunctive therapy for all intubated patients with

TABLE 9.8—*Toxin/mediator removal*

Animal

Author	Animal	Model	Technique	Survivors/total Treatment	Control
Muraji[50]	Dogs	E	PF	6/6	1/8
Gokul[51]	Rats	P	Column	37/39	0/13
Cohen[52]	Rats	E	PF polymxin	4/4	0/4
Hanasawa[53]	Dogs	E	PF polymxin	10/12	1/8
Natanson[54]	Dogs	L	PF	0/6	4/6

Human

Author	Problems	Survivors/total Treatment	Control
Bjorvatn[55]	Historical control	4/4	12/25
Barzilay[56]	Historical control	7/11	1/9
Van Deuren[57]	Historical control	2/15	4/10
Westertdorp[58]	Historical control	76%	22%
Best[59]	Anecdotal	4/4	—
Morley[60]	Anecdotal	7/8	—
Connett[61]	Anecdotal	0/1	—
Tibby[62]	Anecdotal	15/12	—

E, endotoxin; L, live organism; PF, plasmafiltration; P, plasma infected.

SIRS who are receiving inotropic drugs. Filtration facilitates accurate control of fluid balance and electrolytes in addition to removal of mediators of inflammation. We currently use venovenous plasmafiltration as this method allows a large membrane with a large surface area, controlled high blood flow and therefore high solute clearance. After a two plasma volume exchange in four hours, plasma filtration is continued for 12–24 hours. If renal function is impaired then plasmafiltration is followed by haemofiltration. Recurrence of haemodynamic instability leads to a further 24 hours of plasmafiltration.

On connecting a filtration circuit to a patient with sepsis, it is prudent to increase FiO_2 to 1.0 and double the dose of all inotropic drugs or vasoconstrictors to allow for haemodilution (with the extra circuit volume) and drug binding to the circuit. Usually within 15 min infusion rates of drugs can be gradually decreased to previous levels.

Extracorporeal life support

Although children with sepsis may have normal or increased oxygen delivery and cardiac output, these may be inadequate to meet tissue

TABLE 9.9—*Patient data preextracorporeal membrane oxygenation (ECMO)*

Age (yr)	Organism	PRISM	MAP	FiO₂	Inotropes	Organ failure	Outcome
14	*Staph. aureus*	19	31	1.0	D15,NA,1.0	R,I,K,DIC	D
1.7	*Staph. pneumoniae*	21	34	1.0	S15,A3	R,L,DIC Sz	S
0.8	Parainflu. virus	27	29	0.8	D20,A4,NA4	R,L,K,DIC	S
13.4	Mycoplasma	34	35	1.0	D5,Db15,A9	R,I,K,DIC Sz	S
15.4	*Staph. pneumoniae*	29	33	1.0	D15,A1,NA3	R,I,K,DIC Sz	D
12.3	*Staph. aureus*	27	15	1.0	D10,A5	R,I,K,DIC	S
0.1	*B. pertussis*	28	24	1.0	D5,Dᵦ10,A3	R,L,K,DIC Sz	D
15	*Staph. pneumoniae*	27	24	1.0	D15,NA2	R,I,K,DIC Sz	D
2.5	*N. meningitidis*	37	26	1.0	D5,A10,NA4	R,I,K,DIC	S

PRISM score for 24 hours before ECMO

Abbreviations: MAP, mean airway pressure (cmH₂O); FiO₂, inspired oxygen fraction; D, dopamine; Db, dobutamine; A, adrenaline; NA, noradrenaline; all micrograms per kilogram per minute

Organ failure (in addition to cardiovascular): R, respiratory; L, liver; K, kidney; DIC, disseminated intravascular coagulation; Sz, seizures

S, survived; D, died

requirements. Venoarterial extracorporeal membrane oxygenation (ECMO) can provide both circulatory and respiratory support and, in theory, can assist patients where more conventional medical management is failing. Venovenous ECMO can provide respiratory support and a ventricular assist device can be employed to provide isolated circulatory support.

We have used ECMO in nine children with refractory septic shock.[64] Their median age was 12 years and median weight 45 kg. Median intrope requirements (μg/kg/min) before ECMO were dopamine, 15; dobutamine, 12.5; epinephrine, 4; and norepinephrine, 3.5. Four children received two inotropes concurrently and five received three or more. All nine patients had severe respiratory failure; eight had evidence of other organ system dysfunction, with six having five or more organ system dysfunctions. Median PRISM score was 27 (expected mortality six patients). Median duration of ECMO was 137 hours. Within 24 hours of starting ECMO, seven of nine children had ceased inotropic therapy. Five patients (55%) survived, all of whom are leading normal lives. Individual patient data are shown in table 9.9.

This technique maintains vital organ perfusion to allow recovery from the septic process. It is reasonable therapy in hospitals that have an active ECMO programme; transfer of a child with septic shock to such a hospital, however, is potentially dangerous and must be evaluated on a patient by patient basis.

Summary

Despite advances in our understanding of the pathogenesis of septic shock, the mortality in children remains at approximately 40%. The most favourable outcomes are probably related to early recognition, close monitoring, and immediate resuscitation and therapy. The key aspects of therapy include appropriate antimicrobial drugs and early aggressive volume expansion and inotropic drugs to restore circulation to vital organs. Correction of acid–base and electrolyte abnormalities is also essential. The early use of oxygen and mechanical ventilation offers a number of advantages even in the presence of adequate gas exchange. Adjunctive therapies such as ECMO, plasma exchange, immunotherapy, corticosteroids, and granulocyte transfusion, although unproven, may offer additional benefit either alone or in combination.

1 Naqvi JH, Chundu KR, Friedman AD. Shock in children with gram negative bacillary sepsis and Haemophilus influenzae type B sepsis. *Pediatr Infect Dis* 1986;5:512–15.
2 Bone RC, Balk RA, Cerra FB, *et al.* Definitions for sepsis and organ failure and guidelines for the use of innovative therapies in sepsis. *Chest* 1992;101:1644–55.

3 Jacobs RF, Sowell MV, Moss MN, Fiser DH. Septic shock in children: bacterial etiologies and temporal relationships. *Pediatr Infect Dis J* 1990;**9**:196–8.

4 Saez-Llorens X, McCracken GH. Sepsis syndrome and septic shock in pediatrics: Current concepts of terminology, pathophysiology, and management. *J Pediatr* 1993;**123**:497–508.

5 Proulx F, Fayon M, Farrel CA, Lacroix J, Gauthier M. Epidemiology of sepsis and multiple organ dysfunction in children. *Chest* 1996;**109**:1033–7.

6 Shapiro L, Gelfand JA. Cytokines and sepsis: pathophysiology and therapy. *New Horizons* 1993;**1**:13–22.

7 Livingstone DH, Mosenthal AC, Deitch EA. Sepsis and multiple organ dysfunction syndrome: a clinical-mechanistic overview. *New Horizons* 1995;**3**:257–66.

8 Pollack MM, Ruttimann UE, Getson PR. Pediatric risk of mortality (PRISM) score. *Crit Care Med* 1988;**16**:1110–16.

9 Shann F. Paediatric index of mortality. *Intens Care Med* 1997 (in press).

10 Steihm FR, Damrosh DS. Factors in prognosis of meningococcal infection. *J Pediatr* 1966;**68**:457–67.

11 Gedde Dahl TW, Bjork P, Hoiby SA. Severity of meningococcal disease:assessment by factors and scores and implications for management. *Rev Infect Dis* 1990;**12**:973–90.

12 Sinclair JF, Skeoch CM, Hollworth D. Prognosis of meningococcal septicaemia. *Lancet* 1987;**2**:38.

13 McManus ML, Churchwell KB. Coagulopathy as a predictor of outcome in meningococcal sepsis and the systemic inflammatory response with purpura. *Crit Care Med* 1993;**21**:706–11.

14 Henning RJ, Wiener F, Valdes S, Weil MH. Measurement of toe temperature for assessing the severity of acute circulatory failure. *Surg Gynecol Obstet* 1979;**149**:154.

15 Butt W, Shann F. Core-peripheral temperature gradient does not predict cardiac output or systemic vascular resistance in children. *Anaesth Intens Care* 1991;**19**:84–7.

16 Knight RW, Opie JC. The big toe in the recovery room: peripheral warm-up patterns in children after open-heart surgery. *Can J Surg* 1981;**24**:239–45.

17 Doglio GR, Pusajo JF, Egurrola MA, *et al.* Gastric mucosal pH as a prognostic index of mortality in critically ill patients. *Crit Care Med* 1991;**19**:1037–40.

18 Gutierrez G, Palizas F, Doglio G, *et al.* Gastric intramucosal pH as a therapeutic index of tissue oxygenation in critically ill patients. *Lancet* 1992;**339**:195–9.

19 Wo CCJ, Shoemaker WC, Appel PL, *et al.* Unreliability of blood pressure and heart rate to evaluate cardiac output in emergency resuscitation and critical illness. *Crit Care Med* 993;**21**:21–9.

20 Hazelzet JA, van der Voort E, Lindemans J, ter Heerdt PG, Neijens HJ. Relation between cytokines and routine laboratory data in children with septic shock and purpura. *Intens Care Med* 1994;**20**:371–4.

21 Carcillo JA, Davis AL, Zaritsky A. Role of early fluid resuscitation in pediatric septic shock. *JAMA* 1991;**266**:1242–5.

22 Craig WA. Qualitative susceptibility tests versus quantitative MIC tests. *Diagn Microbiol Infect Dis* 1993;**16**:231–6.

23 Witte MK, Hill JH, Blumer JL. Shock in the pediatric patient. *Adv Pediatr* 1987;**34**:139–73.

24 Carcillo JA, Pollock MM, Ruttimann UE, Fields AI. Sequential physiologic interactions in pediatric cardiogenic and septic shock. *Crit Care Med* 1989;**17**:12–16.

25 Prodham LS, Choffat JM, Frenck N, *et al.* Care of the seriously ill neonate with hyaline membrane disease and with sepsis (sclerema neonatorum). *Paediatrics* 1974;**53**:170–81.

26 Xanthou M, Xypolyta A, Anagnostakis D, Economou-Mavrou C, Matsaniotis N. Exchange transfusion in severe neonatal infection with sclerema. *Arch Dis Child* 1975;**50**:901–2.

27 Tollner U, Pohlandt F, Heinze F, Henrichs I. Treatment of septicaemia in the newborn infant: choice of initial antimicrobial drugs and the role of exchange transfusion. *Acta Paediatr Scand* 1977;**66**:605–10.

28 Pearse RG, Sauer PJJ. Exchange transfusion in treatment of severe infections in newborns and of sclerema neonatorum. *Arch Dis Child* 1978;**53**:262.

29 Belhradsky BH, Roos R, Marget W. Exchange transfusion in neonatal septicemia. *Infection* 1978;**6**:S139.

30 Courtney SE, Hall RT, Harris DJ. Effect of blood transfusions on mortality in early-onset group B streptococcal septicemia. *Lancet* 1979;**2**:462–3.

31 Lemos L. Exchange transfusion in treatment of sepsis. *Paediatrics* 1981;**68**:471–2.

32 Bossi E, Meister B, Pfeninger J. Exchange transfusion for severe neonatal septicaemia. *Paediatrics* 1981;**67**:941.

33 Narayanan I, Mitter A, Gujral W. A comparative study on the value of exchange and blood transfusion in the management of severe neonatal septicemia with sclerema. *Indian J Pediatr* 1982;**49**:519–23.

34 Mathur NB, Subramarian BK, Sharma VK, Puri RK. Exchange transfusion in septicaemic neonates. *Acta Paediatrica* 1993;**82**:939–43.

35 Laurenti F, Ferro R, Isacchi G, *et al.* Polymorphonuclear leukocyte transfusion for the treatment of sepsis in the newborn infant. *J Pediatr* 1981;**98**:118–23.

36 Laurenti F, Ferro R, Isacchi G, *et al.* Granulocyte transfusion in very small newborn infants with sepsis. In: Stern L, ed, *Intensive care in the newborn*. Illinois: Masson, 1981: 175.

37 Christensen RD, Rothstein G, Anstall HB, Bybee B. Granulocyte transfusions in neonates with bacterial infection, neutropenia, and depletion of mature marrow neutrophils. *Paediatrics* 1982;**70**:1–6.

38 Cairo MS, Ricker R, Bennetts GA, *et al.* Improved survival of newborns receiving leukocyte transfusions for sepsis. *Paediatrics* 1984;**74**:887–92.

39 Wheeler JG, Chauvenet AR, Johnson CA, *et al.* Buffy coat transfusions in newborns with sepsis and neutrophil storage pool depletion. *Paediatrics* 1987;**79**:422–5.

40 Baley JE, Stork EK, Warkentin Pl, Shurin SB. Buffy coat transfusions in neutropenic neonates with presumed sepsis: a prospective, randomized trial. *Paediatrics* 1987;**80**: 712–20.

41 Baley JE, Stork EK, Warkentin PL, *et al.* Neonatal neutropenia: epidemiology, etiology and outcome. *Pediatr Res* 1986;**20**:374A.

42 Christman JW, Holden EP, Blackwell TS. Strategies for blocking the systemic effects of cytokines in the sepsis syndrome. *Crit Care Med* 1995;**23**:955–61.

43 Bone RC. A critical evaluation of new agents for the treatment of sepsis. *JAMA* 1991; **266**:1686–91.

44 Natanson C, Hoffman WD, Suffredini AF, Eichacker PQ, Danner RL. Selected treatment strategies for septic shock based on proposed mechanisms of pathogenesis. *Ann Int Med* 1994;**120**:771–83.

45 Knaus WA, Harrell FE, LaBrecque JF, *et al.* Use of predicted risk of mortality to evaluate the efficacy of anticytokine therapy in sepsis. *Crit Care Med* 1996;**24**:46–52.

46 Bernard GR, Luce JM, Sprung CL, *et al.* High-dose corticosteroids in patients with the adult respiratory distress syndrome. *N Engl J Med* 1987;**317**:1565–70.

47 Bone RC, Fisher CJ Jr, Clemmer TP, Slotman GJ, Metz CA, Balk RA. A controlled clinical trial of high-dose methylprednisolone in the treatment of severe sepsis and septic shock. *N Engl J Med* 1987;**317**:653–8.

48 McCracken GH Jr, Lebel MH. Dexamethasone therapy for bacterial meningitis in infants and children. *Am J Dis Child* 1989;**143**:287–9.

49 Odio CM, Faingezicht I, Paris M, *et al.* The beneficial effects of early dexamethasone administration in infants and children with bacterial meningitis. *N Engl J Med* 1991;**324**: 1525–31.

50 Muraji T, Okamoto E, Hoque S, Toyosaka A. A plasma exchange therapy for endotoxin shock in puppies. *J Pediatr Surg* 1986;**21**:1092–5.

51 Gokul KS, Shenep JL, Hildner BK, Stidham GL. Detoxification of plasma containing lipopolysaccharide (LPS). *Crit Care Med* 1988;**16**:414.

52 Cohen J, Aslam M, Pusey CD, Ryan CJ. Protection from endotoxaemia: a rat model of plasmapheresis and specific adsorption with polymyxin B. *J Infect Dis* 1987;**155**:690–5.

53 Hanasawa K, Aoki H, Yoshioka T, Matsuda K, Tani T, Kodama M. Novel mechanical assistance in the treatment of endotoxic and septicemic shock. *ASAIO Trans* 1989;**35**: 341–3.

54 Natanson C, Hoffman W, Danner R, *et al.* A controlled trial of plasmapheresis fails to improve the outcome in an antibiotic treated canine model of human septic shock. *Crit Care Med* 1989;**17**:S57.

55 Bjorvatm B, Bjertnaes L, Fadnea HO, *et al.* Meningococcal septicaemia treated with combined plasmapheresis and leuapheresis or with blood exchange. *BMJ Res Ed* 1984; **288**:439–41.

56 Barzilay E, Kessler D, Berlot G, Gullo A, Geber D, Ben Zeev I. Use of extracorporeal supportive techniques as additional treatment for septic-induced multiple organ failure patients. *Crit Care Med* 1989;**17**:634–7.

57 Van Deuren M, Santman FW, van Alen R, Sauerwein RS, Span LFR, van der Meer JWM. Plasma and whole blood exchange in meningococcal sepsis. *Clin Infect Dis* 1992; **15**:424–30.

58 Westertdorp RGJ, Brand A, van Hinsbergh VWM, Thompson J, van Furth R, Meinders EA. Leukoplasmapheresis in meningococcal septic shock. *Am J Med* 1992;**92**:577–8.

59 Best C, Walsh J, Sinclair J, *et al.* Early hemofiltration in meningococcal septicaemia. *Lancet* 1996;**347**:202.

60 Morley S, DiAmore A, Ross Russell RI. Veno-venous hemodiafiltration in meningococcal septicaemia. *Lancet* 1996;**347**:614.

61 Connett G, Waldren M, Woodcock T. Veno-venous haemodiafiltration in meningococcal septicaemia. *Lancet* 1996;**347**:611.

62 Tibby S, Champion M, Hatherill M, Marsh MJ, Murdoch IA. Veno-venous haemofiltration in meningococcal septicaemia. *Lancet* 1996;**347**:612.

63 Reeves JH, Butt W, Sathe AS. A review of veno-venous haemodiafiltration in seriously ill infants. *J Paediatr Child Health* 1994;**30**:50–4.

64 Butt W, Beca J. Extracorporeal circulatory support in children with septic shock in intensive care. *Crit Care Med* 1993;**21**:S381–2.

Index

267

274